D0086731

# Eternal Diseases:
## Cornea, Conjunctiva, Sclera, Eyelids, Lacriminal System

# EXTERNAL DISEASES:

## CORNEA, CONJUNCTIVA, SCLERA, EYELIDS, LACRIMAL SYSTEM

Associate Editors

**JOHN W. CHANDLER, MD, FACS**
Professor and Head
Department of Ophthalmology and Visual Sciences
University of Illinois at Chicago Eye Center
Chicago, IL

**JOEL SUGAR, MD**
Professor of Ophthalmology
Director of Corneal Surgery and External Diseases
Department of Ophthalmology and Visual Sciences
University of Illinois at Chicago Eye Center
Chicago, IL

**HENRY F. EDELHAUSER, PhD**
Ferst Professor of Ophthalmology
Director of Ophthalmic Research
Emory University Eye Center
Atlanta, GA

**VOLUME 8**

# TEXTBOOK OF OPHTHALMOLOGY

**EDITED BY**

**STEVEN M. PODOS, MD, FACS**
Professor and Chairman
Department of Ophthalmology
Mt. Sinai School of Medicine
New York, NY

**MYRON YANOFF, MD, FACS**
Professor and Chairman
Department of Ophthalmology
Hahnemann University
Philadelphia, PA

**Mosby**

London  St. Louis  Baltimore  Boston  Chicago  Philadelphia  Sydney  Toronto

IV

For full details of all Mosby-Year Book Europe Ltd. titles, please write to
Mosby-Year Book Europe Ltd., Brook House, 2-16 Torrington Place, London WC1E 7LT, England.

LIBRARY OF CONGRESS CATALOGING-IN-PUBLICATION DATA
(Revised for volume 8)

Textbook of ophthalmology.

  Includes bibliographical references and indexes.
  Contents: v. 1. Optics and refraction / v. 8. External diseases / associate editors, John W. Chandler,
     Joel Sugar, Henry F. Edelhauser.
  1.  Ophthalmology.  I. Podos, Steven M.  II. Yanoff, Myron.
RE46.T26 1991        617.7        91-34425
ISBN 1-56375-011-2 (v. 1)
ISBN Set: 0-397-44692-6

BRITISH LIBRARY CATALOGUING-IN-PUBLICATION DATA:
A catalogue record for this book is available from the British Library.

ISBN Volume 8: 1-56375-101-1
ISBN Set: 0-397-44692-6

10 9 8 7 6 5 4 3 2 1

Editorial Director: LEAH KENNEDY
Project Manager: DIMITRY POPOW
Editors: DIMITRY POPOW, SHARON RULE
Art Director and Cover Design: KATHRYN GREENSLADE
Interior Layout: THOMAS TEDESCO, JEFFREY S. BROWN
Illustration Director: CAROL KALAFATIC
Illustrators: GARY WELCH, CAROL KALAFATIC, NICHOLAS GUARRACINO, PATRICIA GAST

Originated in Hong Kong by Bright Arts, Ltd.
Produced by Imago Productions, Pte., Ltd.
Printed and bound in Singapore, 1994.

The right of Chandler, Sugar, and Edelhauser to be identified as authors of this work has been asserted by them in accordance with the Copyright, Design and Patents Act 1988.

COPYRIGHT © 1994 MOSBY-YEAR BOOK EUROPE, LTD. All rights reserved. No part of this publication may be reproduced, stored in a retrieval system, copied or transmitted, in any form or by any means, electronic, mechanical, photocopying, recording or otherwise without written permission from the Publisher or in accordance with the provisions of the Copyright Act 1988, or under the terms of any license permitting limited copying issued by the Copyright Licensing Agency, 33-34 Alfred Place, London, WC1E 7DP.

Any person who does any unauthorized act in relation to this publication may be liable to criminal prosecution and civil claims for damages.

Permission to photocopy or reproduce solely for internal or personal use is permitted for libraries or other users registered with the Copyright Clearance Center, provided that the base fee of $4.00 per chapter plus $.10 per page is paid directly to the Copyright Clearance Center, 21 Congress Street, Salem, MA 01970. This consent does not extend to other kinds of copying, such as copying for general distribution, for advertising or promotional purposes, for creating new collected works, or for resales.

# EDITORS' PREFACE

As we approach the twenty-first century, it is apparent that the half-life of medical knowledge is continuing to shrink and the amount of current dogma is continuing to expand. Packaging today's relevant ophthalmic knowledge is a difficult chore, yet one that periodically demands doing. Every editor or author desires to accomplish this task in a new and unique fashion. This ten-volume series represents our vision of a *Textbook of Ophthalmology* for the 1990s: one that integrates the basic visual science and clinical information of each subspecialty in a separate volume that is edited or written by noted basic scientists and clinicians; one that is manageable, readable, and affordable for the ophthalmic expert as well as the neophyte; and one that contains original diagrams, figures, and photographs—all in full color—designed to depict the necessary knowledge we hope to impart.

We are grateful to our associate editors and authors for sharing their superb expertise in the compilation of this unique ophthalmic resourse, to our assistants Barbara Zoldessy and Roe Brennan for their unstinting efforts in organizing and coordinating this project, and to our wives Wendy Donn Podos and Karin L. Yanoff for their continued patience and encouragement throughout the many phases of this endeavor.

**STEVEN M. PODOS, MD, FACS**
DEPARTMENT OF
OPHTHALMOLOGY
MT. SINAI SCHOOL OF MEDICINE
NEW YORK, NY

**MYRON YANOFF, MD, FACS**
DEPARTMENT OF
OPHTHALMOLOGY
HAHNEMANN UNIVERSITY
PHILADELPHIA, PA

# CONTRIBUTORS

**Frank V. Buffam, BSc, MD, CM, FRCSC**
Oculoplastic and Lacrimal Surgery
The Eye Care Centre
Vancouver, British Columbia, Canada

**John W. Chandler, MD, FACS**
Professor and Head
Department of Ophthalmology and Visual Sciences
University of Illinois at Chicago Eye Center
Chicago, Illinois

**Charles Cintron, PhD**
Senior Scientist
The Schepens Eye Research Institute
Associate Professor of Ophthalmology
Harvard Medical School
Boston, Massachusetts

**Antonio R. de Toledo, MD**
Research Associate
Department of Ophthalmology and Visual Sciences
University of Illinois at Chicago College of Medicine
Chicago, Illinois

**Henry F. Edelhauser, PhD**
Ferst Professor of Ophthalmology
Director of Ophthalmic Research
Emory University Eye Center
Atlanta, Georgia

**David B. Glasser, MD**
Department of Ophthalmology
Columbia Medical Plan
Columbia, Maryland

**Sheridan Lam, MD**
Assistant Professor
Department of Ophthalmology and Visual Sciences
University of Illinois at Chicago Eye Center
Chicago, Illinois

**Mark L. McDermott, MD**
Assistant Professor
Department of Ophthalmology
Wayne State University
Detroit, Michigan

**Stephen D. Rheinstrom, MD**
Visiting Associate Professor
Corneal Surgery and External Diseases
University of Illinois at Chicago Eye Center
Chicago, Illinois

**Joel Sugar, MD**
Professor of Ophthalmology
Director of Corneal Surgery and External Diseases
Department of Ophthalmology and Visual Sciences
University of Illinois at Chicago Eye Center
Chicago, Illinois

**Richard W. Yee, MD**
Associate Professor
Department of Ophthalmology
University of Texas Health Science Center
San Antonio, Texas

# CONTENTS

# 1 | THE EYELIDS

## Joel Sugar

## ANATOMY OF THE EYELIDS

The eyelids develop embryologically, beginning at 4 to 5 weeks of gestation, from mesenchymal condensations with ectodermal covering. The mesenchyme in the eyelid prominences becomes vascularized and supplied with nerve fibers, and the rudimentary lid tissue proliferates by lateral elongation and vertical growth from above and below the eye. By 10 weeks the lid margins have contacted each other and fused. Cilia begin to appear just before lid fusion. Meibomian gland development begins in the fourth month, and the other sebaceous glands develop soon thereafter. The orbicularis anlage, originating from the second visceral arch, can be seen in the lid mesenchyme at around the time of lid fusion. The lids are held together by desmosomal attachments and separate as meibomian secretions are formed and as the lid margins keratinize at 5 to 7 months. From 7 months to term, maturation of the eyelids proceeds with eyelid movement, degeneration of lanugo hair, and production of meibomian secretions.[1]

The major functions of the eyelids are to protect the eye from external injury and from light, to protect the tear film from excess evaporation, and to spread tears over the anterior portion of the eye and contribute to the tear film. These multiple functions require unique anatomy and physiology. The major landmarks are the brow, the upper and lower folds (superior and inferior palpebral sulci), and the nasojugal fold (Fig. 1.1). The

**1.1** | External eyelid and orbital landmarks.

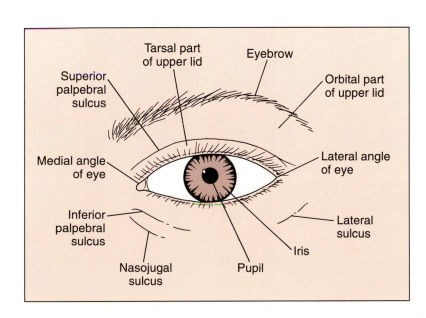

superior and inferior furrows divide the orbital from the tarsal portion of the lid. The upper and lower lids meet medially at the inner canthus and laterally at the outer canthus (angle). The palpebral fissure is the space between the upper and lower lid margins. The typical horizontal opening of the lids is 30 mm, with the vertical opening greatest at the junction of the inner third with the middle third of the lid except in Asians, in whom the opening is greatest at the center of the palpebral fissure. The lid margin is divided into a ciliary portion, bearing the lashes, and a lacrimal portion, which has a rounded rather than a squared contour and overlies the lacrimal caruncle and the plica semilunaris rather than directly overlying the globe. The lacrimal punctum opens in the center of the lacrimal papilla into the lacrimal canaliculus. The punctum sits at the lateral portion of the lacrimal lid margin.

The lid structure in cross-section consists of four layers: the skin and subcutaneous tissue, the orbicularis muscle, the septum and tarsal plates, and the conjunctiva (Fig. 1.2).

The lid skin is very thin, allowing unrestricted movement with blinking, lid closure, and vertical eye movements. Normal skin appendages are present in the eyelid skin, and lid pigmentation is dependent on melanin supplied to the keratinocytes by dendritic melanocytes scattered throughout the basal layer of the epidermis. The cilia protrude from the anterior lid margin and their follicles extend deep into the subcutaneous tissue to the level of the orbicularis and the tarsus. Associated with the hair follicles are the sebaceous glands of Zeis and the sweat glands of Moll, which open into the follicles. In addition, sweat glands beneath the epidermis open into the lid skin; these sweat glands consist of a basal coil, a duct (syrinx), and a duct opening (acrosyringium).

The orbicularis muscle (Fig. 1.3) is an elliptical, flat, striated muscle that lies just below the skin of the lids. The palpebral portion can be divided into pretarsal and preseptal segments. The pretarsal portion overlies the tarsal plate, with the portion closest to the lid margin called the ciliary portion or muscle of Riolan. Medially, the ciliary portion disappears in the lacrimal portion of the lid and becomes Horner's muscle. The pretarsal orbicularis arises from the medial canthal tendon and periosteum anterior to the

**1.2** | Normal anatomy. *A:* Cross section of the eyelid shows the inner white tarsal plate, the middle layers of muscle fibers, and the surface epithelium. Note the cilia coming out of the lid margin inferiorly. *B:* Histologic section shows the inner tarsal plate containing the meibomian glands, the middle muscular bundles and the surface epithelium. The cilia exit from the middle portion of the lid margin inferiorly. Apocrine sweat glands, eccrine sweat glands, sebaceous glands of Zeis, and hair follicles of the surface lanugo hairs also are seen in the lids. (*A,* courtesy of Dr. RC Eagle, Jr.; all figures from Yanoff M, Fine BS: *Ocular Pathology. A Color Atlas,* ed 2. New York: Gower Medical Publishing, 1992, 6.2.)

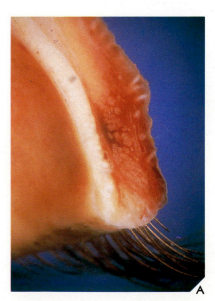

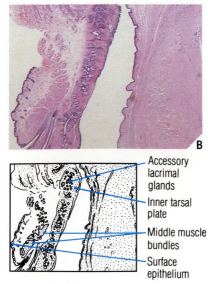

Accessory lacrimal glands

Inner tarsal plate

Middle muscle bundles

Surface epithelium

canaliculus as well as from the posterior lacrimal crest posterior to the canaliculus. The fibers extend laterally to interdigitate at the lateral palpebral raphe. The preseptal portion is similar to the pretarsal but lies beyond the tarsus, while the preorbital portion extends beyond the orbital rim. The muscle of Riolan can be seen through the lid margin as the "gray line,"[2] a clinically important landmark in oculoplastic surgical procedures because an incision here serves to split the orbicularis anteriorly from the tarsus posteriorly (Fig. 1.4). This line also serves to help in anterior–posterior lid margin alignment during repair of lid lacerations.

The orbital septum consists of fibrous tissue arising from the periosteum at the orbital margin and thickening towards the lid margins to form the dense tarsal plates. The septum separates the orbital cavity and the eyelids. The tarsal plates are tethered medially by the medial canthal tendon (medial palpebral ligament), which inserts anterior to the lacrimal sac into the lacrimal crest and maxilla. Laterally, the canthal tendon (lateral palpebral ligament) extends from the tarsal plates to insert on Whitnall's tubercle just posterior to the orbital rim.[3] The aponeurosis of the levator palpebrae superioris sends fibers through the orbital septum to insert on the anterior surface of the upper tarsus and through the orbicularis to insert in the skin forming

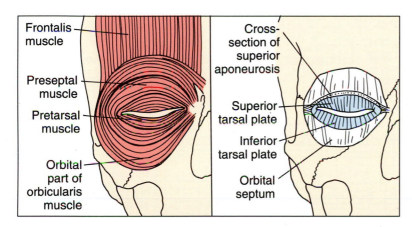

**1.3** | Structures of the normal eyelid. The orbicularis muscle can be divided into three parts but these are not separate anatomically. These are the preseptal, the pretarsal, and orbital parts of the orbicularis muscle. The preseptal and pretarsal parts together form the palpebral section of the orbicularis muscle, which is responsible for blinking, while the orbital part is responsible for forced lid closure. Removal of the orbicularis muscle shows the underlying tarsal plates and orbital septum. The superior aponeurosis is the tendon of the levator muscle which inserts between the orbicularis muscle bundles and is responsible for the skin crease. (From Collin JRO: The Eyelids, in Spalton DJ, Hitchings RA, Hunter PA: *Atlas of Clinical Ophthalmology*. London: Gower Medical Publishing, 2.2.)

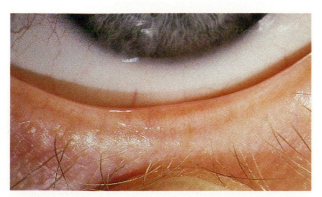

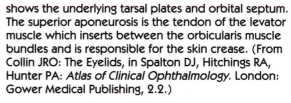

**1.4** | Lid margin anatomy. Note the position of the cilia, gray line, and meibomian orifices.

the superior lid crease. The skin insertion of the levator aponeurosis as well as that of the tarsus is much closer to the lashline in Asians than in whites, creating the lower or even absent Asian lid fold. In the lower lid, the capsulopalpebral fascia is the analogue of the levator aponeurosis. It arises from the inferior rectus tendon sheath and inserts in the inferior tarsal margin. Smooth muscle arises from the levator aponeurosis in the upper lid and extends to the superior margin of the upper tarsus as Müller's muscle. The inferior tarsal muscle arising from the inferior rectus sheath and inserting in the inferior margin of the lower tarsus is analogous.

The tarsus contains 30 to 40 Meibomian glands above and somewhat fewer below (Fig. 1.5). These glands are holocrine modified sebaceous glands whose oily secretion forms the most superficial layer of the tear film, stabilizing it and preventing its evaporation. The semi-rigid structure of the tarsus also serves to spread the tear film evenly.

The most posterior layer of the lid is the conjunctiva, which is densely adherent to the tarsal plates. The conjunctiva arises at the mucocutaneous junction at the posterior lid margin or slightly down on the posterior lid surface, not at the gray line as is commonly taught.[2]

The vascular supply to the eyelids is rich and widely anastomotic. Marginal and peripheral arterial arches extend from the medial and lateral palpebral arteries across the upper and lower lids. The medial arises from the ophthalmic artery in the region of the trochlea, whereas the lateral arises from the lacrimal artery. The conjunctiva is supplied by the conjunctival arteries, which are branches of the anterior ciliary arteries. Venous drainage is to the ophthalmic and angular veins medially and the superficial temporal vein laterally. Lymphatic drainage is to the preauricular superficial parotid nodes from the lateral two thirds of the lids and to the submandibular nodes from the medial portion of the lids.

Motor innervation to the lids comes to the orbicularis from the temporal and zygomatic branches of the facial (VII) nerve, while the levator is supplied by the oculomotor (III) nerve. The smooth Müller's muscle and inferior tarsal muscle are supplied by sympathetic fibers arising from the superior cervical ganglia, damage to which causes the ptosis of Horner syndrome. Sensory innervation to the eyelids is from the supra- and infratrochlear, supraorbital, and lacrimal branches of the ophthalmic division of the trigeminal (V) nerve and from the infraorbital nerve from the maxillary division of the trigeminal.

## DIAGNOSTIC TECHINQUES

Diagnosis of lid lesions is primarily dependent on direct observation of lid appearance and function. Lid motility is assessed in primary, up-, and downgaze, as well as with gentle and forced closure. Palpation for masses is

**1.5** | Infrared transillumination photograph of the meibomian glands (courtesy of Dr. Jeffrey Robin). The light radial areas are the meibomian glands while the dark areas are connective tissue. Some of these glands are irregular and dysfunctional.

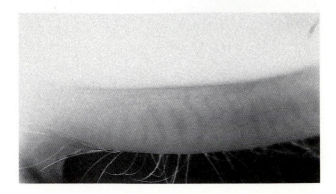

also often helpful. Eversion of the lids for observation of the tarsal surface is readily carried out and is important in complete lid evaluation: the upper lid is everted through gentle traction on the lashes combined with downward pressure on the superior tarsal margin through the lid skin with a fingertip or a probe. The lower lid is everted by combined downward traction on the lid skin and inward pressure on the inferior tarsal margin. Observation of the meibomian glands can be enhanced by transillumination biomicroscopy.[4] Confirmation of diagnosis of many lid lesions requires biopsy and histopathologic evaluation.

## ABNORMALITIES OF THE EYELIDS

The eyelids, consisting of skin, muscle, sebaceous and sweat glands, hair, and mucous membranes, are subject to the disorders seen in these tissues elsewhere in the body as well as to lesions unique to the eyelids. Because many functional deficits and lesions involving the lids are treatable by plastic surgery, Volume 4 (*Orbit and Oculoplastics*) should be consulted for many of these problems.

## INFECTIONS

Infections of the eyelids run the full gamut of human infectious diseases. Bacterial infections are also included in the discussion of chronic blepharitis because of the frequent combination of infectious blepharitis with other forms of blepharitis.

Preseptal cellulitis is a purulent inflammation of the subcutaneous tissues of the eyelid anterior to the orbital septum. This typically occurs after trauma to the lids, with or without an evident break in the skin. It is characterized by marked lid swelling, erythema, and heat, often with fluctuance on palpation. The patients are usually only mildly systemically ill, with low if any fever and leukocytosis. Visual acuity and ocular motility are normal, in contrast to orbital cellulitis in which patients are more ill, acuity may be decreased, and motility is restricted (Fig. 1.6). *Staphylococcus aureus, Streptococcus* species, and *Haemophilus influenzae* in children are the most frequent causative organisms, but anaerobes and gram-negative bacteria can be involved, and cultures are therefore important. Treatment consists of incision and drainage of abscesses and appropriate antibiotic therapy: intra-

### Figure 1.6. Comparison of Orbital and Preseptal Cellulitis

|  | PRESEPTAL | ORBITAL CELLULITIS |
| --- | --- | --- |
| Lid edema and erythema | Present | Present |
| Heat | Present | Present |
| Proptosis | Absent or minimal | Present |
| Chemosis | Absent or mild | Marked |
| Visual acuity | Normal | May be reduced |
| Ocular motility | Normal | Limited |
| Pain on motion | Absent | Present |
| Fever | Absent | Present |
| Leukocytosis | None or mild | Moderate to marked |

(After Jones DB: Microbial pre-septal and orbital cellulitis, in Wilson LA (ed): *External Diseases of the Eye.* Hagerstown, MD: Harper & Row, 1979, 343.)

venous for severe infections or those where orbital extension is possible, or oral agents in less severe cases.

Erysipelas is a form of preseptal cellulitis caused by group A streptococci, characterized by marked redness and well-defined lid swelling. Intravenous antibiotic treatment is appropriate. Impetigo is a cutaneous infection with group A beta-hemolytic streptococci and secondary growth of *S. aureus*, which commonly involves the face and may involve the eyelids. A papular lesion with surrounding erythema becomes vesicular and at times pustular and then ruptures to leave a thick, honey-colored crust. Marked lid swelling occurs when the lesions are periocular, and regional adenopathy is commonly present. The lesions are often in different stages of development, unlike those of *Herpes simplex* in which crops of lesions occur. Cultures and smears help to distinguish the two. Treatment is with local hygiene, topical antibiotics, and systemic antibiotics.

Viral infections of the lids include *Herpes simplex*, *H. zoster*, molluscum contagiosum, and verrucae. *H. simplex* may occur on the lids either as a manifestation of primary disease or as a form of recurrent disease. Primary disease represents the first encounter between the virus and the host that causes clinical disease. This presents as a vesicular eyelid or lid margin eruption with multiple lesions, which are usually unilateral (Fig. 1.7). The vesicles occur in crops, often with preauricular adenopathy, and there may be an associated follicular conjunctivitis and corneal epithelial disease. The vesicles crust, dry, and heal without scarring (Fig. 1.8). In patients with underlying skin disease such as eczema, primary herpes may present as a more diffuse eruption (Fig. 1.9). Immunosuppressed patients may also develop more generalized disease. Diagnosis can be confirmed by culture or more readily and

**1.7** | *A:* Primary *Herpes simplex* blepharitis. Note the vesicles in various stages of development and crusting. *B:* Recurrent *Herpes simplex* orofacial and eyelid involvement in a patient with a history of recurrent keratitis.

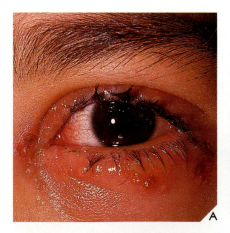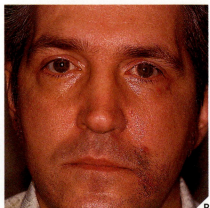

### Figure 1.8. *Herpes Zoster* and *Herpes Simplex* Blepharitis

| | HERPES ZOSTER OPHTHALMICUS | HERPES SIMPLEX | |
| --- | --- | --- | --- |
| | | PRIMARY | RECURRENT |
| Unilateral | Yes | Yes (usually) | Yes |
| Preauricular nodes | Yes | Yes | No |
| Follicular conjunctivitis | Sometimes | Yes | No |
| Scarring | Yes | No | No |
| Vesicles | Numerous | Numerous | Usually few |

inexpensively, by Tzanck scraping of the base of the vesicle to demonstrate multinucleated giant cells (Fig. 1.10) or Papanicolaou staining to demonstrate intranuclear inclusions. Treatment of skin lesions usually requires only local hygiene, although conjunctival and corneal involvement may prompt topical ocular use of antiviral agents. Neonates with herpetic skin disease may have herpes viremia and are at risk for visceral or cerebral involvement. These patients therefore require systemic antiviral treatment.

Recurrent *H. simplex* on the skin is often referred to as a "cold sore," because recurrence may be triggered by fever as well as by trauma, stress, and sunlight. These lesions, when they involve the lid, are usually less numerous than in primary disease, cause less inflammation, and are not associated with adenopathy or follicular conjunctivitis. When there is no ocular involvement, treatment is both unnecessary and ineffective.

*Herpes zoster* is the recurrent form of *Varicella* virus infection. Typically, a single dermatome is involved. This appears to take place because latency is established in the satellite cells in the ganglion. Activation leads to infection of all the cells in the ganglion rather than, as in *H. simplex*, activation of virus in a single nucleus or a small group of cell nuclei leading to more localized recurrences.[5] *Herpes zoster* ophthalmicus refers to the recurrence of *H. zoster* in the dermatomal distribution of the first (ophthalmic) branch of the V cranial nerve. Burning discomfort without skin lesions may initiate involvement, followed by the sequential development of erythematous papules, vesicles, pustules, and then crusted lesions (Fig. 1.11). The lesions heal spontaneously but often with scarring, which may lead to cicatricial ectropion and corneal exposure.

Cutaneous erythema may persist for a prolonged period of time and patients may develop post-herpetic neuralgia, with pain that is sometimes severe in the dermatome previously involved by active infection. Appropriate treatment of the cutaneous eruption is with oral acyclovir, 800 mg five times daily for 10 days. This reduces the duration of the cutaneous eruption and the acute discomfort.[6] Post-herpetic neuralgia, however, is not affected and is often difficult to treat. Post-herpetic neuralgia may respond to various oral analgesic agents such as carbamazepine (Tegretol®), but the response is

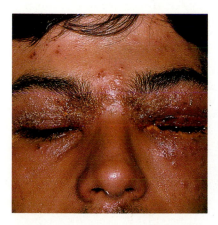

**1.9** | Primary *Herpes simplex* in a patient with atopic eczema (Kaposi's varicelliform eruption).

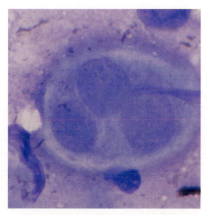

**1.10** | Multinucleated giant cell from Tzanck scraping of *Herpes simplex* lid vesicle. This finding does not distinguish *Herpes simplex* from *Herpes zoster*.

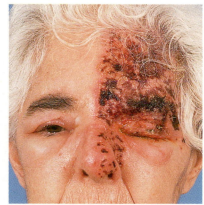

**1.11** | *Herpes zoster* ophthalmicus in the crusting phase. Note the dermatomal distribution and the bilateral lid swelling.

unpredictable and often disappointing. Topical capsaicin (Zostrix®) applied to the skin may provide relief of pain. This agent, the "hot" from hot peppers, appears to deplete substance P from sensory nerves and is often effective when used chronically.

Molluscum contagiosum is a viral eruption caused by a poxvirus. Disease is usually spread by direct contact or fomites in children and is sexually transmitted in adults. Involvement of the eyelids is characterized by single or multiple dome-shaped, umbilicated lesions (Fig. 1.12). In immunosuppressed patients the lesions may be numerous and even confluent. Although the lesions are often self-limited and disappear without scarring, lesions near the lid margin may be associated with a follicular conjunctivitis, punctate keratopathy, and even corneal vascularization. Treatment consists of excision, cryotherapy, or incision and curettage.[7]

Common warts, verruca vulgaris (Fig. 1.13), caused by papillomavirus, may involve the lid margin and can cause a papillary conjunctivitis and punctate keratopathy. The lesions may spontaneously regress or can be treated with surgical excision and cryotherapy.

Fungal eyelid infections are uncommon. *Candida albicans* can cause an ulcerative blepharitis with granulomatous margins in immunosuppressed individuals or with chronic antibiotic use. Diagnosis is made by scraping and culture, and treatment is with topical antifungal agents. The dermatophytes, the classic ringworm organisms, can involve the lids with lesions similar to those seen elsewhere on the skin. Diagnosis and treatment, again, consist of scraping, culture, and topical antifungal agents.

North American blastomycosis is a rare disorder caused by the fungus *Blastomyces dermatitidis*. Eyelid involvement shows the chronic presence of an elevated, crusted lesion with sharp margins and a healed center, often

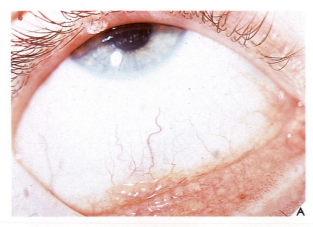

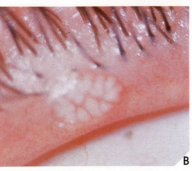

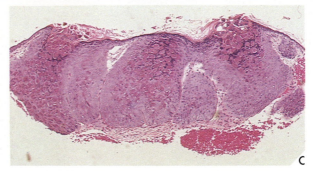

**1.12** | Molluscum contagiosum. *A:* A follicular conjunctivitis is present in the inferior, bulbar conjuctiva. Note the small lesion on the margin of the superior eyelid that is responsible for the follicular conjunctivitis. *B:* Increased magnification demonstrates an umbilicated lesion that contains whitish packets of material. *C:* Histologic section shows that the epithelium is thickened by intracytoplasmic molluscum bodies that are small and eosinophilic in the deep layers but become enormous and basophilic near the surface. After breaking through the surface epithelium, the molluscum bodies may be shed into the tear film where they cause a secondary, irritative, follicular conjunctivitis. (*A* and *B,* courtesy Dr. WC Frayer; all photographs from Yanoff M, Fine BS: *Ocular Pathology. A Color Atlas,* ed 2. New York: Gower Medical Publishing, 1992, 6.5.)

with multiple dark spots within the area of involvement caused by bleeding beneath the lesion. Diagnosis is made by demonstration of yeast forms on biopsy and cultures. Treatment is with both topical and systemic antifungal agents.[8]

Parasitic infections of the eyelids include phthiriasis (infestation with the pubic louse *Phthirus pubis*).[9] This 2-mm louse tends to infest relatively widely spaced hairs (Fig. 1.14). Therefore, pubic, chest, axillary, and facial hair, as well as the eyelashes, become involved. Head and body lice (*Pediculus humanus* var. *corporis* and var. *capitis*) are less likely to affect the lashes.[9] Patients with phthiriasis complain of intense itching of the lids, and both the adult organisms and their eggs or nits may be seen on the lashes. Transmission is by sexual contact or from contaminated clothing or bedding. Treatment can be mechanical with trimming the lashes and removal of nits and organisms at the slit lamp, smothering of the organisms and hatching nits with frequent application of a bland ointment to the lashes for 10 days, or the use of a pediculicide. Lindane (Kwell®) shampoo is toxic to the cornea and may be absorbed through the lids, and also causes central nervous system toxicity, so this agent is not recommended. Permethrin cream rinse (Nix®, Elimite®) can be applied to the scalp and lids, as can pyrethrins shampoo (Rid®). Clothing and bedding should be washed in hot water, and louse-killing sprays can be used on inanimate objects that cannot be readily washed. Patients should be reexamined in 1 to 2 weeks in case nits have survived treatment and infestation is continuing.

*Demodex folliculorum* and *D. brevis* are mites commonly found in the eyelash follicles and the meibomian glands, respectively. Because they are present in almost all adults, they normally do not require treatment. With marked infestation, however, their products can be seen as clear sleeves around lashes, and the organisms themselves contribute to lid margin debris.

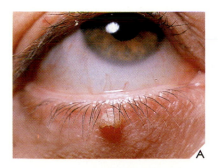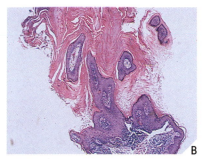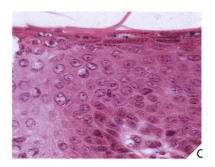

1.13 | Verruca vulgaris. *A:* Clinical appearance of lesion. *B:* Histologic section shows marked hyperkeratosis. Note that the rete ridges are elongated and bent inward, a rather typical finding. *C:* Another area shows deeply basophilic inclusion bodies and vacuolated cells. (From Yanoff M, Fine BS: *Ocular Pathology. A Color Atlas*, ed 2. New York: Gower Medical Publishing, 1992, 6.6.)

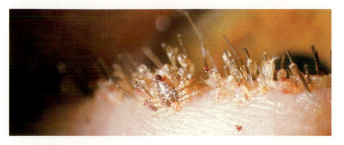

1.14 | Lice infestation. It is not uncommon to find the lashes infested with lice and nits. (From Kirkness CM: *Ophthalmology*. London: Gower Medical Publishing, 1985, 10.)

A granulomatous reaction to the organism has also been seen in chalazia.[10] Treatment is the same as for blepharitis, as discussed below. Ether scrubs have also been recommended.

## BLEPHARITIS

Blepharitis is the general term used to refer to inflammations involving the eyelids and particularly to those involving the lid margins. Blepharitis is a very common presenting problem to the general ophthalmologist, and a classification of blepharitis is helpful in approaching therapy. One classification approach divides inflammation into anterior and posterior lid disease, separating disease involving the anterior lid margin and lashes from that involving the meibomian glands. Another useful approach to classification is that of McCulley and co-workers,[11] which categorizes anterior lid margin disease as staphylococcal, seborrheic, or mixed; posterior lid margin disease as primary meibomitis; and combined disease as seborrheic with meibomian seborrhea or seborrheic with secondary meibomitis. Yet others[12] have classified meibomian disease as meibomian gland dysfunction with sub-categories as discussed below.[13] Additional forms of blepharitis occur in association with other disorders.

Staphylococcal blepharitis is a disorder that predominantly affects young to middle-aged women, with exacerbations and remissions of disease. These patients have lid margin erythema with fine ulceration at the base of the lashes, and collarettes or cuffs of fibrin extending from the base of the lash as a sleeve along the lash. Lashes may be absent or broken. Recurrent hordeolae and chalazia may occur, and bulbar injection with inferior corneal punctate staining, marginal corneal infiltrates, and phlyctenular keratoconjunctivitis may also be present. Lid crusting and mattering are common. Keratoconjunctivitis sicca is a common association.

Seborrheic blepharitis is seen in a somewhat older age group, with a fairly equal incidence in men and women. Patients complain of burning discomfort, some lid mattering, and foreign body sensation which tends to have a more chronic course than does staphylococcal disease, with less severe exacerbations and fewer remissions. Greasy scales are present on the lid margins and around the lashes, and are referred to as "scurf." Telangiectatic lid margin vessels are common and many patients have associated meibomian seborrhea, with excess oily meibomian secretion and foamy tears (Fig. 1.15) or with frank meibomitis with meibomian gland inflammation. Patients with seborrheic blepharitis may have more diffuse changes of seborrhea with dandruff of the scalp, scaling of the brows, scaling behind the ears and at the base of the nose, and greasy scales on the chest. The cause of seborrhea is unknown.

**1.15** | Seborrheic blepharitis. Note the foam at the posterior lid margin from meibomian seborrhea.

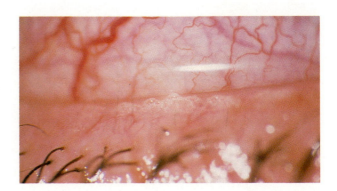

Mixed staphylococcal/seborrheic blepharitis has components of both types, with lid margin scurf as well as collarettes around the lashes.

Primary meibomitis or obstructive meibomian gland dysfunction is manifest as episodic inflammation of the posterior lid, with plugged and pouting meibomian orifices with thick secretions which are difficult to express (Fig. 1.16). The glands may appear enlarged and distorted or there may be "drop-out" of glands over time. Rosacea is a common associated disorder in patients with primary meibomian gland inflammation. Rosacea is a disorder of unknown cause, consisting of facial erythema with telangiectases over the cheeks and nose, a papular and pustular skin eruption, and sebaceous gland hypertrophy typified by rhinophyma (Fig. 1.17). Many patients with meibomitis also have seborrhea, as discussed above.

Chalazia and hordeolae can be seen with any of the forms of blepharitis discussed thus far. An external hordeolum is inflammation and or infection in the ciliary sebaceous glands of Zeis. These usually present as acute swelling with anterior pointing on the skin surface of the lid, with focal tenderness (Fig. 1.18). They may spontaneously point and drain or gradually resolve. A chalazion is a similar process involving the tarsal meibomian

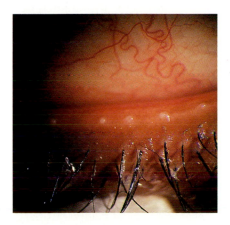

**1.16** | Meibomitis. Note the thick meibomian secretions.

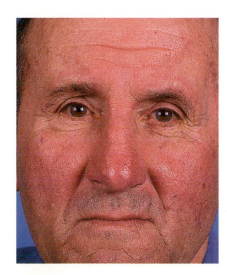

**1.17** | Facial rosacea. Note the facial telangiectases and the prominent pores and mild rhinophyma on the nose. The patient also has rosacea blepharitis.

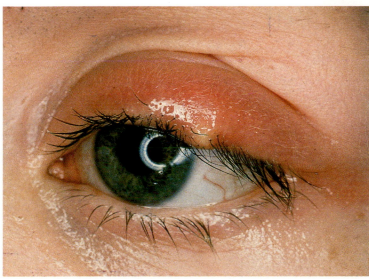

**1.18** | External hordeolum. Note the focal, perifollicular pustule and the more diffuse surrounding edema and erythema. (From Lambert HP, Farrar WE: *Infectious Diseases Illustrated.* London: Gower Medical Publishing, 1982, 11.2.)

glands, with gland obstruction followed by inflammation and granuloma formation (Fig. 1.19).

The pathophysiology of chronic blepharitis appears to be related to the interaction of lid margin secretions, especially lipids, lid-margin organisms, and the tear film. Some investigators have found meibomian secretions to be abnormal in patients with chronic blepharitis.[14] Bacterial lipases may further degrade sebaceous secretions into irritating fatty acids, and bacterial organisms may produce irritating toxins.

Treatment of blepharitis consists of both general treatment, appropriate for all forms, and specific treatment, dependent on the type of blepharitis (Fig. 1.20). Lid hygiene is the mainstay of all blepharitis treatment. Warm moist compresses serve both to loosen lid margin debris and to soften and help remove secretions from the perifollicular and the meibomian glands. After the use of compresses, usually for 5–10 minutes, mechanical scrubbing of the lid serves to remove the loosened and liquified material. A corner of the washcloth or a cotton-tipped applicator with soap or shampoo applied, or commercially available pads soaked in a detergent, can be used for this purpose. Warm compresses and lid scrubs are usually adequate to relieve symptoms in a high proportion of patients, but sometimes additional specific treatment is necessary. For staphylococcal blepharitis the addition of a broad-spectrum antibiotic, such as bacitracin or erythromycin, applied to the lashes and lid margins in ointment form, may be helpful. Lid margin cultures are occasionally necessary and are likely to yield *S. aureus*, *S. epidermidis*, or *Propionibacterium acnes*. Seborrheic blepharitis patients may benefit from the use of keratolytic or tar extract-containing shampoos applied to the face and brows as well as to the scalp. Patients with significant meibomian gland dysfunction may benefit from eyelid massage and expression of meibomian gland secretions. Patients with chronic meibomitis, especially those with rosacea, often respond well to oral antibiotics, such as tetracycline 250 mg four times daily on an empty stomach for 3–4 weeks and then tapered, or doxycycline or minocycline once or twice a day. All patients should be reminded of the chronicity of these diseases and the need to increase or decrease the aggressiveness of therapy depending on the degree of disease activity. It is important to recognize that tear insufficiency is a frequent concomitant disorder in patients with blepharitis. This association may be caused by tear film abnormalities induced by eyelid disease, leading to tear film instability and more rapid tear film evaporation. In turn, aqueous tear insufficiency may reduce the normal rinsing of lid margin debris and thus lead to blepharitis. In either event, it is important to treat the tear insufficiency as well as the blepharitis.

**1.19** | *A:* Chalazion—external appearance of bilateral eyelid lesions. *B:* Granuloma—seen on eyelid eversion.

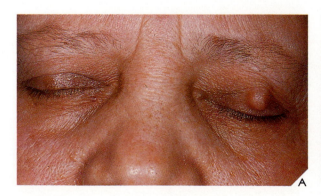
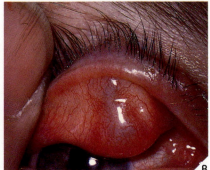

Initial treatment of the chalazia and hordeolae that commonly accompany chronic blepharitis consists of warm compresses. I also prefer to inject intralesional corticosteroids at the time of the initial examination, using 10 mg/ml triamcinolone. Lesions that persist may respond to repeat injection or may require surgical treatment. Persistent hordeolae can be treated with incision and drainage through either the cutaneous or the conjunctival side of the lid. Chalazia are treated by excision of the granuloma through a tarsal conjunctival incision, often followed by intralesional steroid injection. [15] Although skin depigmentation has been reported with intralesional steroid injection in highly pigmented individuals, this is infrequent and is reversible over time.

Other forms of blepharitis include that seen with atopy, in which there is often erythema, edema, hyalinization, or increased wrinkling (Fig. 1.21), and fissuring of the eyelid skin. These patients complain of itching and often have associated conjunctival and/or corneal inflammation.[16] Treatment consists of removal of the allergens when possible, antihistamines, and judicious steroid use. Similar changes are seen with contact dermatitis, which may be induced by skin contact with ophthalmic medications, cosmetics, or glasses frames (Fig. 1.22). Treatment consists of removal of the allergen and, when

## Figure 1.20. Treatment of Chronic Blepharitis

| Blepharitis Type | Treatment Modality | | | | |
|---|---|---|---|---|---|
| | Warm Compresses | Lid Massage | Lid Scrubs | Topical Antibiotics | Systemic Tetracycline |
| Anterior | | | | | |
|   Staphylococcal | Yes | No | Yes | Yes | No* |
|   Seborrheic | Yes | No | Yes | ± | No |
| Mixed | | | | | |
|   Seborrheic and meibomian seborrhea | Yes | Yes | Yes | ± | No |
|   Seborrheic with meibomitis | Yes | Yes | Yes | ± | Yes |
| Posterior | | | | | |
|   Primary meibomitis | Yes | Yes | Yes | ± | Yes |

± = Sometimes.
* Yes, in phlyctenulosis.

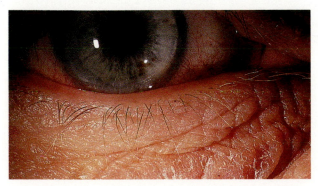

**1.21** | Atopic blepharitis. Note the scaling and thickening of the eyelid skin secondary to chronic inflammation.

necessary, brief use of topical corticosteroids. Urticaria (hives) causes localized swelling, often of unknown cause, and erythema of the skin that responds to antihistamines and adrenergic drugs. Blepharochalasis is an uncommon disorder of unknown cause, characterized by recurrent eyelid swelling in young people and leading to redundant eyelid skin, ptosis, and canthal stretching. Symptoms of recurrent edema decrease into adulthood, and treatment consists of plastic surgery to the lids after the bouts of swelling have abated.[17]

Angular blepharitis is an infectious form of blepharitis usually involving the lateral and/or medial canthal region. Although *Moraxella lacunata* was a common causative agent in the past, staphylococcal organisms now appear to predominate. Treatment is with lid hygiene and topical antibiotics if necessary. Zinc sulfate has also been used for *Moraxella*, and has been presumed to act by inhibition of bacterial proteases that cause skin maceration, although this hypothesis has been questioned.

Madarosis is the loss of eyelashes. The many causes cover the full spectrum of eyelid disease. In addition to the forms of blepharitis mentioned earlier, madarosis may be seen with cutaneous diseases such as alopecia areata or universalis, psoriasis, and systemic lupus erythematosus; infectious diseases including leprosy, tuberculosis, and syphilis; and endocrinopathies such as thyroid disease. Lash loss has also been reported with "crack" cocaine abuse[19] and with various topical ophthalmic medications. An interesting presentation of madarosis is in trichotillomania, a psychogenic disorder of habitual hair removal that occurs most commonly in teenaged girls who repeatedly pluck their lashes. Usually the patient denies this, but the demonstration of multiple broken lashes in the face of otherwise normal lids usually confirms the diagnosis.

## DERMATOLOGIC DISEASE

Many cutaneous diseases affect the eyelid skin and often the conjunctiva and cornea as well. Many, such as Stevens–Johnson syndrome, epidermolysis bullosa, and pemphigoid, are more appropriately discussed with the conjunctiva and cornea. Others, however, predominantly involve the skin and only secondarily affect the eye itself. Psoriasis, a scaling cutaneous disorder with rapid turnover of epidermal cells and the development of thickened red plaques with overlying silver-white scales, may affect the eyelids (Fig. 1.23)

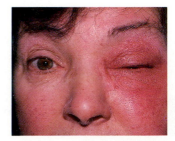

**1.22** | Allergic reaction (contact dermatitis). The well-circumscribed erythema and indurated skin usually present no problem in diagnosis. The conjunctiva is frequently edematous and injected, and a history of local application of eye drops or ointment is obtained. A gradual subsidence of signs occurs with cessation of the exciting agent. (From Kirkness CM: *Ophthalmology*. London: Gower Medical Publishing, 1985, 10.)

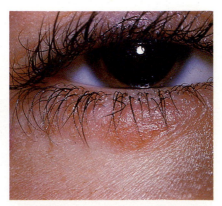

**1.23** | Psoriatic blepharitis. Note the scaly plaque on the eyelid skin.

and may cause blepharitis, but rarely causes keratoconjunctivitis and uveitis. Treatment of the lid disorder is that of the systemic disease. The use of psoralens (drugs that sensitize the skin to ultraviolet light) and ultraviolet light of 320–400 nm (UVA) to treat psoriasis may increase the risk of cataract formation, and ocular protection during and for a period after treatment is important to reduce ocular side effects.

Ichthyosis is a group of inherited cutaneous disorders that cause scaling of the skin. Ichthyosis vulgaris has little ocular consequence. X-linked ichthyosis is associated with corneal opacities and corneal erosions. Lamellar ichthyosis, which is transmitted as an autosomal recessive, is associated with marked hyalinization and scaling of the skin. Involved individuals may have ectropion present in infancy or at birth as "collodion babies," with a thick, almost glassy-appearing membrane covering the skin. They also may develop ectropion as they grow older (Fig. 1.24), and aggressive treatment of this with skin hydration and topical retinoids and surgical treatment when needed may prevent the consequences of corneal exposure.

Ectodermal dysplasia refers to a group of disorders characterized by abnormal or absent development of skin appendages including hair, glands, nails, or teeth. One of these disorders, EEC syndrome, consists of ectodermal dysplasia, claw hand deformity (ectrodactyly), and clefting of the lip and palate. These patients, who have markedly reduced or absent meibomian glands, develop blepharitis and a keratopathy that may be secondary to the blepharitis or a manifestation of ectodermal dysplasia. Treatment is difficult and relies on lid hygiene and ocular lubrication.

## TUMORS

Eyelid tumors are common. They range from the benign, everyday lesions of xanthelasma and seborrheic keratosis to malignant melanoma and sebaceous gland carcinoma. The full spectrum of dermatologic neoplasms can involve the lids. Rather than performing an exhaustive review of all possible eyelid lesions, I will review those commonly encountered or those less frequently encountered but important to recognize. (See Volume 4, Chapter 6.)

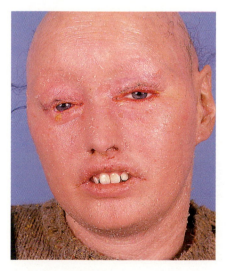

**1.24** | Facial and eyelid changes in patient with lamellar ichthyosis. Note the hair loss, scaling of the skin, and ectropion despite multiple eyelid surgical procedures.

## BENIGN EYELID LESIONS

A variety of cysts can arise from the adnexal glands of the skin, including the glands of Zeis and Moll (Figs. 1.25, 1.26) or, more commonly, the perifollicular glands (Fig. 1.27), as sebaceous cysts. The usual treatment is local excision if the patient desires.

**1.25** | Cyst of Zeis.

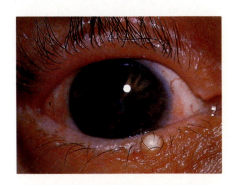

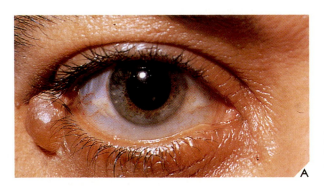

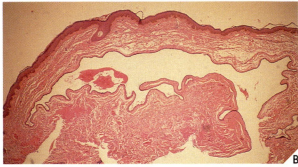

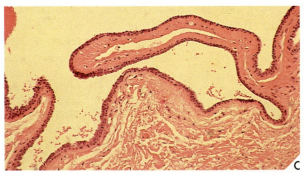

**1.26** | *A:* Ductal cyst noted near outer margin of the right lower lid. *B:* The multiloculated cyst is lined by a double-layered epithelium, shown with increased magnification in *C.* (From Yanoff M, Fine BS: *Ocular Pathology. A Color Atlas*, ed 2. New York: Gower Medical Publishing, 1992, 6.8.)

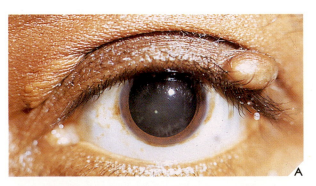

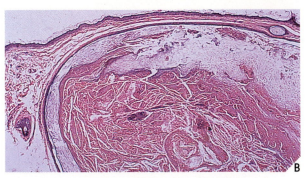

**1.27** | Epithelial inclusion cyst. *A:* The patient has a large, epithelial inclusion cyst of the outer third of the left upper lid. Note the xanthelasma at the inner corner of the left upper lid. *B:* The cyst is lined by stratified squamous epithelium that desquamates keratin into its lumen. (From Yanoff M, Fine BS: *Ocular Pathology. A Color Atlas*, ed 2. New York: Gower Medical Publishing, 1992, 6.7.)

Seborrheic keratoses (basal cell papillomas) are "stuck-on"-appearing lesions with a greasy appearance and a range of pigmentation (Figs. 1.28, 1.29). Proliferation of basal cells and enlargement of the prickle-cell layer are seen, with no involvement of the dermis.

Squamous papilomas are sessile or pedunculated benign lesions (Fig. 1.30), which may form cutaneous horns.

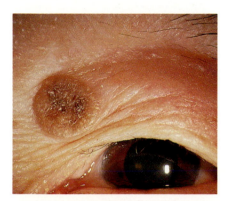

**1.28** | Typical seborrheic keratosis.

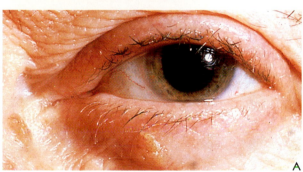

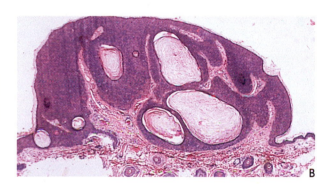

**1.29** | Seborrheic keratosis. *A:* A "greasy" elevated lesion is present in the middle, nasal portion of the left lower lid. Biopsy showed this to be a seborrheic keratosis. The smaller lesion just inferior and nasal to the seborrheic keratosis proved to be a syringoma. *B:* Histologic section shows a papillomatous lesion that lies above the skin surface and is blue in color. The lesion contains proliferated basaloid cells and keratin-filled cysts. (From Yanoff M, Fine BS: *Ocular Pathology. A Color Atlas*, ed 2. New York: Gower Medical Publishing, 1992, 6.10.)

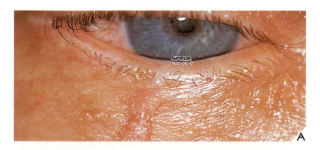

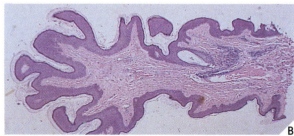

**1.30** | Squamous papilloma. *A:* A skin tag is noted in the middle portion of the lower lid. *B:* Histologic section shows a narrow-based papilloma that contains many finger-like processes called fronds. The fronds are covered by an acanthotic, hyperkeratotic epithelium and contain a fibrovascular core. (From Yanoff M, Fine BS: *Ocular Pathology. A Color Atlas*, ed 2. New York: Gower Medical Publishing, 1992, 6.10.)

Senile keratosis typically involves sunlight-exposed areas, including the forehead and eyelids (Fig. 1.31A). Mitotic activity is high, with dysplastic changes (Fig. 1.31B,C), and this benign lesion may be a precursor of squamous-cell carcinoma. Treatment includes local excision, protection from sunlight and, for diffuse involvement, the use of topical antimetabolites.

Keratoacanthoma is a rapidly growing benign lesion that may become quite large but then usually spontaneously regresses after 2 to 3 months (Fig. 1.32).

Inverted follicular keratosis is a benign lesion that may clinically simulate a malignant lesion and appears as an isolated nodule. Histopathologic examination reveals swirling epithelial cells with proliferation of the prickle-

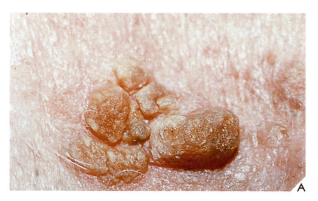

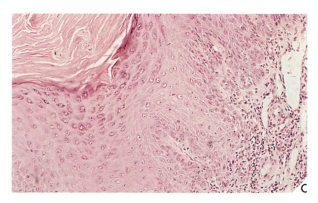

**1.31** | Actinic keratosis. *A:* The clinical appearance of a lesion involving the left upper lid. *B:* Histologic section shows a papillomatous lesion that is above the skin surface, appears red in color, and has marked hyperkeratosis and acanthosis. *C:* Although the squamous layer of the skin is increased in thickness (acanthosis) and the basal layer shows atypical cells, the normal polarity of the epidermis is preserved. (From Yanoff M, Fine BS: *Ocular Pathology. A Color Atlas*, ed 2. New York: Gower Medical Publishing, 1992, 6.9.)

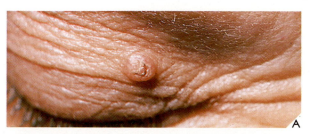

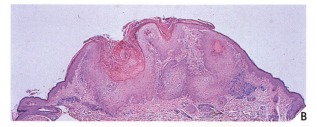

**1.32** | Keratoacanthoma. *A:* This patient had a 6-week history of a rapidly enlarging lesion. Note the umbilicated central area. *B:* Histologic section shows that the lesion is above the surface epithelium, has a cup-shaped configuration, and a central keratin core. The base of the acanthotic epithelium is blunted (rather than invasive) at the junction of the dermis. (From Yanoff M, Fine BS: *Ocular Pathology. A Color Atlas*, ed 2. New York: Gower Medical Publishing, 1992, 6.11.)

cell layer (acanthosis). Other similar lesions with resemblance to neoplasms are often categorized as pseudoepitheliomatous hyperplasia.

The adnexal tissues of the skin, in addition to the cysts mentioned above, may also form neoplasms. Those that differentiate to form immature hair follicles are called trichoepitheliomas (Figs. 1.33, 1.34), while nevoid proliferations of sweat gland ducts are called syringomas (Fig. 1.35). Sebaceous adenomas are benign proliferations of meibomian gland cells in the tarsal plate.

Many other benign lesions, including those of vascular origin (Figs. 1.36, 1.37), may involve the lids and are discussed more completely elsewhere.

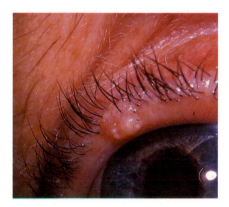

**1.33** | Trichoepithelioma.

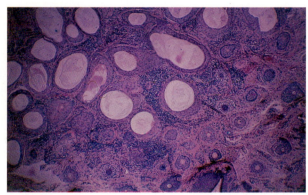

**1.34** | Histopathology of previous patient. Note the numerous hair follicles and cysts with a keratin core surrounded by basal cells.

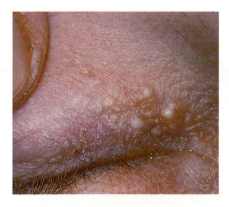

**1.35** | Multiple syringomas.

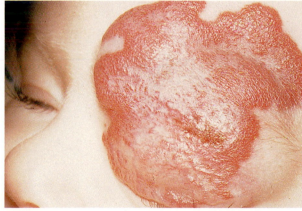

**1.36** | Cavernous hemangioma of the eyelid. Note the marked ptosis caused by the lesion.

**1.37** | Hemangioma of the lid. Different sized, thin-walled spaces are filled with blood. These vascular spaces are lined by endothelium. The intervening fibrous septa show variable thickness. (Courtesy of Dr. Myron Yanoff.)

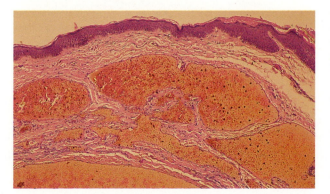

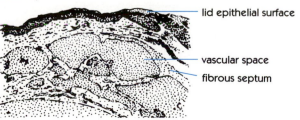

lid epithelial surface

vascular space

fibrous septum

## Figure 1.38. Common Eyelid Malignancies

Basal cell carcinoma
Squamous cell carcinoma
Sebaceous gland carcinoma
Malignant melanoma
Metastatic carcinoma
Kaposi's sarcoma
Other

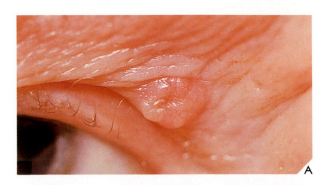

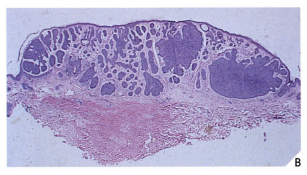

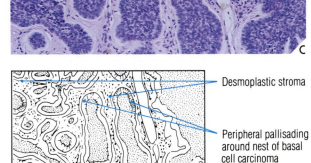

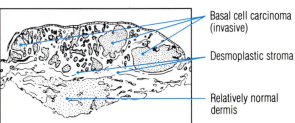

Basal cell carcinoma (invasive)

Desmoplastic stroma

Relatively normal dermis

Desmoplastic stroma

Peripheral pallisading around nest of basal cell carcinoma

**1.39** | Basal cell carcinoma. *A:* A firm, indurated, painless lesion had been present for about 8 months. *B:* Excisional biopsy shows epithelial proliferation arising from the basal layer of the epidermis. The proliferated cells appear blue and are present in nests of different sizes. Note the sharp demarcation of the pale, pink area of stroma supporting the neoplastic cells from the underlying (normal) dark pink dermis. This stromal change, called desmoplasia, is characteristic of neoplastic

lesions. *C:* The nests are composed of atypical basal cells and show peripheral palisading. Mitotic figures are present. Again, note the pseudosarcomatous change (desmoplasia) of the surrounding supporting stroma which is light pink and contains proliferating fibroblasts. (*A,* courtesy of Dr. HG Scheie; all photographs from Yanoff M, Fine BS: *Ocular Pathology. A Color Atlas,* ed 2. New York: Gower Medical Publishing, 1992, 6.12.)

The eyelid is a common site of cutaneous malignancy and is the most frequent location of malignancies encountered in ophthalmic practice. These lesions will be discussed in order of their relative frequency of occurrence (Fig. 1.38).

Basal cell carcinoma is the most common human malignancy. It most often involves the head and neck and frequently affects the eyelids.[20] Not surprisingly, this is by far the most common eyelid malignancy. Most lesions involve the lower lid or inner canthal region and, less frequently, the outer canthus or upper lid. The most common lesion is nodular, with prominent surface vessels. As the lesion enlarges the margins become pearly and remain elevated, while the center of the lesions may ulcerate and become depressed. Clinical and histopathologic variations exist (Figs. 1.39–1.41). Although many methods have been used for removal of these lesions and simple excision is appropriate for small lesions, the safest approach includes microscopic control of tissue resection that ensures tumor-free margins.[21]

Squamous cell carcinoma of the eyelid has often been thought to be a common malignancy, but in reality it accounts for only about 9% of eyelid malignancies[22] and as little as 0.5% of eyelid tumors.[23] Squamous-cell carcinomas (Figs. 1.42, 1.43) are seen in sunlight-exposed areas and are more common on the lower eyelid. These lesions may arise de novo or from actinic keratoses. They progress from a scaly area to ulceration with thick-

# MALIGNANT EYELID LESIONS

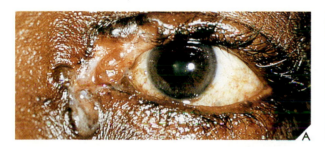

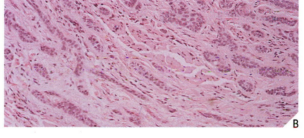

**1.40 | Basal cell carcinoma. A:** The inner aspect of the eyelids is ulcerated by the infiltrating tumor. **B:** Histologic section shows the morphea-like or fibrosing type, where the basal cells grow in thin strands or cords, often only one cell layer thick, closely resembling metastatic scirrhous carcinoma of the breast ("indian file" pattern). This uncommon type of basal cell carcinoma has a much worse prognosis than the more common types, i.e., nodular, ulcerative, and multicentric. (From Yanoff M, Fine BS: *Ocular Pathology. A Color Atlas*, ed 2. New York: Gower Medical Publishing, 1992, 6.13.)

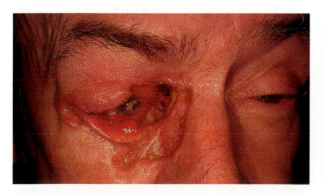

**1.41 |** Basal cell carcinoma with direct extension into the orbit and the ethmoid sinuses.

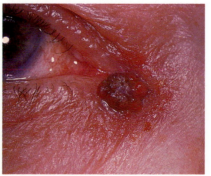

**1.42 |** Squamous cell carcinoma with a papillomatous appearance.

ened margins, or may present as benign-appearing papillomatous lesions or nodules or as horn-like lesions. Spread is by local invasion and extension to regional nodes, although metastasis is infrequent with appropriate treatment. Microscopically controlled complete excision of lesions is the treatment of choice, although favorable responses can in some instances be achieved with radiation or cryotherapy. When orbital invasion is present, exenteration is indicated.

Sebaceous gland carcinoma may well be as common a cause of eyelid malignancy as squamous cell carcinoma, accounting for 1% to 5.5% of malignant lesions.[24] These tumors arise from sebaceous adnexal glands, most commonly the meibomian glands or the perifollicular glands of Zeis, or from other lesser adnexal sebaceous glands (Fig. 1.44). Women are more commonly involved than men, and the upper eyelid is the most usual site. The usual presentation is a firm, nodular lid mass, initially involving the deeper lid structures. Its resemblance to chalazion is sufficient to prompt histopathologic evaluation of recurrent chalazia. Extension of tumor cells into the conjunctival epithelium by pagetoid spread may lead to a chronic unilateral conjunctivitis that clinically resembles squamous cell carcinoma or to chronic blepharoconjunctivitis. Biopsy is essential to confirm the diagnosis; when sebaceous gland carcinoma is suspected, fresh-frozen tissue should be submitted for fat stains. Treatment consists of local excision with wide margins, along with map biopsy of the conjunctiva and other eyelid areas, because of the multicentric origin and pagetoid spread of many of these tumors. Extensive involvement may require orbital exenteration. Local cryotreatment of conjunctival involvement has also been suggested.[25] Despite aggressive local treatment, recurrence is not unusual. Spread is to the orbit and regional lymph nodes, and sometimes to the systemic viscera.

Other neoplasms that may involve the lids include malignant melanoma (Figs. 1.45, 1.46), which can arise de novo, from a preexisting

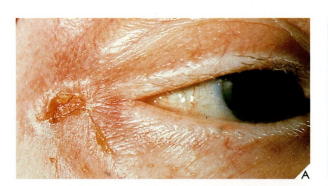

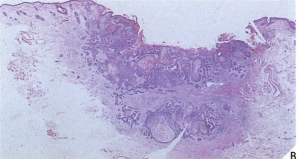

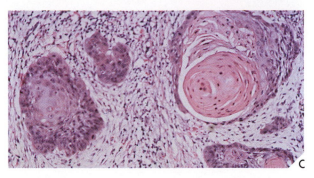

**1.43** | Squamous cell carcinoma. *A:* The patient has an ulcerating lesion of the lateral aspect of the eyelids that had increased in size over many months. *B:* Histologic section of the excisional biopsy shows epithelial cells, with an overall pink color, which infiltrate the dermis deeply. The overlying region is ulcerated. *C:* Increased magnification shows the squamous neoplastic cells making keratin (horn cyst) in an abnormal location (dyskeratosis). Numerous mitotic figures are present. Note the pseudosarcomatous (dysplastic) change in the surrounding stroma. (From Yanoff M, Fine BS: *Ocular Pathology. A Color Atlas,* ed 2. New York: Gower Medical Publishing, 1992, 6.13.)

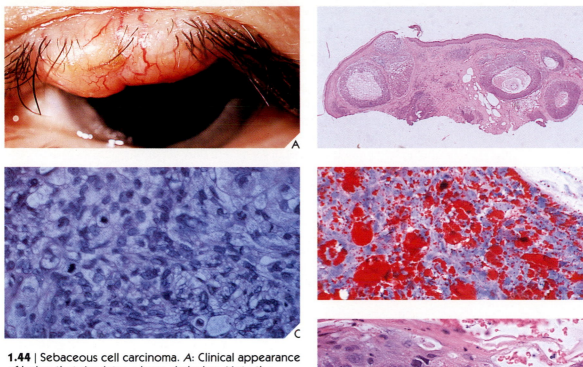

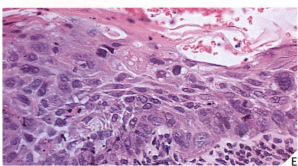

**1.44** | Sebaceous cell carcinoma. *A*: Clinical appearance of lesion that simulates a large chalazion. Note the characteristic loss of hair over the lesion. *B*: Histologic section shows large tumor nodules, most of which exhibit central necrosis, in the dermis. *C*: Increased magnification shows that numerous cells resemble sebaceous gland cells. A number of mitotic figures are present. *D*: Many of the cells stain positively for fat. Any recurrent or suspicious chalazion should be biopsied. *E*: In another case, large tumor cells are scattered throughout the epithelium, resembling Paget's disease and called pagetoid change. The cancerous invasion of the epithelium can cause a chronic, nongranulomatous, blepharoconjunctivitis (masquerade syndrome). (*D*, oil red-O.) (From Yanoff M, Fine BS: *Ocular Pathology. A Color Atlas,* ed 2. New York: Gower Medical Publishing, 1992, 6.14.)

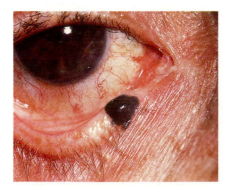

**1.45** | Malignant melanoma of the eyelid.

nevus, or can represent metastasis from other skin lesions. Treatment is the same as for malignant melanoma elsewhere on the skin.

Metastatic spread of neoplasms to the eyelid is rare and accounts for less than 1% of eyelid malignancies.[26, 27] The most common primary sources appear to be breast, gastrointestinal tract, respiratory system, skin, and the genitourinary system. Diagnosis requires biopsy to be performed.[28]

Lymphoma involving the eyelids is uncommon, accounting for only 8% of Jakobiec and Knowles' series of 108 patients with ocular adnexal lymphoma.[29] Unlike conjunctival and orbital lymphomas in which nonocular lymphoma was present or developed in only about one third of patients, two thirds of patients with eyelid lymphoma had or developed lymphoma elsewhere.[29] For localized lesions, treatment is irradiation after systemic evaluation has been carried out.

Kaposi's sarcoma as part of the acquired immune deficiency syndrome (AIDS) may present as a purple or red cutaneous lesion involving the eyelid skin and often the conjunctiva. This is readily recognized as part of the AIDS syndrome.

Merkel cell carcinoma is a rare tumor of a normally occurring dendritic form of epithelial cell found in the skin, especially around appendages. These tumors often involve the eyelid and present as a smooth, bulging red nodule. Treatment consists of wide local excision, and radiation may also play a role. Recurrence is common and these tumors may spread to regional nodes. Systemic spread may cause death.[30]

The large number of benign and malignant lesions that can involve the eyelids warrants an awareness of the possible causes and should prompt biopsy and histopathologic evaluation when there is clinical uncertainty.

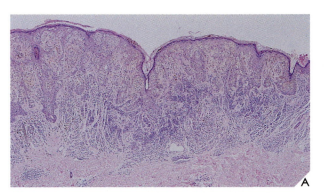
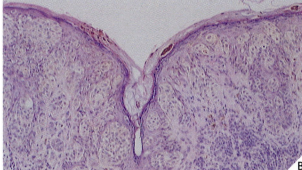

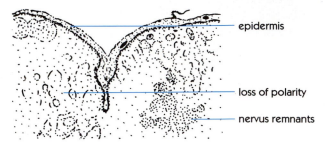

**1.46** | Malignant melanoma of skin. *A*: The melanoma has arisen from a preexistent nevus. *B*: Increased magnification shows remnants of a nevus, especially on the right half, in the deeper layers. On the left half, however, the normal polarity of a nevus (larger cells towards the surface and smaller, more spindly cells towards the bottom) is lost. Also, both individual and nests of melanoma cells are invading the epidermis. (Courtesy of Dr. Myron Yanoff.)

epidermis

loss of polarity

nervus remnants

# 2 THE CONJUNCTIVA

## Stephen D. Rheinstrom

## ANATOMY AND EMBRYOLOGY

The conjunctiva is the thin, flexible layer of tissue that covers the inner surface of the eyelids and the anterior sclera. Although it is a continuous membrane, convention divides it into three portions: palpebral, fornical (cul de sac), and bulbar. The elasticity of the conjunctiva enables eye movements to be unencumbered without an excessive redundancy of tissue. It contributes to the tear film by the production of mucus, and in the cul de sac areas acts as a reservoir and mixing area for tears. In addition, the conjunctival epithelium and its secretions form an important barrier to foreign matter and infection. The conjunctiva is also important in ocular wound healing. Conjunctival wounds heal rapidly with little formation of scar tissue. The conjunctival and corneal limbal epithelia may be involved in the maintenance of the corneal epithelium.[1,2]

Embryologically, the ectodermal and subectodermal tissues overlying the optic vesicle provide the epithelial and subepithelial components of the cornea, conjunctiva, and eyelid. Differentiation of the conjunctival epithelium from the eyelid skin and cornea can be seen as early as the tenth week of fetal life when goblet cells become visible in the tissue. Invagination of epithelium of the upper temporal fornix heralds the formation of the palpebral and orbital portions of the lacrimal gland (at week 8), and later invaginations of the upper and lower fornical and palpebral conjunctivae (at 12 weeks) begin the formation of the accessory glands of Krause and Wolfring.

The caruncle arises from the medial portion of the lower lid fold and is separated from the lid as the lower canaliculus develops. The caruncle develops to be covered with nonkeratinized stratified epithelium in which fine hairs with sebaceous glands are found. Just lateral to the caruncle, the semilunar fold (plica semilunaris) is formed as a soft fold of the bulbar conjunctiva, and is the equivalent of the nictitating membrane seen in other mammals.

The palpebral conjunctiva begins at the mucocutaneous border of the lids, and extends to cover the tarsal plates of the

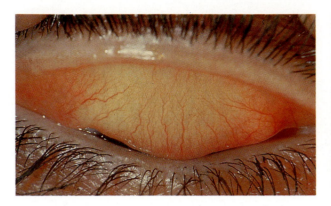

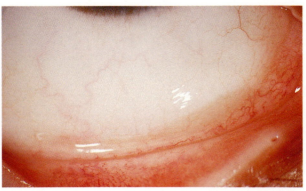

**2.1.** | Normal palpebral conjunctiva overlying the superior tarsal plate seen by everting the upper lid.

**2.2** | Inferior fornix, showing folds and abundant lymphoid tissue.

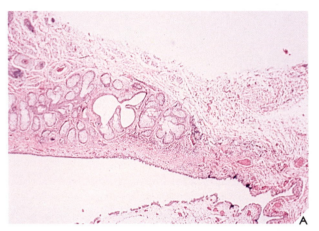

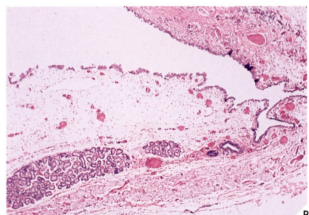

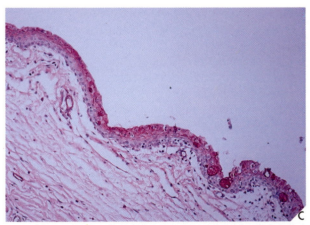

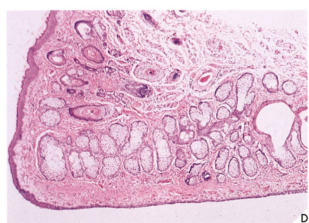

**2.3** | Conjunctiva. *A:* The normal conjunctiva, a mucous membrane composed of nonkeratinizing squamous epithelium intermixed with goblet cells, rests on a connective tissue substantia propria. It is divided into three zones: palpebral, fornical, and bulbar. *B:* Increased magnification shows the tight adherence of the substantia propria of the palpebral (tarsal) conjunctival epithelium to the underlying tarsal connective tissue and the loose adherence of the substantia propria of the bulbar conjunctival epithelium to the underlying tissue. *C:* The goblet cells of the bulbar conjunctiva are easily seen with PAS stain. *D:* The tarsal conjunctiva becomes keratinized as it becomes continuous with the keratinized squamous epithelium of the skin on the intermarginal surface of the the lid near its posterior border. (From Yanoff M, Fine BS: *Ocular Pathology. A Color Atlas,* ed 2. New York: Gower Medical Publishing, 1992, 7.2.)

lids (Fig. 2.1). It has a smooth surface containing crypts (of Henle) lined with epithelium that range from 0.1–0.5 mm in diameter.[3] These openings are also found in the fornix and bulbar conjunctiva.

The conjunctiva of the fornix is loosely attached to the underlying tissue (Fig. 2.2). It is perforated by ducts of the lacrimal gland in the temporal upper fornix and by ducts of the accessory lacrimal glands of Krause and Wolfring in both upper and lower fornices (Fig. 2.3).

The bulbar conjunctiva (Fig. 2.4) continues from the fornix to the corneal limbus to complete the coverage of the anterior segment of the eye.

The conjunctiva is similar to other mucous membranes and is composed of epithelium and stroma. The epithelium has stratified squamous cells at the limbus and at the palpebral margins but otherwise consists of two or more layers of stratified columnar epithelium. Melanocytes are present in the basal layer, and melanin pigment granules can be seen in adjacent basal and overlying wing cells (a common finding in darkly pigmented individuals). The basal cells have a thin basement membrane with few hemidesmosomes. The cells have deep interdigitations and intercellular attachments that mimic those in the corneal epithelium. The superficial cells are very flattened and have microplicae and microvilli analogous to the corneal surface.[4]

Goblet cells can be found throughout most of the conjunctival epithelium but are most numerous in the inferonasal portion of the bulbar conjunctiva.[5] These cells have abundant mucin-containing granules and appear to be deficient in dry-eye syndromes.[6] Vitamin A plays a role in conjunctival differentiation. In vitamin A deficiency, loss of goblet cells and keratinization of the conjunctival epithelium can be documented with impression cytology.[7]

Other superficial conjunctival epithelium contains mucous vesicles, and this is thought to be the "second mucous system."[8,9] This portion of the mucus overlies the epithelial surface, and the outer layer of mucus (from the goblet cells) is believed to function in lubrication of the globe and lids and to aid in wetting of the hydrophobic conjunctival and corneal epithelium.[8]

The stroma possesses fibrovascular connective tissue containing blood vessels, nerves, and lymphatics. The palpebral portions are more compact and become looser in the cul de sac and bulbar areas, thinning again at the limbus.

The palpebral conjunctiva and the eyelids share a common blood supply from the distal branches of the ophthalmic artery along with contribu-

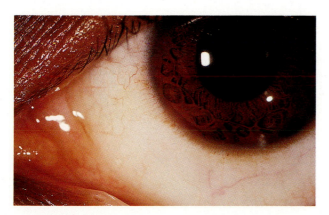

**2.4** | Bulbar conjunctiva, closely applied to the sclera. Both conjunctival and episcleral blood vessels can be easily seen through the transparent tissue. The fine terminal branches of the posterior conjunctival and anterior ciliary arteries combine to form the limbal arcade, which normally extends slightly into the cornea. The limbal insertion of the bulbar conjunctiva marks the beginning of Bowman's corneal membrane.

tions from branches of the facial artery. The bulbar conjunctiva is nourished by twigs of the anterior ciliary artery. The fornix receives its arterial supply from both bulbar and palpebral sources. Venous drainage of the bulbar conjunctiva adds to the episcleral venous plexuses. The palpebral veins merge with the post-tarsal eyelid veins and fill into the orbital veins as well as the branches of the anterior facial vein and pterygoid plexus.

Lymphatic connections of the conjunctiva parallel those of the eyelids. The medial third of the upper lid/conjunctiva and the medial two thirds of the lower lid/conjunctiva drain to the submandibular lymph nodes. The lateral two thirds of the upper and the lateral third of the lower lid/conjunctival drain to the preauricular lymph nodes.

The V cranial nerve supplies sensory branches to the conjunctiva. Other components of the stroma include melanocytes, fibroblasts, and inflammatory cells. Inflammatory cells are absent at birth and begin to appear after 1 month of age. Concentrations of lymphocytes can normally be seen in the fornix, some of which have germinal centers.

## PHYSIOLOGY AND BIOCHEMISTRY

Few studies of conjunctival physiology have been performed. Maurice[10] found an electrical potential similar to that reported for the cornea. The permeability of the conjunctival epithelium is more than five times that of the cornea. Active aerobic metabolism occurs in conjunctiva. High levels of tricarboxylic acid cycle, glycolytic, and respiratory chain enzymes are found, and large numbers of mitochondria are present.[11]

## DIAGNOSTIC TECHNIQUES

Problems relating to the conjunctiva are a frequent reason for the patient to present to an ophthalmologist. As is often the case, a detailed history is the best foundation on which to base any diagnostic conclusions. Specific questioning as to when the condition was first noted, type and quantity of any discharge, and any associated pain can help to confirm a clinical impression.

A detailed external and slit-lamp biomicroscopic examination of the affected tissues, including eversion of the lids to expose the palpebral conjunctiva, is an absolute necessity. A correct clinical judgment based on the history and the physical examination often eliminates the need for further tests. When to do laboratory studies is a difficult decision and is made much easier by a detailed understanding of the possible pathology. A thorough knowledge of the spectrum of presentations of cases of viral conjunctivitis will make bacteriologic investigations unnecessary in these cases. However, viral cultures, immunofluorescent stains, and/or antibody titers can still be done when confirmation is essential.

After the examination, the clinician must determine if any further tests are needed to confirm or to make a definitive diagnosis. Most viral and all vernal conjunctivitides are identifiable on clinical grounds, and supplementary investigation is not cost effective. When the disease is not so easily pigeonholed, laboratory tests may be helpful, as in cases of follicular conjunctivitis [to distinguish among trachoma inclusion conjunctivitis (TRIC), adenovirus, and *Herpes simplex* virus]. Cultures can also be diagnostically helpful in cases of persistent blepharoconjunctivitis unresponsive to therapy. Laboratory tests are indicated when the findings suggest bacterial or fungal infection (e.g., to rule out *Neisseria gonorrhoeae* in a markedly purulent acute conjunctivitis) and in infectious conjunctivitis of the newborn. Investigations are also needed in any moderately severe long-standing conjunctivitis and in Parinaud oculoglandular syndrome.

Microbiologic cultures of the conjunctiva are typically done only on blood and chocolate agar (for cultivation of *Haemophilus* and *Neisseria* species). The use of additional media is dictated by the clinical impressions [e.g., Lowenstein–Jensen medium for *Mycobacterium* and *Nocardia* species, Sabouraud's dextrose agar (without cycloheximide—an inhibitor of saprophytic fungi) in oculoglandular conjunctivitis].

Viral cultures are rarely used because of expense and low yield. However, if a viral culture is done early in the infective course, recovery of isolates is higher. Direct transfer of an inoculum to an appropriate cell line in tissue culture is rarely possible. A transport medium is used to hold the inoculum viable until it can be placed in tissue culture. If this cannot be done within 2 h or less, the transport medium should be deep frozen. The participation of a virologist in the selection of the tissue culture is most helpful. Even under the best of circumstances, recovery rates can be 50% or less.

Cytologic examination can be very helpful in the differential diagnosis of conjunctivitis. Kimura platinum spatula scrapings of the conjunctiva are often more useful than examinations of smears of conjunctival exudates, as recognizable organisms are often not seen in the smears of exudate. A scraping of conjunctiva spread in a thin layer on a glass slide stained by the Gram method will often show organisms in bacterial conjunctivitis.

Cytologic response can be tested with a Giemsa stain. This is best done with the Kimura spatula, scraping the upper pretarsal conjunctiva. With mild pressure, epithelium and surface cells are removed. Excessive pressure results in bleeding, which will make the examination of the slide difficult. The scraping should be smeared on a clean glass slide and immediately placed in methyl alcohol to prevent any drying effects and preserve cell morphology.

The Papanicolaou stain technique can be useful with certain epithelial tumors or with *H. simplex* (intranuclear inclusion bodies). These slides are made in a similar fashion but are immediately placed in alcohol–ether solution.

Cytological studies may be helpful in assessing acute and chronic conjunctivitis but are not diagnostic. (Fig. 2.5)

An impressive use of ocular cytology is a Giemsa-stained scraping of

### Figure 2.5. Cytology of Conjunctival Scrapings

| CELL TYPE | PROBABLE CONJUNCTIVITIS |
| --- | --- |
| Polymorphonuclear leukocytes | Bacterial |
| | Acute viral |
| | Acute chlamydial |
| | Acute fungal |
| | Drug reaction |
| Mixed PMN and lymphocytes | Chlamydial |
| | Intermediate viral |
| Lymphocytes | Viral |
| | Drug reaction |
| Eosinophils | Allergic |
| Multinucleated giant cells | *Herpes simplex, Herpes zoster,* rubella, tuberculosis |

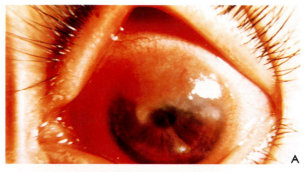

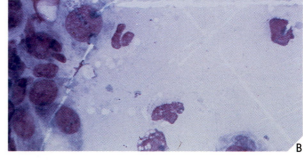

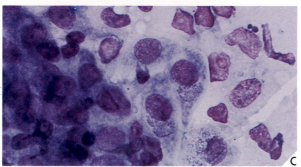

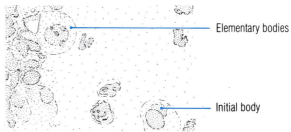

Elementary bodies

Initial body

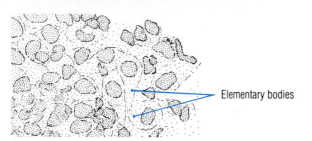

Elementary bodies

**2.6** | Trachoma. *A:* The patient has a trachomatous pannus growing over the superior cornea. With healing, the follicles disappear from the peripheral cornea, leaving areas filled with a thickened, transparent epithelium called Herbert pits. The palpebral conjunctiva scars by the formation of a linear white horizontal line or scar near the upper border of the tarsus, called a von Arlt line. (Photo courtesy of Dr. AP Ferry.)
*B:* Conjunctival smear from a trachoma patient showing a large cytoplasmic basophilic initial body. Small cytoplasmic elementary bodies are seen in other cells.
*C:* Small cytoplasmic elementary bodies are seen in several cells of this scraping. (From Yanoff M, Fine BS: *Ocular Pathology. A Color Atlas,* ed 2. New York: Gower Medical Publishing, 1992, 7.6.)

the conjunctiva in suspected cases of chlamydial infection, looking for intra-cytoplasmic inclusion bodies, although this is less reliable in adults, especially if tetracycline has already been administered.

Polymorphonuclear leukocytes (PMN) predominate in Giemsa-stained scrapings of any inflammatory membranous conjunctivitis, bacterial and fungal conjunctivitis, and in ocular Stevens–Johnson syndrome. Zinc sulfate, cocaine, and silver nitrate cause a PMN conjunctival response when instilled into the eye. Inclusion conjunctivitis of the newborn has a mainly PMN response, but in adults an equal lymphocytic–PMN response is noted. This balanced PMN–lymphocyte response is also seen in trachoma, with macrophages, multi-nucleated cells with four nuclei or less, and fewer plasma cells (Fig. 2.6).

A cell response consisting of a majority of lymphocytes is commonly seen in viral infection. Toxic follicular conjunctivitis from drugs (such as idoxuridine or miotics) or lid margin lesions (molluscum contagiosum or verruca vulgaris) also cause this mononuclear response.

Eosinophils in any number suggest allergic conjunctivitis, vernal catarrh, or giant papillary conjunctivitis (Fig. 2.7).

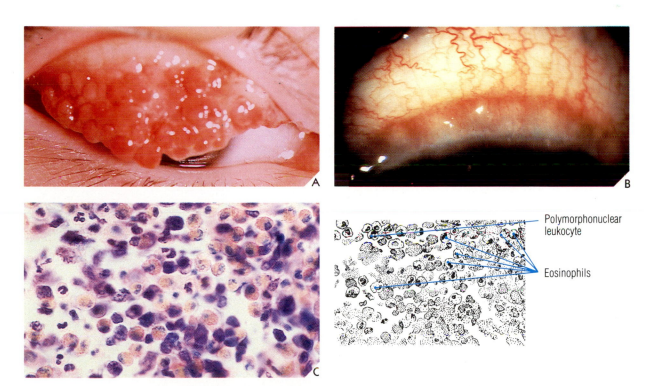

**2.7** | Vernal catarrh. *A:* Clinical appearance of the papillary reaction of the palpebral conjunctiva. *B:* Clinical appearance of the less commonly seen limbal reaction. *C:* Histologic examination of a conjunctival smear shows the presence of many eosinophils. (From Yanoff M, Fine BS: *Ocular Pathology. A Color Atlas,* ed 2. New York: Gower Medical Publishing, 1992, 7.7.)

## THE ABNORMAL CONJUNCTIVA
### CONGENITAL ABNORMALITIES
#### DERMOIDS

Dermoids are common congenital lesions that have little growth potential. Three types of conjunctival dermoids are described: the solid limbal dermoid, the more diffuse dermolipoma, and the complex choristoma and ectopic lacrimal gland. The limbal dermoids are compact pale-yellow growths that typically develop at the lower temporal limbus, with penetration into cornea and sclera as well as conjunctiva (Fig. 2.8). This is a choristoma, as it contains epithelial and dermal elements not normally found in conjunctiva.

Most limbal dermoids are superficial and only minimally involve the cornea and sclera. The occasional coincidence of lid colobomas with limbal dermoids has led to postulates that the dermoid may result from incomplete fusion of the lids, with displacement of skin elements into the dermoid.

Dermolipomas are less dense and contain more adipose tissue. The typical location of these lesions is superior temporally. Extension posteriorly between the lateral and superior recti towards the orbit, with close approximation to the lacrimal gland, and anterior extension towards the limbus can be seen (Fig. 2.9).

Treatment of dermoids is careful surgical excision. Care must be taken to isolate the dermoid from the surrounding structures. Occasionally lamellar keratoplasty is necessary for limbal dermoids that have deep penetration

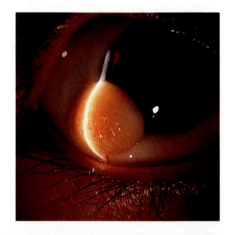

**2.8** | Conjunctival dermoid. Limbal dermoid cysts are benign choristomas most often seen at the lower temporal limbus, where they typically involve the cornea, conjunctiva, and sclera. Treatment (usually on cosmetic grounds) consists of careful surgical excision and possibly an anterior segment reconstruction with a lamellar keratoplasty.

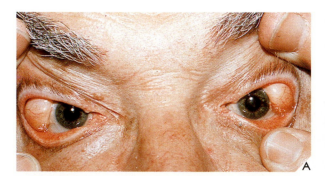
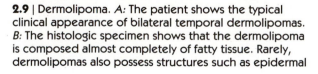
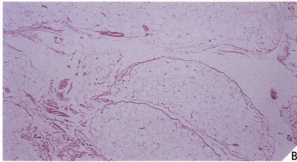

**2.9** | Dermolipoma. *A:* The patient shows the typical clinical appearance of bilateral temporal dermolipomas. *B:* The histologic specimen shows that the dermolipoma is composed almost completely of fatty tissue. Rarely, dermolipomas also possess structures such as epidermal appendages and fibrous tissue. The differential diagnosis for this condition is prolapsed orbital fat. (From Yanoff M, Fine BS: *Ocular Pathology. A Color Atlas,* ed 2. New York: Gower Medical Publishing, 1992, 7.3.)

into the stroma of the cornea. The surgeon must be prepared for these recon-structions.

     Bilateral limbal dermoids or dermolipomas are found in many children with Goldenhar's syndrome (oculoauriculovertebral dysplasia).[12] The other features of first branchial arch syndrome are preauricular skin tags, blind-ended preauricular fistulas, and vertebral anomalies. Hypoplasia of facial bones is also seen. Colobomas of the upper lid may also be present unilater-ally in this syndrome.[13]

EPITHELIAL CYSTS

Inclusion cysts can be found in bulbar and palpebral conjunctiva. They are filled with clear fluid, lined with epithelium, and are usually symptom free (Fig. 2.10). Treatment, if needed, is simple excision.

DEGENERATIONS

The conjunctival degenerative processes are listed in Figure 2.11.

XEROSIS

Xerosis refers to drying of the conjunctiva and corneal epithelium in associa-tion with several systemic disorders or with localized ocular disorders. These are discussed in detail in Chapter 14.

PINGUECULUM

Pinguecula are degenerative lesions of the bulbar conjunctiva that resemble the histology of skin with chronic exposure to sunlight. They appear as yel-low-white subepithelial deposits of amorphous material nasal and sometimes

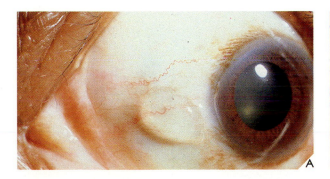

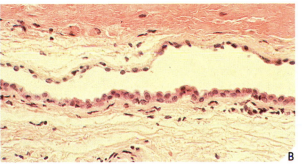

**2.10** | Conjunctival cyst. *A:* A clear cyst is present just nasal to the limbus. *B:* Histologic section of another clear conjunctival cyst shows that it is lined by a double layer of epithelium, suggesting a ductal origin. (From Yanoff M, Fine BS: *Ocular Pathology. A Color Atlas,* ed 2. New York: Gower Medical Publishing, 1992, 7.11.)

### Figure 2.11. Degenerations of the Conjunctiva

Xerosis
Pingueculum
Pterygium
Amyloidosis
Spheroidal degeneration
Lipid deposits

temporal to the limbus in the interpalpebral zone of the bulbar conjunctiva of older patients, with gradual enlargement over time (Fig. 2.12).

The subepithelial collagen fibers of a pingueculum become fragmented and basophilic on H&E staining. The tissue also stains positive for elastic tissue, although elastic elements are lacking. This change is called elastoid or elastotic degeneration.[14] Calcification can also occur. Removal for cosmesis or chronically inflamed tissue is by excision.

PTERYGIUM

Pterygia are similar to pinguecula in histology and in relationship to the effects of actinic exposure. However, a pterygium extends from the conjunctiva to invade the peripheral cornea, with penetration of Bowman's layer by fibrovascular ingrowth (Fig. 2.13). The epithelium may be of variable thickness and can exhibit dyskeratosis.[15]

Because of the potential for recurrence, surgery is indicated only when a severe cosmetic defect is evident or when vision might be affected by ptery-

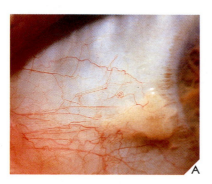

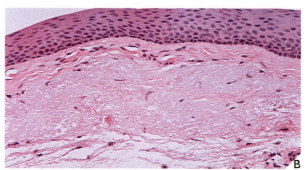

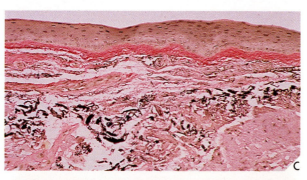

**2.12** | Pinguecula. *A:* A pingueculum characteristically involves the limbal conjunctiva, most frequently nasally, and appears as a yellowish-white mound of tissue. *B:* Histologic section shows basophilic degeneration of the conjunctival substantia propria. *C:* Another case shows even more marked basophilic degeneration that stains heavily black when the Verhoeff elastica stain is used. (From Yanoff M, Fine BS: *Ocular Pathology. A Color Atlas,* ed 2. New York: Gower Medical Publishing, 1992, 7.10.)

**2.13** | Pterygium. Similar to a pingueculum in histology, a pterygium is an overgrowth of bulbar conjunctiva that invades the cornea, with resultant effects on vision as the leading edge of the growth nears the visual axis. This case of active growth was a recurrence of a pterygium removed 1 year before this photograph, and was affecting vision. Discomfort is another reason for surgical removal. A casual approach to the surgical excision of pterygium is not wise because of the high rate of recurrence.

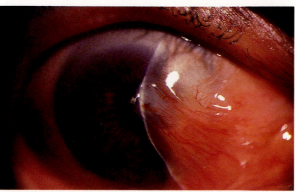

gial ingrowth into the visual axis. A 1-mm ingrowth onto the cornea that appears to be stable with no recent growth should be watched, whereas an actively growing pterygium should be removed before it can further encroach towards the corneal center.

Medical treatment of pterygium has little value as a primary therapy but is often an essential adjunct to surgical removal. Strontium-90 (a beta-radiation source) and thiotepa have been useful in preventing recurrence, but recent multiple reports have demonstrated that topical mitomycin-C, an antimetabolite–antibiotic agent, may be more effective in preventing both short- and long-term recurrence.[16–18] Significant toxicity, however, warrants caution with this agent.

There is considerable discussion in the ophthalmic literature concerning the best surgical approach and whether removal should be combined with lamellar keratoplasty, conjunctival autograft, or postoperative supplementary treatments. We prefer the bare sclera type of excision plus antimetabolite treatment, as there is evidence that this approach is more effective than other strategies.[16] We can still reserve the use of lamellar keratoplasty for cases with multiple recurrences and therapeutic failures.

## AMYLOIDOSIS

The uninflamed and mostly avascular deposition of noncollagenous protein in conjunctiva, cornea, intraocular, and/or adnexal tissues constitutes amyloid degeneration. Amyloid stains positive with Congo red and exhibits dichroism and birefringence when examined with polarized light, shows metachromasia when stained with crystal violet, fluoresces in UV light when stained with thioflavine T, and has a filamentous appearance by transmission electron microscopy. In the cornea and conjunctiva, amyloid is usually subepithelial, with a yellow-white to salmon color. Classification is either (i) primary (idiopathic) or secondary to a chronic disease such as trachoma or systemic multiple myeloma, or (ii) localized or systemic.[19]

Most common is primary localized amyloidosis of the conjunctiva with the appearance of a plaque of amyloid, usually in the palpebral conjunctiva (Fig. 2.14 ).

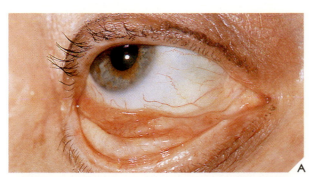
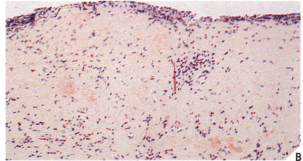

**2.14** | Amyloidosis. *A:* The patient has a smooth "fish-flesh" redundant mass in the inferior conjunctiva of both eyes, present for many years. The underlying cause was unknown and the patient had no systemic involvement. Clinically this could be lymphoid hyperplasia, lymphoma, leukemia, or amyloidosis. The lesion was biopsied. *B:* Histologic section shows an amorphous pale hyaline deposit in the substantia propria of the conjunctiva that stains positively with Congo red stain. The scant inflammatory cell infiltrate consists mainly of lymphocytes, plasma cells, and mast cells. (From Yanoff M, Fine BS: *Ocular Pathology. A Color Atlas*, ed 2. New York: Gower Medical Publishing, 1992, 7.10.)

Conjunctival concretions are epithelial inclusion cysts filled with epithelial and keratin debris. They are seen in elderly patients or in patients with chronic conjunctivitis such as trachoma[20] (Fig. 2.15).

## INFECTIONS AND INFLAMMATIONS

The conjunctiva is prone to a variety of primary and secondary sources of inflammatory change owing to its anatomic association with its surrounding structures and the potential for exposure to extrinsic organisms and toxic agents (Fig. 2.16). The inflammation varies in intensity and clinical features according to cause and duration. Knowledge of these presentations is funda-

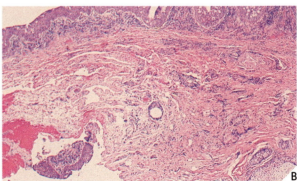

**2.15** | Concretions are the small, hard, yellowish bumps on the palpebral conjunctiva of elderly people or in cases of chronic inflammatory disease. These inclusion cysts of keratin and epithelial debris rarely cause any symptoms. If large enough to protrude through the conjunctival surface, they are easily removed with a needle under topical anesthesia. This is a case of concretions in old trachoma. (Courtesy of Dr. HS Sugar.)

## Figure 2.16. Inflammations of the Conjunctiva

| ACUTE CONJUNCTIVITIS | CHRONIC CONJUNCTIVITIS | ALLERGIC CONJUNCTIVITIS |
|---|---|---|
| Bacterial | Blepharoconjunctivitis | Atopic conjunctivitis |
| Acute viral | Chlamydia | Allergic dermatoconjunctivitis |
| Neonatal conjunctivitis | Parinaud oculoglandular syndrome | Microbiallergic conjunctivitis |
| | Toxic conjunctivitis | Vernal conjunctivitis |
| | Ligneous conjunctivitis | Giant papillary conjunctivitis |

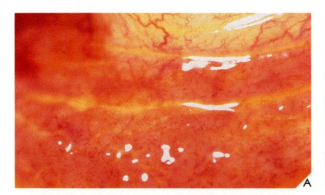

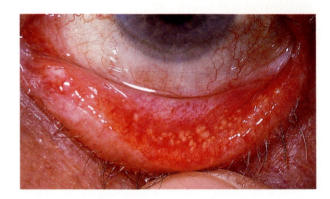

**2.17** | Papillary conjunctivitis. *A:* The surfaces of the papillae are red because of many tiny vessels, whereas their bases are pale. *B:* Histologic section of the conjunctiva demonstrates an inflammatory infiltrate in the substantia propria and many small vessels coursing through the papillae. The inflammatory cells are lymphocytes and plasma cells. (From Yanoff M, Fine BS: *Ocular Pathology. A Color Atlas*, ed 2. New York: Gower Medical Publishing, 1992, 7.5.)

mental in the differential diagnosis of the red eye. It seems most logical to divide these changes into acute and chronic.

The conjunctiva may respond to infections and inflammations with the formation of collections of inflammatory cells within the conjunctival stroma–papillae and/or follicles. These may be present in both subacute and chronic conjunctival infections, and can also be associated with allergic conjunctivitis.

A papillary reaction creates a fine "cobblestone" appearance of the conjunctiva overlying the tarsal plates and is composed of inflammatory cells and transudate (Fig. 2.17). With more spread and the influx of lymphocytes and plasma cells, a breakdown of the fibrous connections between the epithelium and tarsus occurs, and coalescence of papillae results in giant or "paving-stone" papillae (Fig. 2.18).

Follicles are aggregates of lymphocytes or active germinal centers of lymphocyte production in the stroma of the conjunctiva. Unlike the papillary response, these bumps are whitish, with a red look to the bases as vessels surround the bottom of the follicle (Fig. 2.19). The adjacent tissue often shows lymphocyte infiltration, along with some plasma cells.

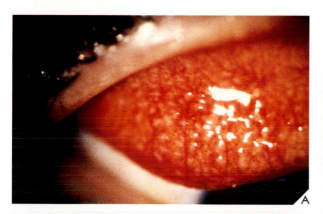
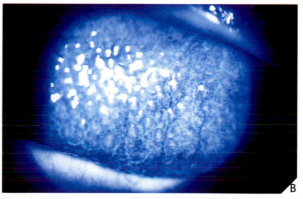

**2.18** | Giant papillae. Also described as "cobblestone" in appearance, giant papillae form from a coalescence of smaller papillae. This is a case of giant papillary conjunctivitis. (From Weinstock FJ: *Contact Lens Fitting*. New York: Gower Medical Publishing, 1989, 3.12.)

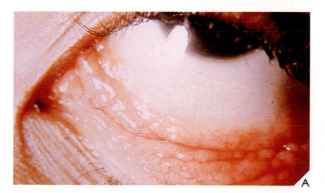
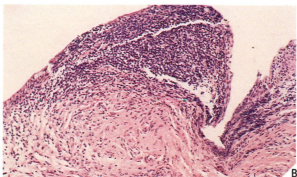

**2.19** | Follicular conjunctivitis. *A:* The surfaces of the follicles are pale, whereas their bases are red. *B:* Histologic section of the conjunctiva shows a lymphoid follicle in the substantia propria. (From Yanoff M, Fine BS: *Ocular Pathology. A Color Atlas*, ed 2. New York: Gower Medical Publishing, 1992, 7.5.)

ACUTE CONJUNCTIVITIS

Acute conjunctivitis is characterized by rapid onset of tearing, engorgement of conjunctival blood vessels (redness), edema (from transudation of fluid and cells into the perivascular space), and production of an exudate of mucus, epithelial cells, and inflammatory cells (Figs. 2.20 and 2.21). If the inflammation is severe enough, chemosis or diffuse swelling of the bulbar and fornical conjunctiva results.

The combination of inflammatory cells and mucous secretions with the protein and fibrin in the exudate can form an inflammatory membrane. When loosely adherent to the conjunctival epithelium, it is called a "pseudomembrane," as it can be removed from the eye without any bleeding. With more intense inflammation, the epithelial cells become necrotic, and a "true mem-

**2.20** | Acute conjunctivitis. The hyperemia diminishes in severity towards the cornea (the opposite is true for iritis). (From Lambert HP, Farrar WE: *Infectious Diseases Illustrated.* London: Gower Medical Publishing, 1982, 11.5.)

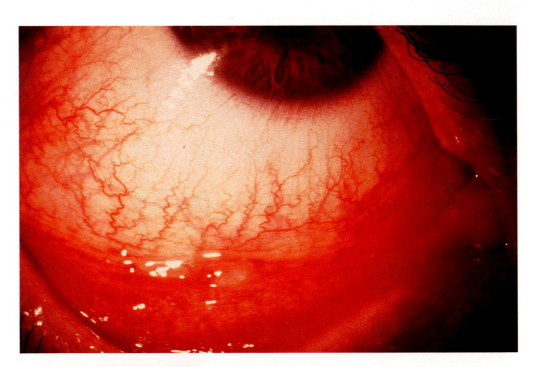

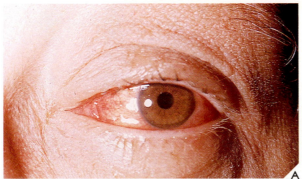

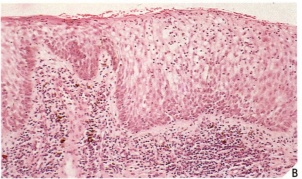

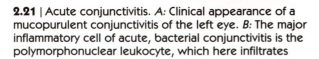

**2.21** | Acute conjunctivitis. *A:* Clinical appearance of a mucopurulent conjunctivitis of the left eye. *B:* The major inflammatory cell of acute, bacterial conjunctivitis is the polymorphonuclear leukocyte, which here infiltrates the swollen, edematous epithelium and the substantia propria. (From Yanoff M, Fine BS: *Ocular Pathology. A Color Atlas,* ed 2. New York: Gower Medical Publishing, 1992, 7.3.)

brane" of coagulum with firm adhesions to the epithelial layer of the conjunctiva is formed. When this membrane is removed, the underlying epithelium is torn and a raw, bleeding surface is left behind (Figs. 2.22 and 2.23).

The cellular composition of the exudate varies according to the cause and severity of the inflammation. Bacterial infections and toxic agents cause PMN leukocytes to predominate, whereas a monocyte response to viral infection, and eosinophils and basophils in the exudate of allergic reactions, are typical.

The character of the discharge is very helpful in the diagnosis. A watery discharge is usually the case in viral illness, a more mucoid discharge is seen in allergic reaction, and a thick, ropy, fibrinous secretion is common in bacterial conjunctivitis.

## Figure 2.22. Inflammatory Membranes

True membrane
    When removed, epithelium is also removed, leaving a bleeding surface.
    Seen in epidemic keratoconjunctivitis (EKC), *Corynebacterium diphtheriae*, *Streptococcus pneumoniae*, *Staphylococcus aureus*, and Stevens–Johnson syndrome.

Pseudomembrane
    When removed, epithelium is not disturbed.
    Seen in EKC, *Corynebacterium diphtheriae*, *Streptococcus haemolyticus*, pharyngoconjunctival fever, vernal conjunctivitis, ligneous conjunctivitis, and alkali burns.

(Adapted from Yanoff M, Fine BS: *Ocular Pathology. A Color Atlas*, ed 2. New York: Gower Medical Publishing, 1992, 7.4.)

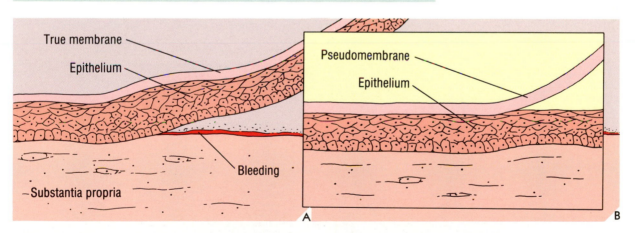

**2.23** | Inflammatory membranes. *A:* In a true membrane, when the membrane is stripped off, the epithelium is also removed and a bleeding surface is left. *B:* In a pseudomembrane, when the membrane is stripped off, it comes off the epithelium, leaving the epithelium intact with no bleeding. (From Yanoff M, Fine BS: *Ocular Pathology. A Color Atlas*, ed 2. New York: Gower Medical Publishing, 1992, 7.4.)

### Bacterial Conjunctivitis

Isolated bacterial infections of the conjunctiva are rare; most also involve the lid margins (Fig. 2.24). The infection is most often characterized by a rapid onset, with lid hyperemia and discharge. Exogenous infection from airborne bacteria or existing opportunistic conjunctival flora is the most common cause of this type of conjunctivitis. Endogenous spread of a systemic disease, such as syphilis, is less frequent. Most infections become bilateral. However, if one eye is more susceptible to infection owing to injury, lid malposition, decreased tear production, or exposure, a unilateral infection is usual.

Many bacteria can cause conjunctivitis, and the clinical features of the infection may not be specific to the particular "bug." However, clues can be helpful.

An acute "hyperpurulent" conjunctivitis, sometimes requiring hospitalization and treatment with parenteral antibiotics, can be seen with *Neisseria gonorrhoeae* and *N. meningitidis*. Prompt attention to this infection is critical because these organisms have the potential to infect the cornea and cause perforation within 24 h after symptoms appear.[21–23]

Acute mucopurulent conjunctivitis does not exhibit the same outpouring of exudate as the hyperpurulent cases, and is usually caused by *Streptococcus pneumoniae*, coliforms, *Staphylococcus*, and other *Streptococcus* species. *Haemophilus aegyptius* and *H. influenzae*, as well as *Corynebacterium diptheriae*, may also cause a purulent conjunctivitis. Treatment is with appropriate topical antibiotics.

### Acute Viral Conjunctivitis

Viral infections of the conjunctiva are among the most common presenting complaints of acute care, whether at an emergency room or a private office. This class of infection is of manifest importance in the red-eye differential diagnosis. Although it is possible to culture viruses from the conjunctiva during active infection, the expense and the low recovery rate make this a rarely used tool. The diagnosis of viral conjunctivitis is made on the grounds of typical history and clinical presentation. Most viral conjunctivitides will resolve without sequelae in a matter of days to weeks. Many different viruses can cause infection of the conjunctiva.

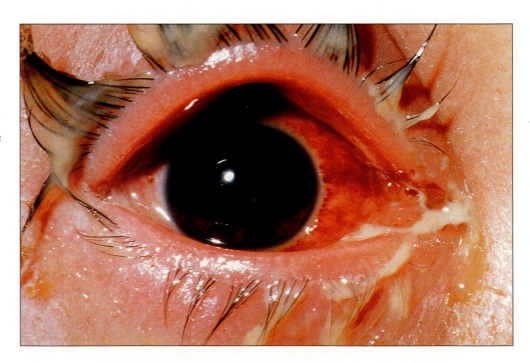

**2.24** | Purulent conjunctivitis. Beads of purulent fluid are exuding from the eye. This is a common feature in bacterial conjunctivitis. (From Lambert HP, Farrar WE: *Infectious Diseases Illustrated.* London: Gower Medical Publishing, 1982, 11.5.)

Primary cases of nonneonatal *H. simplex* conjunctivitis are relatively rare to see and document, and many cases go undiscovered. Most cases occur in children under the age of 5 years, who display signs of ocular irritation, watery discharge, and follicular response (Fig. 2.25). Preauricular lymph node swelling is usually present, and periocular epidermal lesions of vesicular eruption are also possible. Corneal involvement may occur, characterized after 7 days by punctate and/or dendritic changes of the epithelium. Resolution is spontaneous in most cases, but the use of topical antivirals is a logical step if the patient has lid vesicles.

Epidemic keratoconjunctivitis (EKC) is an uncomfortable and relatively severe irritation with serotypes 8 and 19 of adenovirus found most often on culture. The acute syndrome lasts 7 days to 3 weeks, with a mixed papillary and follicular response in the conjunctival stroma. A watery discharge, a high degree of hyperemia and chemosis, regional lymphadenopathy, and pronounced discomfort are common prominent features (Figs. 2.26 and 2.27).

Membrane formation occurs in about a third of cases, and subconjuntival hemorrhages are frequent. The corneal aspect of this infection usually shows by the seventh to the thirteenth day in the form of punctate epithelial elevations, with subepithelial opacities developing at day 14 in 20% to 50% of cases (Fig. 2.28). These opacities can be visually disabling and may persist for

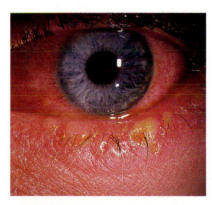

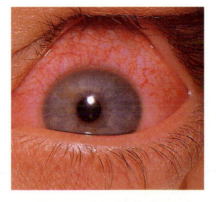

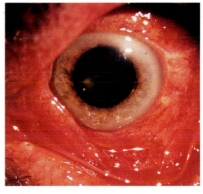

**2.25** | Primary *Herpes simplex*. Most cases of primary *H. simplex* go unrecorded, occurring before age 5. When seen, these cases have a watery discharge and a follicular conjunctivitis. Rarer still is a primary *H. simplex* in an adult, as seen in this photograph.

**2.26** | Epidemic keratoconjunctivitis, early adenovirus infection. The acute stage of EKC is characterized by a watery discharge, marked hyperemia and chemosis, and considerable discomfort.

**2.27** | Epidemic keratoconjunctivitis. The conjunctiva responds to EKC with a mixed papillo–follicular reaction, and subconjunctival hemorrhages are frequent.

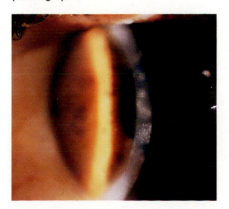

**2.28** | Epidemic keratoconjunctivitis. Twenty to 50% of cases of EKC will go on to develop corneal findings, beginning with punctate epithelial elevations as early as day 7. Subepithelial infiltrates, as seen in this case, can be seen by day 14. Depending on location, these opacities can be very detrimental to clarity of vision, but most will resolve without scarring in a matter of weeks (to as long as several years).

months to years, but most resolve without scarring or vascularization. Transmission is by direct spread (respiratory tract to eye, eye to hand to eye), and instruments (such as a Goldmann tonometer tip) can act as vectors.[24] The incubation period is 2–14 days, and the other eye usually becomes involved within the first week.

Pharyngoconjunctival fever is another adenovirus infection, with serotypes 3, 4, and 7 most likely. As its name implies, it is a combination of pharyngitis, fever, and conjunctivitis, characterized by a predominately follicular response. A scant watery discharge from the eyes, hyperemia and chemosis, and a fine epitheliopathy of the cornea are the ocular features of this infection. Preauricular lymph node enlargement is seen in about 90% of cases (Fig. 2.29).

Acute hemorrhagic conjunctivitis is also known as Apollo disease, because its first appearance in Ghana was at the same time as the lunar landing mission in 1969. Two picornaviruses, enterovirus 70 and Coxsackie virus A24, have been identified as the usual causative agents. The rapid onset of a mild to severe papillary conjunctivitis with chemosis in the first 24 h and the development of minute subconjunctival hemorrhages that can coalesce into larger spots are characteristic. Corneal involvement is rare and is confined to a fine subepithelial keratitis and/or erosions.[25] It usually last 10 days or less and resolves without sequelae.

Other less common viral conjunctival infections are associated with infectious mononucleosis (Epstein–Barr virus), paramyxovirus (RNA viruses that cause Newcastle's disease in poultry workers and measles), and poxviruses (variola, vaccina, and molluscum contagiosum).

## Neonatal Conjunctivitis (Ophthalmia Neonatorum, Neonatal Ophthalmia)

Conjunctivitis of the newborn is defined by the World Health Organization as any conjunctivitis within the first 4 weeks of an infant's life with clinical signs of erythema and edema of the eyelids and the palpebral conjunctiva, and/or purulent eye discharge with one or more polymorphonuclear cells per oil immersion field on a Gram-stained conjunctival smear. Indeed, conjunctivitis is the most common reported infection during this period of life.[26]

**2.29** | Pharyngoconjunctival fever. Caused by any of several different strains of adenovirus, PCF results in a conjunctivitis associated with pharyngitis and fever. This photograph shows the diffuse injection and a pseudomembrane on the lower palpebral conjunctiva. (From Lambert HP, Farrar WE: *Infectious Diseases Illustrated.* London: Gower Medical Publishing, 1982, 11.4.)

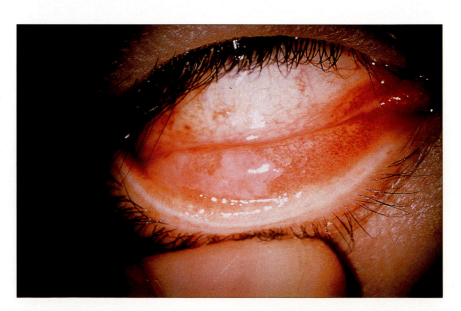

Ophthalmia neonatorum (ON) can be caused by bacterial, viral, or chlamydial infection, or by toxic response to topically applied chemicals. The frequency of each cause depends on a variety of factors, including maternal infections, time of rupture of the amniotic sac, prophylaxis used (if any) at the time of delivery, and postdelivery exposure to microorganisms. As one might expect, these factors vary throughout the world.

*Cause*

The bacteria that cause ophthalmia neonatorum can be classified according to their mode of infection. A host of organisms, such as *Staphylococcus aureus*, *Streptococcus pneumoniae*, *Streptococcus viridans*, and *Haemophilus* species, are probably transmitted through the air to the infant soon after delivery. These infections are often uncomplicated and are treated with lid hygiene and topical antibiotics. *E. coli, S. pneumoniae, Branhamella catarrhalis, H. influenzae* and *H. parainfluenzae, Pseudomonas aeruginosa, Proteus mirabilis,* and *Klebsiella pneumoniae* can also present as an acute purulent conjunctivitis. These must be distinguished from *Neisseria* infection and treated appropriately.

Typical cases of bacterial conjunctivitis related to delivery present 2 to 4 days after birth. Later presentations have been reported, and early infections are sometimes seen in cases of premature rupture of amniotic membranes.

*Neisseria* species (in particular *N. gonorrhoeae*) are usually transmitted from the mother to the infant during delivery. These species produce a severe conjunctivitis with lid swelling, chemosis, and watery or serosanguinous discharge that quickly becomes copious with pus. The more severe the infection, the greater the likelihood of corneal involvement. This assumes great importance because *Neisseria* is among the few bacteria that can perforate an intact cornea. Septicemia and meningitis are other possible sequelae.

Viral conjunctivitis of the newborn is rare but can be associated with significant morbidity and mortality. *Herpes simplex* virus type I and II infections of the conjunctiva occur within 2 weeks of birth and may be followed by herpetic keratitis or keratouveitis. Vitritis, retinitis, retinal detachment, optic neuritis, and cataract have been reported in association with a neonatal ocular herpes. Pneumonitis, septicemia, and meningitis are other possible sequelae. Rare cases of cytomegalovirus and adenovirus infections have also been seen in neonates.

When good prenatal care is available, the incidence of herpetic infections of the newborn is greatly reduced by early diagnosis of pregnant women who have herpetic genital lesions.

Chemical conjunctivitis resulting from institution of the Credé prophylaxis is a very frequent cause of neonatal conjunctivitis. About 90% of infants that receive 1% $AgNO_3$ solution have a mild, transient conjunctival injection and tearing that resolves in 24–48 h. A toxic response to tetracycline or erythromycin ointment is rare.

The more severe injuries of lid edema, chemosis, and corneal and/or conjunctival scarring from the caustic effects of more concentrated silver nitrate solutions occurred when 1% solutions were made in stock bottles and used multiple times. Over time, some of the silver nitrate would settle out of solution, and the bottom of the bottle would therefore have a much more concentrated solution. This problem has been eliminated with single-use ampules.

Neonatal inclusion conjunctivitis is now the most common form of ophthalmia neonatorum, affecting up to 3% of all newborns.[27] Passage of the child through an infected cervix leads to neonatal inclusion conjunctivitis in 30%–40% of cases.

The incubation period is from 4 to 12 days after birth, and the infection presents as a unilateral or bilateral mucopurulent conjunctivitis with lid edema, pseudomembrane formation, and a papillary response. If the disease becomes chronic, the patient develops follicles and preauricular adenopathy after 6–12 weeks. Mild conjunctival scarring can be seen in some patients who have developed membranes. Superficial epithelial keratitis and superior micropannus are occasional findings. In addition, affected infants are at risk for pneumonitis, which is associated with 10%–20% of cases.[28]

*Diagnosis*   Ophthalmia neonatorum (ON) represents an ocular emergency that requires a detailed history of both the infant and the mother, physical examination, and laboratory studies.

The mother should be questioned about the extent of her prenatal care, any history of sexually transmitted diseases, and whether there was premature rupture of the amniotic membrane. The baby's history should note the time of onset of the conjunctivitis after birth and the use of any ocular prophylaxis or antibiotic treatment. It is also mandatory to be aware of any ongoing infections in the newborn nursery.

Physical examination of the infant should focus on temperature (both current and prior chartings), respiratory rate and evidence of respiratory difficulty (including auscultation of the lungs), and examination of the skin for lesions suggestive of septicemia or herpes.

The eye exam should detail the extent of eyelid erythema and edema; the degree of conjunctival injection; the type of discharge (watery, mucopurulent, pus); the condition of the cornea (presence of dendrites, infiltrates, ulceration, perforation); and any indication of uveitis, cataract, retinitis, or retinal detachment.

Conjunctival smears are a routine and integral part of the neonatal conjunctivitis workup. Gram and Giemsa stains help make the preliminary diagnosis of the causative agent. In suspected cases of HSV infection, a Papanicolaou smear is useful.

Cultures for aerobic bacteria and gonococcus should be taken, without the use of topical anesthetic, by prewetting the culture swab in sterile liquid medium (which will increase the yield of bacterial growth). Reduced blood agar, cooked meat or thioglycolate broth, and either chocolate agar in $CO_2$ or Thayer–Martin medium, are recommended for neonatal conjunctivitis cultures.

The high inxcidence of neonatal inclusion conjunctivitis throughout the world indicates the need for a reliable test for *Chlamydia trachomatis*. The McCoy cell culture stained with fluorescent monoclonal antibodies to *Chlamydia* is a test that is expensive, not widely available, and slow (2–3 days). Two rapid diagnostic tests are available in the United States for suspected cases of chlamydial infection. An enzyme-linked immunoassay (ELISA) test gives 93% sensitivity, 98% specificity, and predictive values of 97% positive, 95% negative. This test takes several hours and has an objective endpoint measured on spectrophotometry. A direct immunofluorescent monoclonal antibody stain (DFA) for *Chlamydia* screens for chlamydial antigens on conjunctival smears. DFA has 100% sensitivity, 94% specificity, and predictive values of 94% positive and 100% negative. This test can identify chlamydial infection not seen with culture techniques. DFA can be read immediately, but requires a trained observer and a fluorescence microscope.[29]

Viral cultures are done only when there is reason to suspect a viral cause. Collections are made from the eyes, skin, and mucous membrane vesicular lesions. In addition, the mother's oropharynx, genitalia, and cervix are examined for lesions. The absence of antibody to HSV in both the mother and infant does not eliminate the possibility of herpes infection.

*Therapy*

Specific treatment of neonatal conjunctivitis is based on the findings of the history, physical examination, and stained smears. ON caused by prophylactic chemical usage requires no therapy.

Treatment of bacterial ON is directed to either Gram-positive (tetracycline 1% or erythromycin 0.5% ointment) or Gram-negative (gentamicin 0.3% or tobramycin 0.3% ointment) coverage, and is used every 4 hours for 7 days.

Therapy for intracellular Gram-negative diplococci is a separate issue. Aqueous penicillin G, 100,000 U/kg/day, in four divided doses IV for 7 days, or benzathine penicillin (50,000 U/kg IM) is used without the need for topical therapy in many cases. However, gonorrheal ophthalmia treatment has changed because of the prevalence of penicillinase-producing strains. These should be treated with ceftriaxone 25–50 mg/kg IV or IM once a day for 7 days, or gentamicin 5 mg/kg/day IM in two divided doses for 7 days.[30] Current Public Health Service recommendations should be sought and followed.

The treatment of neonatal inclusion conjunctivitis involves the use of erythromycin syrup 50 mg/kg/day orally in four divided doses for 14 days. The use of topical tetracycline, erythromycin, or sulfacetamide ointment is not necessary. Persistent chlamydial conjunctivitis occurs in 7%–19% of patients taking oral erythromycin, but most cases resolve with retreatment. It is very important to treat the parents at the same time.

Herpetic ON is treated with trifluridine 1% solution every 2 hours for 7 days or until the epithelium is healed. Acyclovir, 10 mg/kg or 500 mg/m$^2$ IV every 8 h for 10 days, should be used also to decrease the likelihood of systemic involvement.

The baby should be assessed for efficacy of therapy in 2 to 3 days, and reexamined one week after cessation of medication. Most cases of bacterial ON respond to an appropriate regimen, and it is necessary to distinguish ON from the conjunctivitis associated with a blocked nasolacrimal duct.

The incidence of gonococcal ON constituted a major public health problem of the 19th century, with reports ranging from 1%–14%.[31] Estimates suggested that 20%–79% of children in institutions for the blind had gonococcal ophthalmia neonatorum as a cause of their disability.[32] In 1881, Credé in Leipzig reported a reduction in the rate of gonococcal ON with the use of a two-part prophylactic regimen: mechanical cleaning of the newborn's eyelids before the eyes opened and instillation of an antiseptic agent into the conjunctival sacs as soon as possible after birth.[33] He initially recommended a 2% aqueous AgNO$_3$ solution but this was changed to a less irritating 1% concentration. The prophylaxis reduced the incidence of gonococcal ophthalmia neonatorum from 13.6% to 0.5%.

Recently, the routine prophylactic use of 1% AgNO$_3$ drops to prevent neonatal ophthalmia has become controversial. The side effects of chemical conjunctivitis and incomplete protection against *Chlamydia* have caused concern. Some states have changed their laws to allow the substitution of erythromycin or tetracycline ophthalmic antibiotics for the silver nitrate. Some countries, such as Sweden and the United Kingdom, no longer require the routine use of any prophylaxis for ophthalmia neonatorum.

The assumption that any neonatal ocular prophylaxis will entirely prevent chlamydial neonatal conjunctivitis is questionable. Among infants exposed to maternal infection with *Chlamydia trachomatis* in Nairobi, Kenya, chlamydial conjunctivitis developed in 10.1% of AgNO₃ patients and in 7.2% of tetracycline-treated patients (not statistically significant), although both agents significantly reduced the incidence of both gonococcal and chlamydial conjunctivitis when compared to historical controls.[34]

Another study in New York found no significant difference in the development of chlamydial ON between topical prophylactic use of silver nitrate, tetracycline, or erythromycin.[35] A Swedish study (with no prophylaxis) demonstrated that all treatment of neonatal chlamydial conjunctivitis failed with topical chloramphenicol and succeeded with oral erythromycin ethylsuccinate.[36]

Neonatal conjunctivitis would have the lowest incidence in babies (i) born to mothers with good prenatal care and surveillance for evidence of chlamydial, gonococcal, or herpetic infection and (ii) whose eyes were cleaned with cotton immediately after birth, followed by instillation of a topical antimicrobial prophylaxis. These considerations are not mutually exclusive but are complementary. Ocular prophylaxis is imperative in cases where prenatal care has not been received and/or when the mother is at risk for sexually transmitted disease. The Kenyan study by Laga and associates makes a point of timing the ocular prophylaxis immediately after birth.[34] This may be a factor in the resulting degree of reduction of both gonococcal and chlamydial ocular infections in the days following birth that many other studies fail to show.

Diagnosis and treatment of gonorrheal, chlamydial, or herpetic infections in pregnant women obviously represent the best approach to prevention of ophthalmia neonatorum. However, this is often not possible because of expense and lack of access to quality prenatal care. Such treatment should definitely be used for those at high risk for contracting sexually transmitted diseases.

The issue of universal prophylaxis is still controversial. The need for prophylaxis is clear for all exposed infants, but how can we be certain that we catch all in this group and do not miss some cases? Because there is no long-term morbidity from any of the prophylactic agents, and because gonococcal ON is a blinding condition, there is no reason to adopt a universal policy of no ocular prophylaxis.[37] The choice between single-dose wax ampules of 1% AgNO₃ drops, 0.5% erythromycin ointment, or 1.0% tetracycline ointment can be made on the basis of considerations of cost, availability, and prevalence of cause of ON in the area. An alternative topical ocular prophylaxis may be povidone-iodine, as pointed out by a recent in vitro study, but further testing is required of the potential of this broad-spectrum disinfectant in ON.[38]

A final consideration that requires mention is that the antibiotic ointments cause some temporary blurring of vision, and this may interfere somewhat in bonding between the infant and parents. This particular issue is not settled, but there seems to be better ON prophylaxis when the agents are used immediately after birth.

## CHRONIC CONJUNCTIVITIS

Any conjunctivitis that lasts beyond 2 weeks should be regarded as chronic. By this, we do not mean any long-term sequelae, such as the subepithelial infiltrates of EKC, but rather the continued and active process of a disease that may have had an acute onset but has persisted. Some chronic conjunctivitis develops insidiously and may continue for months to years.

The changes in chronic conjunctivitis are often nonspecific, related to recurring or constant low-level infection of the lid margins, chronic conjunctival exposure (from proptosis or ectropion of the lid), decreased tear production, chronic allergies, medicamentosum response to topical medication, or to a foreign body (eye cosmetics) or neoplasm. All can cause epithelial hypertrophy with infoldings (pseudoglands of Henle) that may become subepithelial retention cysts. The secretions of these cysts may form calcified concretions. Stromal inflammation results in the formation of papillae and follicles.

**Blepharoconjunctivitis**

Chronic bacterial infections of the conjunctiva can smolder on for weeks to months. They represent a challenge to diagnose and treat properly. Most cases are associated with blepharitis and are caused by *Staphylococcus, Moraxella, H. influenzae,* or coliforms.

Chronic staphylococcal infections may produce marginal corneal infiltrates and ulcerations owing to production of an extremely powerful exotoxin that causes an allergic hypersensitivity.

*Moraxella* organisms are another common cause of chronic conjunctivitis, manifesting either as a chronic follicular conjunctivitis or as an angular blepharoconjunctivitis with ulceration of the lateral lid margins and lateral conjunctival injection.

Treatment must address the lid component of the "blepharoconjunctivitis" with lid scrubs, use of effective antibiotics, and use of steroids for control of the inflammatory response.

***Chlamydia* Conjunctivitis**

In the United States, chlamydial disease is often overlooked as a diagnostic possibility. As an obligate intracellular parasite, it is often classed with viruses, but it has organelles, both RNA and DNA, and a cell wall, and can be killed by antibiotics. Two species, *Chlamydia trachomatis* and *C. psittaci,* cause chlamydial disease, although the latter infects nonhumans, especially birds.

Trachoma is endemic in some regions of the globe, characterized by a surreptitious onset and significant sequelae. Caused by serotypes A–C of *C. trachomatis,* this disease can lead to cicatricial changes of the conjunctiva with corneal scarring and resulting blindness. The chronic follicular conjunctivitis of the initial infection is usually more prominent on the upper palpebral conjunctiva, with limbal follicles a possibility as well. Conjunctival papillary hyperplasia and pannus invading the superficial cornea, with a fine epithelial keratitis, are early findings. Some degree of light sensitivity, a mucopurulent discharge, and pain are other common features.

The evolution of the disease into four phases was described by MacCallan in 1908: Stage I, early lymphoid hyperplasia with follicular conjunctivitis, diffuse punctate keratitis, and early pannus; Stage II, florid inflammation with increase in pretarsal papillary and follicular hypertrophy, and increasing pannus; Stage III, beginning of scarring and cicatrization; Stage IV, no active inflammation, replacement of papillae and follicles with scar, resolution of pannus.

Subsequent proliferation of connective tissue in the conjunctiva results in scar formation and cicatrization of these scars leads to lid deformities. Arlt's line is a characteristic finding, a horizontal line of scar most often at the junction of the posterior two thirds and anterior one third of the pretarsal conjunctiva (Figs. 2.6 and 2.30).

Cicatrization of limbal follicles results in filling of the defect with epithelium, the clear cavities known as Herbert's pits (see Fig. 2.6). The pannus also regresses, with a diffuse haze persisting.

The complications of trachoma typically arise in Stage IV. Lid deformities, trichiasis, distichiasis, and keratitis sicca all contribute to further corneal damage, leading to a scarred, vascularized cornea or to ulceration and perforation of the cornea[39] (Fig. 2.31).

Trachoma on an individual basis responds well to oral tetracycline, 1.0–1.5 g daily for 4 weeks. Oral triple sulfa can be substituted in patients who are resistant to tetracycline. Topical tetracycline, sulfisoxazole, and erythromycin can have an additive effect.

Community-wide utilization of systemic antibiotics to eradicate trachoma in an endemic area is not a safe solution to such a public health problem because of the potential side effects. The main thrust is to try to prevent the scarring of the conjunctiva by use of topical antibiotics. Tetracycline or erythromycin ointment used twice daily for 5 days and repeated monthly for 6 months is the most common regimen today. This is not sufficient to treat and eradicate the infection, but it definitely reduces or prevents blinding complications of the disease.

The serotypes D–K of *C. trachomatis* are responsible for inclusion conjunctivitis (these had the prior designation of *C. oculogenitale*). The adult infection is usually classed as a chronic follicular conjunctivitis, and the neonatal infection as an acute infection (see above). The transmission of the adult disease is venereal or hand to eye, and neonates become infected as they pass through the birth canal.

Adult inclusion conjunctivitis initially presents unilaterally, with a red eye that has a mild or moderate mucopurulent discharge and a follicular response (Fig. 2.32).

A membranous reaction is not a feature of this disease, and there is no scarring of the conjunctiva. The cornea may show a superficial punctate epitheliopathy with a superior limbal micropannus. Subepithelial infiltrates can develop. These infiltrates are smaller than those typically seen with EKC and last 1–2 years if untreated.

Preauricular lymph node enlargement is common. Basophilic intracytoplasmic epithelial inclusions seen on Giemsa staining of conjunctival scrapings are a clear indicator of the disease (Fig. 2.33). Immunofluorescent testing of the scraping can also help to establish the diagnosis.

**2.30** | Conjunctival scarring from trachoma Stage IV. This typical Arlt's line is caused by a contracture of dense scar tissue of the upper lid conjunctiva (see also Fig. 2.6).

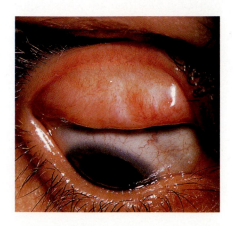

Because of the venereal nature of the disease, the treating physician must look for urethritis or vaginitis in both the patient and his or her sexual partners.

Treatment consists of tetracycline 250 mg q.i.d. for 4 weeks (or erythromycin in the case of pregnant women). All sexual partners should be treated to avoid the possibility of reinfection.

This rare and mild follicular conjunctivitis was first described in French orphanages, and since then has been reported by various boarding schools. The disease does not produce conjunctival scarring or corneal changes and therefore has been classed as a separate entity, although it appears to be similar to very mild trachoma cases seen in Native American boarding schools. Trachoma-type treatment with oral tetracycline is recommended.[40]

**Axenfeld's Chronic Follicular Conjunctivitis**

Thygeson described an epidemic of follicular conjunctivitis with associated mild keratitis in a California high school, with healing in 4–5 months. Most of the cases involved girls who shared eye makeup. Since these patients were not tested with modern immunofluorescent cytology or current culture techniques, this also may be a mild form of trachoma.[41]

**Thygeson and Merrill's Chronic Follicular Conjunctivitis**

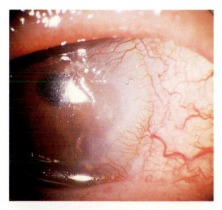

**2.31** | Corneal changes from trachoma. The complications of trachoma come from a combination of contracture of conjunctival scarring, distortion of lid architecture, and destruction of the sources of tear production. This in turn leads to marked corneal scarring, pannus, and decreased vision, as in this case of old trachomatous scarring of the cornea.

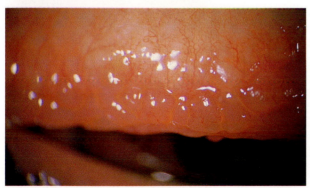

**2.32** | Adult inclusion conjunctivitis. Inclusion conjunctivitis, formerly known as TRIC conjunctivitis, is caused by serotypes D–K of *Chlamydia trachomatis.* It is a chronic follicular conjunctivitis in adult patients and is transmitted by venereal or hand-to-eye contact. This photo shows the typical large follicle formation.

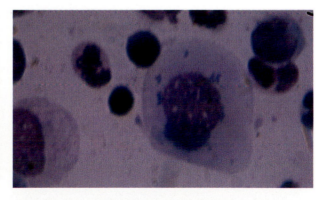

**2.33** | Adult inclusion conjunctivitis. Basophilic intracellular inclusion bodies (Halberstaedter–Prowazek bodies) are seen within the epithelial cells in a Giemsa stain of a conjunctival scraping (see also Fig. 2.6).

Parinaud Oculoglandular Syndrome

First described in 1899, this disease is characterized by focal conjunctival granulomas that may be surrounded by follicles, combined with visibly enlarged lymph nodes (usually preauricular). Ulceration of the conjunctiva may also be seen, but there is variation in corneal involvement depending on the etiology of the disease.

A common cause of oculoglandular syndrome is cat-scratch disease (CSD), from contact with cats by a scratch or bite, via an open wound, or direct contact with mucous membranes. Person-to-person vectors are not seen. Identical Gram-negative pleomorphic bacilli have been found in lesions in the conjunctiva, skin, and lymph nodes of patients with Parinaud oculoglandular syndrome. These cat-scratch disease bacilli are similar in location, size, and shape to the earlier descriptions by Verhoeff and others of the Gram-negative filamentous bacterium *Leptothrix*, which had been thought to be the cause of cat-scratch disease. It is not yet clear whether CSD bacillus and *Leptothrix* are the same organism or only very similar.[42] Recently, Brenner and co-workers classified the presumed agent of cat-scratch disease as a new genus named *Afipia*, of which only one species is associated with cats—*Afipia felis*.[43]

After skin infection, within 3–5 days a papule develops. This becomes vesicular and crusts, leaving a macular appearance like that of chickenpox. If the conjunctiva is the site of entry, a palpebral granuloma evolves in 7–14 days, surrounded by follicles. The ocular involvement is usually unilateral, with associated injection, chemosis, and watery discharge.

Irritation, foreign-body sensation, and photophobia can be noted. Nontender enlargement of the regional lymph nodes is also seen in 1–2 weeks, with slow resolution. Suppuration of these nodes may occur (10%–30%).

Most patients have a mild rise in temperature, with symptoms of aching, loss of appetite, and vague malaise. Antibiotics (such as intravenous gentamicin) may be helpful in patients with systemic cat-scratch disease.[44]

Other common causes of the uncommon Parinaud syndrome are *Franciscella tularensis* (tularemia; necrotizing conjunctivitis with tender lymphadenopathy) and *Sporotrichum schenckii* (sporotrichosis; ulcerative nodules in eyelid skin with painful lymphadenopathy). Tuberculosis, syphilis, coccidioidomycosis, lymphogranuloma venereum, leprosy, and *Yersinia* have also been reported to cause this syndrome.[45]

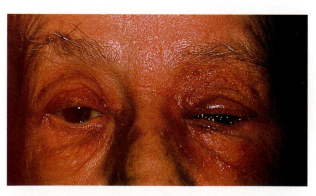

**2.34** | Toxic conjunctivitis. Allergic response to atropine in a patient after corneal transplant.

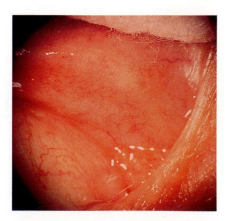

**2.35** | Toxic conjunctivitis. Chronic conjunctivitis and occluded puncta secondary to IDU usage.

Chronic follicular conjunctivitis with a trachomatous appearance (but without scarring) is a side effect associated with the use of several different drugs, often over extended periods. An additional finding of an epithelial keratitis with pannus and keratinization can be discerned in some cases. Atropine (Fig. 2.34), gentamicin, tobramycin, neomycin, antivirals [such as idoxuridine (IDU) or trifluorothymidine] (Fig. 2.35), and antiglaucoma agents (such as eserine, diisopropyl fluorophosphate, pilocarpine, and epinephrine) have all been implicated as causes of follicular conjunctivitis. The preservatives used in ophthalmic preparations such as benzalkonium chloride and thimerosal can also be inciting agents. The toxic response of idoxuridine is classic for this type of conjunctivitis, but this is not often seen today because this drug is not frequently used. Treatment consists of stopping the drug, and resolution occurs over several weeks.

Molluscum contagiosum virus with lid lesions causes a similar toxic response in the conjunctiva but with the potential for scarring. The conjunctivitis is eradicated by excision of the lid lesion that is shedding the virus.

First described in the early 1960s, superior limbic keratoconjunctivitis (SLK) is a chronic inflammation of unknown cause that involves the superior pretarsal and bulbar conjunctivae.[46] The disease is usually bilateral but may be asymmetric in severity. In 20%–50% of patients with SLK there is associated thyroid disease, but correct care of the thyroid problem has little or no effect on the SLK. A dry-eye syndrome is a common association.

The superior bulbar conjunctiva shows a segmental papillary reaction with injection. The conjunctival epithelial cells exhibit keratinization, acanthosis, dyskeratosis, and infiltration with polymorphonuclear cells. In addition, there are increased numbers of goblet cells and boggy edema of the pretarsal conjunctiva. The hyperemia and associated punctate staining of the superior bulbar conjunctiva extends 8–10 mm above the limbus and from 10:30 to 1:30 o'clock (Fig. 2.36).

The symptoms are nonspecific, with foreign-body sensation, tearing, photophobia, blepharospasm, and pain. The cornea has a micropannus with fine punctate staining of the superior portions of the cornea at the limbus. A filamentary keratitis is present in 50% of cases. The superior conjunctiva and superior cornea will stain with fluorescein and Rose Bengal.

**Toxic Conjunctivitis**

**Superior Limbic Keratoconjunctivitis of Theodore**

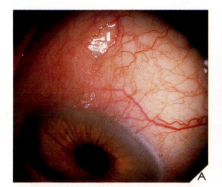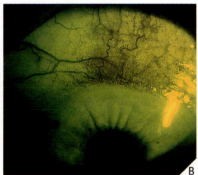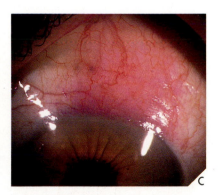

**2.36** | Superior limbic keratoconjunctivitis of Theodore. *A:* Injection pattern of the superior bulbar conjunctiva, with edema extending about 10 mm from the limbus, and about 3 clock hours wide. *B:* Viewed with a green filter, the dilated vessels are easily seen. *C:* Rose Bengal staining pattern in the same patient, demonstrating the localized area of drying and irritation.

Treatment of this condition is often difficult, and patients who also have dry-eye syndrome respond less well to therapy. The disease has a variable course, with periods of exacerbations and remissions. Many different modalities have been tried, with inconsistent results. Artificial tears can help a little but the use of topical steroids is usually ineffective.

Silver nitrate is a very common treatment for SLK. The use of 0.25%–1% silver nitrate solution can improve many SLK patients and may be repeated if needed. The mechanism of improvement may be the removal of abnormal keratinized epithelium.[47] It is very critical that the solution be freshly made (I have the pharmacy make 1–2 ml of a 0.5% solution), as higher concentrations of $AgNO_3$ are caustic. Specifically, one cannot use the 75% $AgNO_3$ "ARZOL" applicator sticks used in emergency rooms and ENT offices for nasal bleeding cauterization in the treatment of SLK, as this causes intense pain and severe but usually not permanent damage to the conjunctiva and cornea.

For patients in whom the use of 0.5% $AgNO_3$ solution is ineffective, thermocauterization of the superior bulbar conjunctiva with a disposable ophthalmic cautery has been utilized and found to be about 70% effective.[48] Another surgical approach is conjunctival resection of the superior bulbar conjunctiva. This seems to work better in patients who have a normal Schirmer test.[49]

## Ligneous Conjunctivitis

A rare unilateral or bilateral condition of unknown etiology, ligneous conjunctivitis consists of a "woody" induration of the lid associated with a membranous or pseudomembranous conjunctivitis of acute onset and chronic course. Ligneous conjunctivitis is probably related to acute infection or mild trauma, with systemic signs and symptoms preceding or concurrent with the onset of the eye process. These possibilities include fever, upper respiratory infections, urinary tract infections, otitis media, and infections of the sinuses, vagina, and cervix. In the chronic phase, recurrent chronic, non-

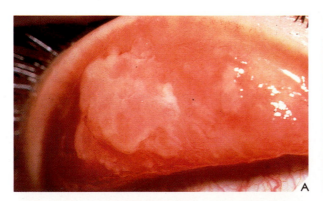
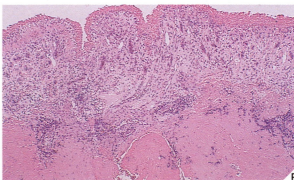

**2.37** | Ligneous conjunctivitis. *A:* A thick membrane covers the upper palpebral conjunctiva. *B:* Biopsy shows a thick, amorphous material contiguous with an inflammatory membrane composed mostly of mononuclear inflammatory cells (mainly plasma cells and some lymphocytes). (Case presented by Dr. J.S McGavic at the Verhoeff Society, 1986.) (From Yanoff M, Fine BS: *Ocular Pathology. A Color Atlas,* ed 2. New York: Gower Medical Publishing, 1992, 7.4.)

specific inflammation, usually of the upper pretarsal conjunctiva, develops (and may also include the lower palpebral and bulbar conjunctiva). This becomes compacted and invaded by granulation (Fig. 2.37).

In a study of 17 patients with ligneous conjunctivitis, long-term follow-up showed that three patients had other areas of mucous membrane involvement.[50] Removal of the conjunctival membrane is difficult and recurrence is commonplace. Surprisingly, extensive conjunctival scars were not seen in these patients, even with multiple recurrence and surgeries. Occasionally, there can be secondary involvement of the cornea with scarring and vascularization, and keratomalacia and perforation are possible.

Hyperpermeability of the blood vessels is a local feature of this disease. Fibrin is a major component of the membrane, and albumin and immunoglobulins are also present. The causes of the vascular changes (abnormal blood vessels with wide spaces between endothelial cells and degeneration of these cells) is unknown.

An immunohistochemical analysis of ligneous conjunctival lesions showed an inflammatory response characterized by new blood vessels, plasma cells, activated T-lymphocytes, and B-lymphocytes. IgG was a major component of the amorphous hyaline material that is often seen in these lesions.[51]

Many different therapies have been tried. Alpha-chymotrypsin, hyaluronidase, antibiotics, topical steroids, antiviral agents, cautery, beta- and x-ray radiation have all been attempted with little success. Hidayat and Riddle found cryotherapy not helpful despite a previous article reporting improvement with cryosurgery.[50,52] Six of 17 patients in the AFIP study showed spontaneous resolution, and in these cases a variety of treatments were tried.

Cyclosporine used as a 2% topical solution can be very helpful in treating this rare and difficult disease. Because of the immunohistologic features and the inability of many other therapies to resolve the condition, cyclosporine was successfully used in conjunction with topical steroids after excisional biopsy by Holland and co-workers on two patients.[53] They postulated that the cyclosporine interfered with the T-lymphocyte's ability to produce the lymphokine interleukin-2 (IL-2) or to respond to IL-2 through the blockage of formation of new IL-2 receptors. This would block the main path for recruitment and activation of new T-cells. Cyclosporine 2% topical solution has been used successfully in conjunction with topical steroids to suppress an episode of reactivation of ligneous conjunctivitis in one patient.[54] Further studies are needed to evaluate the usefulness of cyclosporine in this and other conditions.

The acute form of atopic conjunctivitis is an immediate type of allergic response and is mediated by IgE. It is caused by a spectrum of agents that also cause the upper respiratory allergic response (e.g., dust, molds, animal dander, pollens, spores). The patient experiences sudden hyperemia and edema, followed by development of chemosis and a watery, sometimes mucoid discharge (Fig. 2.38). There is often a family history of atopy. Cyto-

## ALLERGIC CONJUNCTIVITIS
Atopic Conjunctivitis

logic examination of a conjunctival scraping will reveal eosinophils. Treatment of this type of conjunctivitis involves the use of topical vasoconstrictors and/or 4% disodium cromoglycate (Opticrom), with steroids used in more severe cases. Elimination of the allergen would be ideal but is often impossible. Desensitization has variable success.

Chronic atopic conjunctivitis is characterized by the same itching, burning, tearing, and photophobia as its acute cousin, but exhibits a pale edema with papillary hypertrophy and a mucopurulent discharge. Scraping will reveal many eosinophils.

### Allergic Dermatoconjunctivitis

A very common form of allergic conjunctivitis, most contact dermatoconjunctivitis is caused by localized drug reactions or reactions to cosmetics, plastics, animal or vegetable products, or chemicals. The patient complains of itching (not as severe as in atopic reactions), followed by the development of a papillary reaction and a mild mucoid or more mucopurulent discharge. The conjunctival involvement is more marked inferiorly but can become diffuse. Punctate epithelial keratitis and erosions dot the lower third of the cornea. Eczema of the skin of the eyelids develops. Keratinization can ensue, and punctal edema, stenosis, and occlusion may evolve. Making the diagnosis is difficult until the characteristic skin changes occur—itching, hyperemia, and flaking of the skin, with scales, vesicles, crusts, and edema.

Cytology of these cases reveals monocytes, PMNs, and mucus, with mild keratinization of the epithelial cells. Eosinophils may be present.

The drugs commonly associated with these cases are neomycin, gentamicin, IDU, atropine, thimerosal, penicillin, and phenylephrine.[55] Treatment consists of stopping the drug or chemical and the use of topical steroids.

The immune reaction in these cases is a type IV delayed hypersensitivity. The drug or chemical acts as a partial antigen or hapten and combines with tissue proteins (carriers) to form complete antigens (conjugates). These antigens combine with T-lymphocytes, with release of lymphokines resulting in inflammation. Sensitization can be as short as 5–10 days or up to years later.

### Microbiallergic Conjunctivitis

Protein that is the product of bacterial tissue destruction can be converted by allergy into a toxic response. For the eyes, the most common cause of this reaction is staphylococcal blepharoconjunctivitis. The conjunctivitis is a result of the toxic response and is a type IV hypersensitivity. There is usually no history of allergy, but a chronic infection is necessary to allow sensitization to the products of the microbe. Culture of the conjunctiva is negative for *Staphylococcus*. Marginal infiltrate of the cornea can also be associated with this presentation (Fig. 2.39).

Phlyctenular keratoconjunctivitis is another manifestation of micro-

**2.38** | Atopic conjunctivitis. Immediate type of allergic response caused by a ragweed allergy. Sudden hyperemia and edema have been followed by extensive inferior chemosis. The appearance is alarming but there is usually a rapid spontaneous resolution. Topical vasoconstrictor/antihistamine can help to relieve the discomfort.

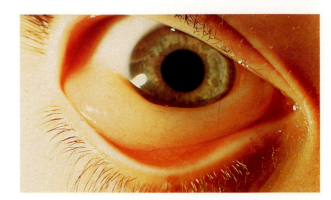

biallergic conjunctivitis. In years past, this was commonly associated with tubercular disease, but today is seen most often with *Staphylococcus* (Fig. 2.40). Other possible sources are *Candida albicans, Coccidioides immitis,* lymphogranuloma venereum, and nematodes. This condition is characterized by the formation of slightly raised, small pinkish-white or yellow nodules near the limbus, with invasion into cornea. These nodules are surrounded by dilated vessels. The nodule ulcerates and heals without a scar on the conjunctiva. A type IV delayed hypersensitivity in the cornea and conjunctiva to a foreign antigen is the likely explanation.

The treatment of these conditions requires an attempt to identify the microbiologic organism responsible and eradicate it. In chronic staphylococcal blepharoconjunctivitis, eradication of the organism is very difficult, if not impossible. Symptomatic improvement can often be obtained with the use of a 50%–50% mixture of water and baby shampoo as a lid scrub (for mechanical debridement of mucus, debris, and bacteria) plus topical antibiotics. In more persistent cases, systemic antibiotics such as tetracycline (250 mg PO q.i.d. for 2 weeks, then a maintenance dose of 250 mg daily for several months) or doxycycline or minocycline (once or twice a day) can be beneficial.

Topical steroids are again useful in treatment of the localized toxic effects on the eye. We tend to use steroids only when really needed in the treatment of chronic blepharoconjunctivitis, and early in the therapy of phlyctenular disease.

## Vernal Conjunctivitis

Vernal conjunctivitis is a fairly rare bilateral inflammation that takes its name from its seasonal predilection for the spring equinox. Onset is common in early spring and summer, with remissions during the cooler months. However, this seasonal pattern is less marked in tropical climates. The condition occurs mainly in children, and boys predominate in a 2:1 ratio. In onset after the age of 20, the male-to-female ratio is equal. The peak incidence is from 11–13 years of age, with most of the cases beginning between 6–14 years of age (and extremes of 1 month to 75 years).

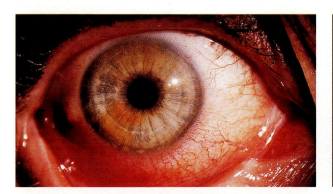

**2.39** | Marginal infiltrates of staphylococcal blepharoconjunctivitis. A chronic staph infection has resulted in sensitization to the proteins of tissue destruction by the bacteria, with a type IV delayed hypersensitivity. Marginal infiltrates are seen at the inferior limbus of this patient with chronic staph blepharoconjunctivitis. Treatment is directed against the causative organism, with topical antibiotics and mechanical debridement with lid scrubs. More resistant cases require the use of systemic antibiotics and topical steroids.

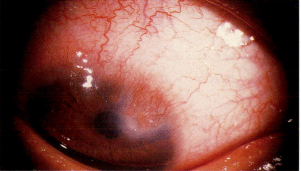

**2.40** | Staphylococcal phlyctenule. A raised whitish to yellow nodule near the limbus with invasion into the cornea is typical for phlyctenular disease, and staphylococcal infection is the most common source of this problem today. There are dilated blood vessels surrounding and within the nodule. The phlyctenule is a type IV delayed hypersensitivity to a foreign antigen and responds well to treatment with topical steroids.

The highest incidence is in the Middle East, areas adjoining the Mediterranean, and Mexico. The lowest frequency is in areas of cool temperate zones, such as Canada, the northern United States, Sweden, and Russia. Three types of vernal conjunctivitis occur: palpebral, limbal, and mixed. All races are affected, with the limbal type more common in blacks and Native Americans. Average duration of this self-limited disease is 4–6 years, and there is usually no permanent scarring.

The most common symptom is itching. Other complaints are photophobia, burning sensation, tearing, a thick, ropy mucoid discharge (usually without crusting), and later development of a mild ptosis (Fig. 2.41). Vessel engorgement causes hyperemia in both the limbal and palpebral forms.

The tissue is infiltrated with lymphocytes, plasma cells, macrophages, basophils, and eosinophils. With further development of the disease, the connective tissue of the substantia propria undergoes hyperplasia and proliferation. Focal proliferation and cellular infiltrate cause giant papillae to form on the tarsal plate or (possibly and) limbal elevation (Figs. 2.42 and 2.43). As more time passes, large, flat-topped cobblestones are seen instead of giant papillae, due to hyalinized avascular connective tissue and epithelial thinning.

The limbal form goes on to develop focal areas of confluent limbal papillae with a gelatinous opaque appearance. Accumulations of eosinophils,

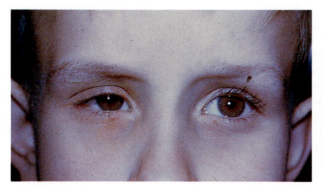

**2.41** | Pseudoptosis in vernal conjunctivitis. The chronic inflammatory changes in the upper conjunctiva result in a droopy right lid in this patient with vernal disease.

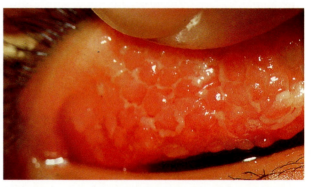

**2.42** | Vernal conjunctivitis. This allergic conjunctivitis is frequently found in patients with a history of atopy. Giant papillae or "cobblestones" develop in the upper pretarsal conjunctiva. The eyes accumulate mucus, and are itchy and watery. The name vernal is somewhat misleading, because cases may be seen at any time of the year (but spring is most common).

**2.43** | Limbal vernal conjunctivitis. Limbal changes in cases of vernal conjunctivitis may occur without the typical pretarsal cobblestones. These opaque, gelatinous limbal papillae can form white, chalky, Horner–Trantas dots, usually at the superior limbus.

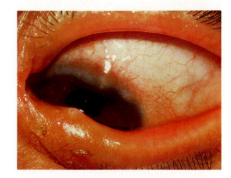

epithelial debris, and granules form the white, chalky Horner–Trantas dots (see Fig. 2.43). The development of intraepithelial cysts results in oval clear spots in the limbus.

Keratitis associated with vernal conjunctivitis occurs in up to 50% of patients. Progression of the conjunctival disease onto the cornea results in a superficial pannus and nodular epithelial hyperplasia. When no limbal extension occurs, keratitis may take the form of diffuse epithelial erosions, or opacities of small gray patches of necrosing epithelium (keratitis epithelialis vernalis of Tobgy) described as a dusting of flour[56] (Fig. 2.44).

Vernal ulcer is an oval (long axis horizontally), shallow, nonvascularized loss of corneal epithelium rarely associated with palpebral vernal conjunctivitis (see Fig. 2.44). Eosinophil major basic protein may be responsible for injury to the corneal epithelium. Superficial stromal infiltration is present, which can be very difficult to treat.

Topical and even systemic steroids have been used to decrease the size of the giant papillae and thus reduce the contact abrasion. Cryotherapy of the upper tarsal conjunctiva and soft bandage lenses to protect the cornea and allow healing can also be tried. Many resolve without scarring, although some may leave a plaque on Bowman's membrane.

The specific cause of this disease is unknown. However, investigations indicate both IgE- and IgG-mediated immune mechanisms are active in patients with vernal conjunctivitis. Type I IgE-mediated hypersensitivity reaction is suggested, with varying reports (26%–86%) of personal and family history of atopy and conjunctival eosinophils. Testing showed increased levels of IgE in tears and patient sera.[57] In addition, increased tear histamine levels can be found in vernal patients.[58] IgG antibodies to pollen in patients that have vernal have also been reported.[59]

Treatment of vernal conjunctivitis must reflect the chronic nature of the illness. Moving to a more temperate climate is often not possible, but cold compresses several times daily can be helpful. Removal of potential allergens with air conditioners and filtering systems to eliminate dust and

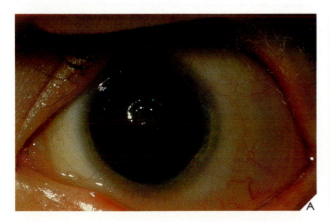
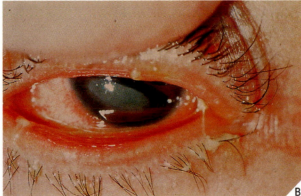

**2.44** | Vernal corneal ulceration. *A:* Beginning as fine, grayish punctate epithelial erosions, a keratopathy from vernal conjunctivitis can become confluent into one large ulcer. *B:* Grayish plaque oval ulceration of the cornea is a shallow loss of corneal epithelium with superficial stromal infiltration. These ulcers can be difficult to treat.

pollens can help, but desensitization seems to be of little use in this problem. Corticosteroids can relieve many of the signs and symptoms of vernal conjunctivitis but must be used with moderation and only for the peak of symptoms. The patients like the comfort, and the steroids are very effective in reducing the size of the giant papillae, but one must remember the potential for cataract development and glaucoma with chronic topical steroid use. Disodium cromoglycate 4% solution is very useful in the chronic treatment of vernal after the majority of symptoms have been alleviated by topical steroids. Severe cases have also been treated with 2% cyclosporine with improvement.[60]

Giant Papillary Conjunctivitis

Very similar in some respects to vernal conjunctivitis, giant papillary conjunctivitis (GPC) is a syndrome seen in users of hard and soft contact lenses, plastic artificial eyes, or with protruding sutures in the conjunctiva. It is seen 10 times more frequently in soft lens users than in hard lens wearers, with an

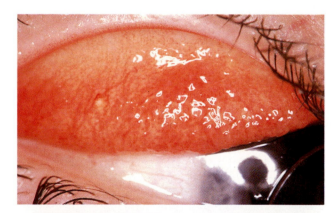

**2.45** | Mild giant papillary conjunctivitis (GPC). Initial symptoms are itching, increased lens awareness, and mucus production. (From Weinstock FJ: *Contact Lens Fitting.* New York: Gower Medical Publishing, 1989, 1.25.)

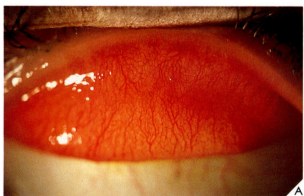

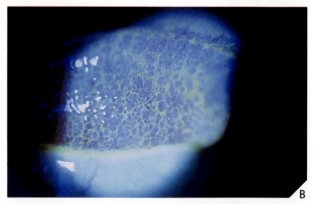

**2.46** | Moderately advanced GPC. *A:* Mild injection of the tarsal plate; papules are seen with white light. *B:* Cobalt blue filter photograph showing large papules (0.75–1 mm).

(From Weinstock FJ: *Contact Lens Fitting.* New York: Gower Medical Publishing, 1989, 10.6.)

average of 8 months minimum time to onset of symptoms in soft users and 8 years in hard wearers. Estimates of prevalence vary from 1%–5% of wearers of soft contact lenses and 1% of hard lens wearers.[61] One study of 200 hard lens wearers for 5 years found 10.5% of the patients to have papillary changes of 0.3 mm or larger in diameter.[62]

Symptoms of GPC appear in advance of the clinical evidence of the process. These include mild itching after lens removal (not nearly as marked as in vernal or atopy), increased mucus on the lens and in the nasal canthus, lens awareness, blurring of vision after hours of lens wear, excessive lens movement, and eventually lens intolerance.

Signs of GPC progress from a generalized thickening of the superior pretarsal conjunctiva and elevation of papillae with hyperemia (Fig. 2.45). With further advancement, the conjunctiva becomes more opaque, with macropapillae (0.3–1.0 mm) (Fig. 2.46), or giant papillae (1.0–2.0 mm) (Fig. 2.47). Trantas dots, mucoid gelatinous nodules at the limbus, can occasionally be seen. Whitish deposits on the soft contact lens are present in almost every case of GPC.

The histology of giant papillary conjunctivitis shows irregular thickened conjunctival epithelium over the papillae. There are many downgrowths into the stroma, and the interpapillary crypts have hyperplastic mucous-secreting elements. Infiltration with eosinophils and basophils is noted but is not as marked as with vernal disease. In addition, PMNs, lymphocytes, and mast cells are found. Eosinophil major basic protein is not increased in the tears of GPC patients.[63] The stroma of the superior palpebral conjunctiva shows lymphocytes, plasma cells, PMNs, eosinophils, basophils, and macrophages, with proliferation of fibroblasts with collagen.

The cause is likely a combination of factors. It is probable that antigens

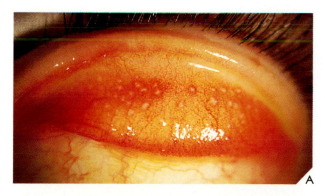 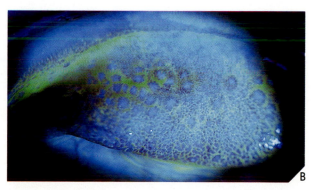

**2.47** | Advanced GPC. *A:* Larger elevated papillary reaction, generalized on the upper lid pretarsal conjunctiva. *B:* Cobalt blue filter photograph with 2% fluorescein, showing large papillae. (From Weinstock FJ: *Contact Lens Fitting.* New York: Gower Medical Publishing, 1989, 10.7.)

from the environment attach to the mucus and protein on the surface of the contact lens (Fig. 2.48).

With the repeated contact of these antigens with the upper tarsal conjunctiva from blinking, and mechanical trauma to the superior tarsal conjunctiva (from the lens, prosthesis, or exposed suture ends), type IV basophil hypersensitivity of the conjunctiva (resembling cutaneous basophil hypersensitivity) occurs. Type I immediate hypersensitivity is also represented in GPC patients.[64]

Treatment of GPC is dictated by the fact that the condition is not dangerous. Whenever possible, we like to have the patient ultimately continue wearing of contact lenses—a desire commonly shared by the patient! Whatever the severity of presentation of the GPC, the first step is stopping lens wear to allow time for recovery. This period is shortened by the use of disodium cromoglyate 4% topically 4 times daily in mild cases, and topical

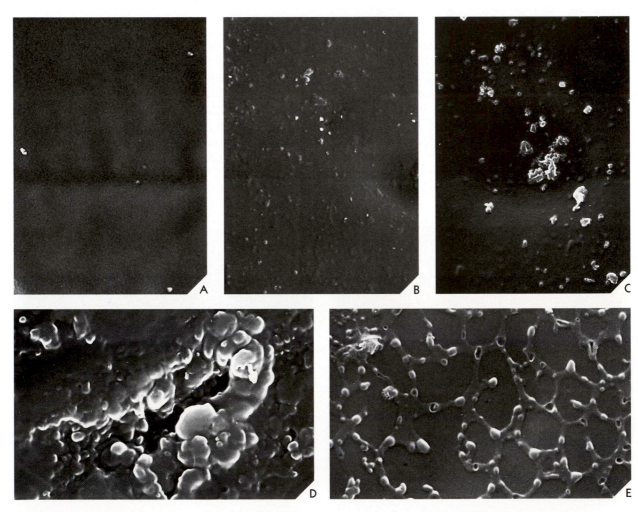

**2.48** | Photomicrographs of lens surfaces. *A:* An unworn lens (x3500). The few spots of debris in the field result from making the photograph. *B:* A lens worn continuously for 1 week (x2500). The lens is almost clean but shows a few scattered protein deposits and debris. *C:* A lens worn continuously for 2 weeks (x3400). The lens has more protein deposits and debris. *D:* A lens worn continuously for 3 weeks (x3400). The lens has prominent thick and thin patches of biofilm. *E:* A lens worn continuously for 3 weeks (x3600). The lens has thick and thin patches of biofilm with bacteria within the matrix. (Photos courtesy of Dr. JW Costerton, University of Calgary.) (From Weinstock FJ: *Contact Lens Fitting.* New York: Gower Medical Publishing, 1989, 3.10.)

steroids in the more severe cases. In some cases we allow the use of new lenses during this period, but it seems to prolong the recovery phase.

The next step is to get new lenses and switch to a system of disinfection that is as much as possible preservative free. For soft contact lens users, we try a fresh set of the same lens type with a hydrogen peroxide method of sterilization. Daily cleaning and frequent use of papain enzyme (at least once a week) are mandatory. Frequent replacement of the lenses can help prevent GPC recurrence.

If the soft lens patient redevelops GPC, use of a different polymer (non-hydroxy-ethylmethacrylate) lens can be useful. Use of a gas-permeable rigid lens may be needed if tolerance to any soft lens cannot be achieved. Cessation of all contact lens use may be necessary in the most refractory of cases.

## SYSTEMIC DISORDERS WITH CONJUNCTIVAL INVOLVEMENT
### CICATRICIAL PEMPHIGOID

Cicatricial pemphigoid (ocular pemphigoid, benign mucous membrane pemphigoid, essential shrinkage of the conjunctiva) is a fairly rare disorder seen in older patients. It is a disease of recurrent bullae of mucous membranes and may involve skin (in about 25% of cases). The conjunctiva is ultimately affected in about 75% of patients. The course of ocular pemphigoid is slow, usually bilateral but often asymmetric, and often unremittingly progressive.

The pathogenesis of cicatricial pemphigoid is thought to be autoantibodies to the basement membrane zone (BMZ) of mucous membranes. These autoantibodies bind to the BMZ, activate complement (evidence of the antigen–antibody reaction at this site), and the resulting inflammatory response leads to scarring and fibrosis.[65,66]

The first ocular symptom of cicatricial pemphigoid is a chronic irritation. Burning and tearing are also common complaints. Secondary bacterial conjunctivitis is a possibility. The conjunctival inflammation and subepithelial fibrosis proceed to conjunctival shrinkage and symblepharon formation. These adhesions from palpebral to bulbar conjunctiva occur first in the inferior fornix (Fig. 2.49). Progression to ankyloblepharon, with complete obliteration of the conjunctival fornices, is the end result (Fig. 2.50).

The conjunctival subepithelial fibrosis results in a secondary dry-eye syndrome, with further contribution to progression of the disease. Because of xerosis and the distortion of the normal lid architecture leading to entropion, trichiasis, and lagophthalmos, the cornea can develop erosions, kera-

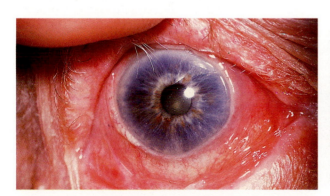

**2.49** | Cicatricial pemphigoid (CP). A rare disease of recurrent bullae of mucous membranes, cicatricial pemphigoid involves the conjunctiva in about 75% of cases. Early findings are a chronic irritation and conjunctival shrinkage with symblepharon formation, usually in the lower fornix.

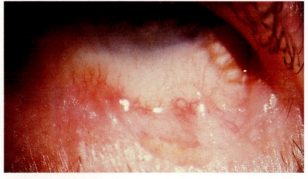

**2.50** | Ankyloblepharon in CP. Obliteration of conjunctival fornices is the result of continued scarring and shrinkage of the conjunctiva.

tinization, neovascularization (leading to opacity), and perforation (with resulting blindness) (Fig. 2.51).

Conjunctival biopsy can be performed to detect immunoglobulin and complement deposition at the basement membrane zone by direct immunofluorescence techniques (positive in 20%–92% of cases).[67,68] Testing of sera for circulating autoantibodies to the BMZ by indirect immunofluorescence methods is less likely to be positive (12% of patients in a recent study).[69]

Several diseases can mimic cicatricial pemphigoid. Other bullous disorders of the skin can cause shrinkage of the conjunctiva. Pemphigoid can be induced by a drug reaction. Radiation, thermal burns, or chemical burns may cause scarring of the conjunctiva and corneal opacity. Severe membranous conjunctivitis with scarring can be confused with cicatricial pemphigoid[70] (Fig. 2.52).

Treatment of this condition is very difficult. Artificial tears help to replace the tear deficit that develops but will not prevent progression of the disease. Topical antibiotics are useful to control secondary infection, and lid scrubs can also be somewhat preventative by controlling bacterial overgrowth. Surgical repair of entropion, cryotherapy for trichiasis, and lysis of symblepharon can be performed when needed but may set off a bout of increased disease activity.

Many different therapy modalities have been tried to effect a solution for this problem. The most promising seems to be the combination of an immunosuppressive agent, cyclophosphamide (Cytoxan), and systemic corticosteroids.[71] Because of the possibility of side effects, all patients on this

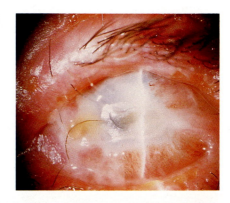

**2.51** | End-stage CP. Continued scarring and shrinkage causes lid distortions, trichiasis, and dry-eye syndrome. Corneal complications include keratinization, neovascularization, opacity, thinning, and perforation.

## Figure 2.52. Diseases that Mimic Cicatricial Pemphigoid

**BULLOUS SKIN DISEASES**
Stevens–Johnson/erythema multiforme
Dermatitis herpetiformis
Epidermolysis bullosa

**DRUG-INDUCED PSEUDOPEMPHIGOID**
Epinephrine
Pilocarpine
Echothiophate iodide
Idoxuridine
Practolol

**ACUTE, NONPROGRESSIVE CONJUNCTIVAL SHRINKAGE**
Radiation
Chemical burns
Thermal burns
Severe membranous conjunctivitis (with scarring)
Adenovirus
*Herpes simplex*
Diphtheria
Beta-hemolytic streptococci

treatment must be followed carefully, preferably in conjunction with an oncologist.

In a study at Johns Hopkins using Cytoxan (1–2 mg/kg/day for 12 months) and prednisone (1 mg/kg/day with a tapering dosage in 2 to 3 months), there was 100% response in 20 patients. Seventeen of the 20 went into remission, with 4 of these patients having a relapse after the end of therapy.[72] Further work is needed to assess these findings.

Erythema multiforme [mucocutaneous syndrome, Lyell's syndrome (toxic epidermal necrolysis), Stevens–Johnson syndrome] is an acute vesiculobullous disorder of the skin and mucous membranes. Erythema multiforme (E-M) has variations in presentation. The minor form typically involves the skin and lasts for 2 to 3 weeks in its acute phase. The more serious variant, also known as Stevens–Johnson syndrome, has skin and mucosal involvement and lasts up to 6 weeks for the acute phase, with a slow recovery. Before the availability of corticosteroids the disease had a 40% mortality.

The cause of erythema multiforme is unknown. Erythema multiforme has been causally related to an unusual toxic response to drugs such as sulfonamides, penicillin, barbiturates, phenylbutazone, phenytoin, mercury, and arsenic. By far the most common single drug class related to this rare deleterious drug reaction is the sulfonamides, especially the long-acting types.[73]

Positive cultures of bacteria, fungi, viruses, and rickettsiae from patients with erythema multiforme that has a toxic course can lead to the assumption of an infectious cause. It has been impossible, however, to document a direct causal relationship between infection and the development of E-M.

Generalized malaise, fever, and arthralgias precede the onset of skin lesions. The lesions affect the entire body and develop rapidly. Different forms can be seen, from small vesicles to maculopapular rings of erythema and pallor to large bullae and loss of the epidermis (Fig. 2.53). The severity of mucous membrane involvement, when present, usually matches the severity of the skin lesions.

The conjunctival involvement may be restricted to a patchy injection and edema with a mucous discharge. The more severe cases exhibit chemosis, vesicles and bullae, membrane formation, and ulceration (Fig. 2.54).

## ERYTHEMA MULTIFORME

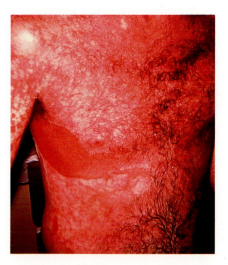

**2.53** | Skin appearance in Stevens–Johnson syndrome. The lesions may affect the entire body and may vary from small vesicles to maculopapular rings of erythema and large bullae with sloughing of the epidermis.

Secondary bacterial infections are a common problem. Therapy with systemic and topical steroids, topical antibiotics, and lysis of adhesions will not prevent the cicatrization that starts near the end of the acute phase and continues during the chronic recovery phase. Symblepharon formation between palpebral and bulbar conjunctiva can occur despite all supportive measures (Fig. 2.55). Dry eye, entropion, and trichiasis can also result, and corneal scarring, vascularization, and ulceration can ensue.

Histology of the lesions shows subepithelial bullae with nonspecific perivascular inflammation of mononuclear cells, eosinophils, and PMNs. Conjunctival pseudomembranes form from the fibrinous exudate, inflammatory cells, and necrotic conjunctival epithelium. True membranes occur with the additional sloughing of the conjunctival epithelial and subepithelial layers into the membrane.

Progression of scarring does not typically occur once the acute phase is over, and the ocular changes are therefore related to the initial damages and their consequences to lid and conjunctival structures (including goblet cell and lacrimal gland destruction), plus any additional scarring if bacterial superinfection had occurred.

There are reported cases of documented episodes of Stevens–Johnson syndrome that have gone on to a progressive and chronic ocular mucosal scarring which appears to be typical for ocular cicatricial pemphigoid. There were linear immune deposits of IgG, IgM, and fibrin at the basement membrane zone. These cases of cicatricial pemphigoid after Stevens–Johnson syndrome represent a small subset of all Stevens–Johnson syndrome patients.[74]

The severity of the presentation of the E-M is the prime determinant of the severity of ocular complications. Local treatment seems to have little influence on ocular outcome. Systemic corticosteroids have been recommended for the treatment of erythema multiforme since the 1950s, but their value and necessity are not proven and a case can be made for not treating

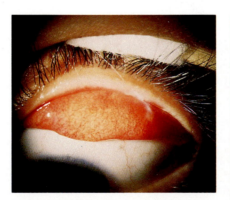

**2.54** | Conjunctival scarring from Stevens–Johnson syndrome. This case resulted from an idiosyncratic response to Dilantin®. With healing, a scar on the upper pretarsal conjunctiva developed, along with a severe dry-eye syndrome.

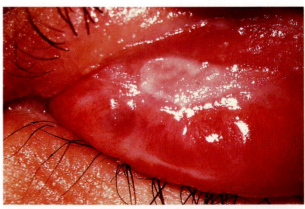

**2.55** | Severe conjunctival scarring from Stevens–Johnson syndrome. Despite all supportive measures during the acute stage, severe conjunctival scarring and shrinkage can occur.

with steroids.[75] Treating the dry-eye syndrome and correcting lid contractures and keratinization, lid malpositions, and trichiasis are the key to the correct management of the ocular component of erythema multiforme.

A rare hereditary disease of the skin and other structures, epidermolysis bullosa can have an autosomal dominant inheritance or an autosomal recessive pattern, and is characterized by bullae formation appearing shortly after birth or associated with mild trauma. Ocular involvement has been reported in the various forms of this disease. Conjunctival vesicles and chronic blepharoconjunctivitis can be seen. Progression to membranous conjunctivitis, symblepharon, and shrinkage of the conjunctiva are documented. The cornea can be involved with a spectrum of mild to severe complications, with bullous changes, keratitis, opacity, vascularization, ulceration, and perforation.[76]

## EPIDERMOLYSIS BULLOSA

A rare disease of bilaterally symmetric grouping of vesicles on erythematous bases, with recurrence and periods of remission, dermatitis herpetiformis has a chronic course of 5–10 years, usually between the second and fifth decades of life. The typical locations are the extensor surface of the knees and elbows, the buttocks and sacral areas, about the shoulder blades, and the scalp.

Ocular involvement is not common, but vesicles in the conjunctiva, erosions, membranes, symblepharon, shrinkage, and keratinization can cause this process to be confused with cicatricial pemphigoid. However, the amount of scarring of the conjunctiva is less in dermatitis herpetiformis.[77]

## DERMATITIS HERPETIFORMIS

Thermal injuries to the face can affect the lids, conjunctiva, and cornea. In addition, injury to the conjunctiva alone can occur with direct contact with hot objects such as hot oil, match heads, or pieces of fireworks. The conjunctiva undergoes a phase of direct tissue destruction, then a reactive phase, and finally a repair phase.

The extent of damage is directly related to the severity of the insult to the tissue. Factors of temperature and length of contact with the conjunctiva, as well as the nature of the causative agent, will influence the extent of the conjunctival burn. Minor thermal injuries are buffered by the tear film and cause mild damage to the conjunctival epithelium, followed by hyperemia of the stromal vessels, swelling, and inflammation. Repair of these mild injuries is by migration of epithelial cells from undamaged areas and by miotic activity of the epithelium for replacement.

More severe injuries, such as from hot foreign bodies that are not immediately cooled by contact with the tears and the conjunctiva, cause the same loss of conjunctival epithelium, but with stromal coagulation and necrosis as well (Fig. 2.56).

Scarring results with healing. If the insulting agent causes significant damage to the conjunctival and episcleral vessels, an anterior ischemia results, with severe consequences to the eye (Fig. 2.57).

## INJURIES
### THERMAL INJURIES

CHEMICAL INJURY    Concentration of the fluid, pH, and time of exposure are major factors in the severity of chemical injury to the conjunctiva. In general, acids cause less injury than alkalis, as they are more readily buffered by the coagulation of the tissue. Alkalis tend to cause severe burns to the eye as they penetrate deep in the conjunctiva, stroma, and cornea (Fig. 2.58). The lipid solubility of the alkali allows quicker and deeper penetration and more difficulty in dilution from the deeper structures of the anterior segment, causing continued damage (Fig. 2.59).

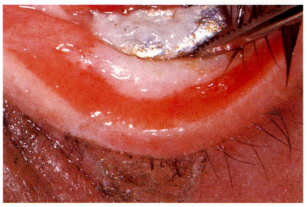

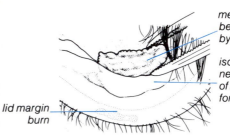

*metal cast being removed by forceps*

*ischaemic necrosis of lower fornix*

*lid margin burn*

**2.56** | Thermal burns. With thermal burns the damage is done at the time of injury; molten metal burns form a cast which must be gently removed with sterile blunt forceps after instilling topical anesthesia. In any severe burn, blepharospasm and marked lid edema may make immediate treatment and subsequent assessment diffi-

cult, and general anesthesia may be required. After completion of the emergency treatment, the extent of damage to the eye and to the surrounding tissues is assessed and future management planned. (From Eagling M, Roper-Hall MJ: *Eye Injuries.* London: Gower Medical Publishing, 1986, 4.2.)

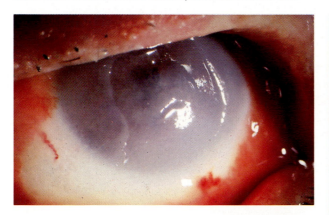

**2.57** | Anterior ischemia from severe thermal burn. The eye does much worse if large areas of tissue ischemia result from the insult. This usually occurs in alkali burns where alkali penetrates the tissues, and rarely in thermal burns (like molten metal). This eye, shown some time after the injury, still shows nearly 90% of limbal ischemia, both conjunctival and episcleral. There is a large epithelial defect, and the induced enzymatic activity (collagenase) is leading to disruption of the collagen fibers (corneal melting). (From Kirkness CM: *Ophthalmology.* London: Gower Medical Publishing, 1985, 27.)

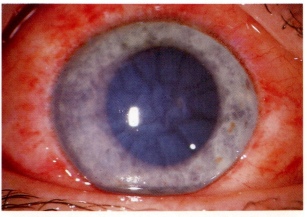

**2.58** | Alkali burns. Lime, sodium or potassium hydroxide or ammonium hydroxide, and other strong alkalis cause severe chemical burns to the eye. Unlike acids, which coagulate tissues, alkalis penetrate deeply, causing conjunctival and limbal ischemia, endothelial damage, trabeculitis, and cataract. Corneal melting may follow. The end result is perforation or a severely vascularized cornea. (From Kirkness CM: *Ophthalmology.* London: Gower Medical Publishing, 1985, 27.)

An initially completely white eye is a bad sign with alkali injury, as it denotes the absence of the normal anterior segment vasculature, and likelihood of the development of anterior segment ischemia (Fig. 2.60).

Conjunctival alkali burns can penetrate to damage episcleral aqueous outflow channels, causing a secondary glaucoma. Scar formation and contracture can cause symblepharon formation, conjunctival shrinkage, trichiasis, and lid distortion. It is very common to have severe problems with a dry-eye syndrome after alkali burns, owing to destruction of the goblet cells of the conjunctiva and damage to the lacrimal glands. The production of collagenase in severe alkali burns compounds the problems, and may cause scleral and corneal melts. Perforation is a definite possibility in these cases, and the eye often has a very poor visual prognosis.

The overriding first principle of treatment of chemical burns to the eye is immediate and copious irrigation. We irrigate even when others have already irrigated the patient, and it is very important to sweep the superior and inferior fornices and evert the lids to remove any retained particles of foreign material.

Topical steroids are used to treat the concomitant uveitis associated with chemical injury, along with cycloplegics and prophylactic topical antibiotics. Artificial tears are also useful in facilitating healing in mild cases.

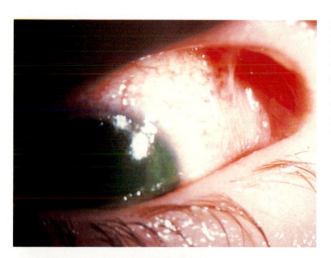

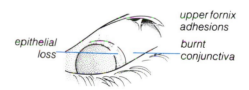

**2.59** | Management of fornix and lid margin burns. Where both the bulbar and palpebral surfaces of the conjunctiva have full-thickness burns, care must be taken to prevent adhesions. Treatment by daily sweeping of the fornices with a glass rod is both painful and traumatic. A contact lens or a fornix shell can help to keep the surfaces apart while healing. (From Eagling M, Roper-Hall MJ: *Eye Injuries.* London: Gower Medical Publishing, 1986, 4.9.)

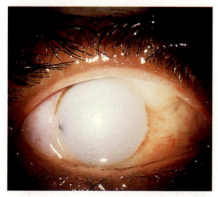

**2.60** | Anterior segment ischemia from severe alkali burn.

Use of acetylcysteine 10%–20% has not proved to prevent the melts of severe burns. Conjunctival transplantation has been used to help patients heal persistent epithelial defects after alkali burns.[78]

## CONJUNCTIVAL TUMORS

### EPITHELIAL TUMORS

#### PSEUDOCANCEROUS LESIONS

##### Hereditary Benign Intraepithelial Dyskeratosis (HBID)

A classification of the origins of conjunctival tumors is presented in Figure 2.61. A list of pseudocancerous epithelial lesions appears in Figure 2.62. HBID is a bilateral abnormal keratinization of the conjunctival epithelium (a surface normally devoid of keratin), with keratinization of the epithelial cells before they become surface epithelial cells. This dyskeratosis is inherited as an autosomal dominant trait and is associated with similar lesions in the oral mucosa. It is a pseudocancerous lesion (Fig. 2.62).

Clinically, there are raised, semicircular, gray-white, highly vascularized elevations of conjunctiva at the nasal and/or temporal limbus of both eyes. The histology of these lesions shows a marked thickening of the squamous epithelium (acanthosis), with dyskeratotic cells in the superficial layers of the epithelium. The subepithelium is very vascular[79] (Fig. 2.63).

### Figure 2.61. Origins of Conjunctival Tumors

| TISSUE OF ORIGIN | BENIGN | MALIGNANT |
|---|---|---|
| Epithelium | | |
|   Surface | Keratoacanthoma<br>Dyskeratosis<br>Papilloma | Carcinoma in situ<br>Squamous cell carcinoma |
|   Glandular | Adenoma | Basal cell<br>  carcinoma (rare) |
| Connective tissue | Fibroma<br>Myxoma<br>Osteoma | Sarcoma |
| Vascular | Hemangioma | Angiosarcoma |
| Reticular | Lymphoid<br>  hyperplasia | Lymphoma<br>Lymphosarcoma |
| Pigmented | Nevus | Melanoma |

### Figure 2.62. Pseudocancerous Epithelial Lesions

Hereditary benign intraepithelial dyskeratosis
Pseudoepitheliomatous hyperplasia
Papilloma
Eosinophilic cystadenoma (oncocytoma)

PEH is a benign reactive acanthosis of the epithelium accompanied by inflammation. The squamous epithelial cells may show some mitotic figures but do not have keratinization or atypia. This mimic of neoplasm is distinguished by the white blood cells, especially PMNs mixed in with the squamous cells. In the subepithelial tissue, a chronic nongranulomatous inflammation is seen. PEH is sometimes seen within a pinguecula or a pterygium, causing sudden growth.

**Pseudoepitheliomatous Hyperplasia (PEH)**

Believed to be of viral etiology, the benign stalk-supported or flat papillomas have smooth, nonkeratinized surfaces. They are often asymptomatic and are usually found in the inferior fornix [although they can be seen at the medial canthus (on the semilunar fold or the caruncle) or pretarsal conjunctiva]. Recurrent lesions and spreading often follow excision. Cryotherapy has been used to treat these cases successfully (Fig. 2.64).

**Pedunculated or Sessile Papilloma**

Limbal papilloma arise from a broad base at or near the limbus, with spread centrally on the cornea and posteriorly on the bulbar conjunctiva. This benign lesion is usually monocular and singular, with a slow growth potential. Biopsy is usually needed to distinguish this lesion from other perilimbal tumors. The histology of these lesions shows a fibrovascular stroma sur-

**Limbal Papilloma**

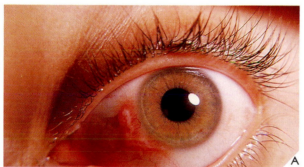
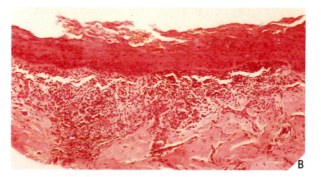

**2.63** | Hereditary benign intraepithelial dyskeratosis (HBID). *A:* The patient has an obvious nasal vascularized, pearly lesion in her left eye. The right eye was quite similar. The patient's mother also had similar lesions. *B:* Histologic section shows an acanthotic epithelium that con-

tains dyskeratotic cells. (*B,* case reported in Yanoff M: *Arch Ophthalmol 1968;79:291.*) (From Yanoff M, Fine BS: *Ocular Pathology. A Color Atlas,* ed 2. New York: Gower Medical Publishing, 1992, 7.11.)

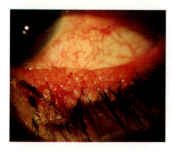

**2.64** | Papillomas. Infection of the conjunctiva with papillomavirus results in papillomata, which may be sessile, as here on the lid margin, or more frond-like. Treatment is difficult and apt to encourage spread. Cryotherapy offers the best prospect of eradication. (From Kirkness CM: *Ophthalmology.* London: Gower Medical Publishing, 1985, 28.)

**2.65** | Limbal papilloma. *A:* A large, sessile papilloma of the limbal conjunctiva is present. *B:* Histologic section shows a papillary lesion composed of acanthotic epithelium and many blood vessels going into the individual fronds. The base of the lesion is quite broad. *C:* Higher magnification shows the blood vessels and the acanthotic epithelium. Although the epithelium is thickened, the polarity from basal cell to surface cell is normal and shows an appropriate transition. (*A*, courtesy of Dr. DM Kozart.) (From Yanoff M, Fine BS: *Ocular Pathology. A Color Atlas,* ed 2. New York: Gower Medical Publishing, 1992, 7.12.)

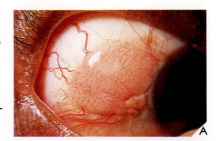

A

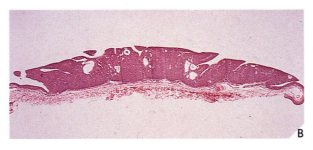

B

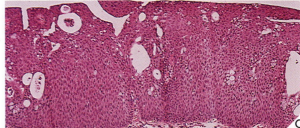

C

**2.66** | Eosinophilic cystadenoma (oncocytooma, oxyphilic cell adenoma). *A:* A fleshy vascularized lesion is present at the caruncle. *B:* Histologic section shows proliferating epithelium around a cystic cavity. *C:* Higher magnification shows large eosinophilic cells which resemble apocrine cells and are forming gland-like spaces. (*A*, courtesy of Dr. HG Scheie.) (From Yanoff M, Fine BS: *Ocular Pathology. A Color Atlas,* ed 2. New York: Gower Medical Publishing, 1992, 7.12.)

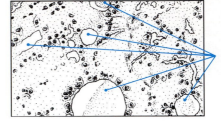

A

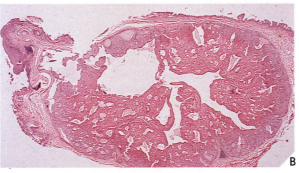

B

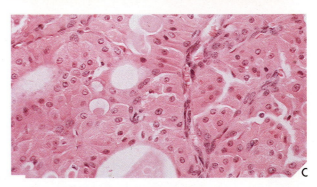

C

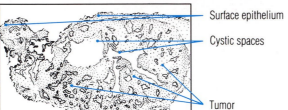

Surface epithelium

Cystic spaces

Tumor

Lumina surrounded by epithelial cells

rounded by acanthotic, mildly pleomorphic epithelium, with intact basal layer (Fig. 2.65).

Keratoacanthoma is a variant of PEH and is a benign lesion more commonly seen on the eyelid. The acanthosis surrounds a central keratin mass.

Keratoacanthoma

Eosinophilic cystadenoma is a rare tumor of the caruncle. Microscopically, one or more cystic cavities are lined with large proliferating eosinophilic epithelial cells that look like apocrine cells (Fig. 2.66).

Eosinophilic Cystadenoma (Oncocytoma)

Dysplasia is a condition in which there is a change in the normal polarity of maturation of epithelial cells, with some atypia but not enough to involve the entire thickness of the epithelium (usually just the deeper layers). Some of these lesions go on to develop into malignancy. Dyskeratotic epithelial cells are also sometimes seen (Fig. 2.67).

PRECANCEROUS LESIONS
Dysplasia

Actinic keratosis of the conjunctiva, like its skin counterpart, is believed to be related to prolonged exposure to ultraviolet light. It often occurs in the

Actinic Keratosis

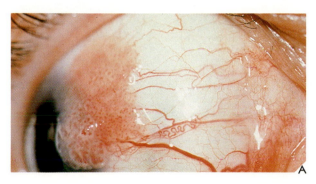

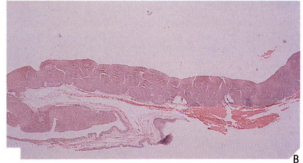

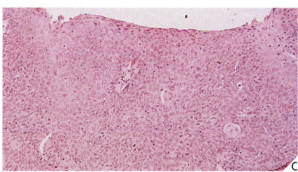

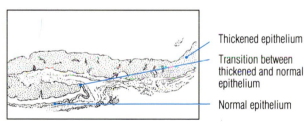

Thickened epithelium

Transition between thickened and normal epithelium

Normal epithelium

**2.67** | Papilloma with dysplasia. *A:* Clinical appearance of a typical limbal sessile conjunctival papilloma. *B:* Histologic section shows a sudden and abrupt transition from normal conjunctival epithelium to a markedly thickened epithelium. The lesion is broad-based and shows many blood vessels penetrating into the thickened epithelium. *C:* Higher magnification shows a tissue with normal polarity but which contains atypical cells and individual cells making keratin (dyskeratosis). Because the polarity is normal, a diagnosis of dysplasia was made. About 8% of conjunctival dysplasias or squamous cell carcinomas will contain the human papillomavirus. (From Yanoff M, Fine BS: *Ocular Pathology. A Color Atlas,* ed 2. New York: Gower Medical Publishing, 1992, 7.13.)

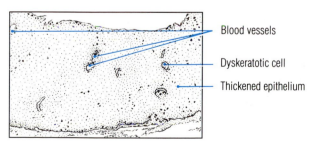

Blood vessels

Dyskeratotic cell

Thickened epithelium

epithelium overlying a pingecula or a pterygium. These lesions can look much like PEH but often have more severe pleomorphism and dyskeratosis.

### CANCEROUS EPITHELIAL LESIONS
#### Carcinoma in Situ

In the malignant category of the World Health Organization classification, conjunctival carcinoma in situ does not behave like a typical malignancy. It is usually confined to the epithelium and rarely invades deeper layers. Recurrence after excision is common but remains intraepithelial. The commonly employed descriptive use of "Bowen's disease" here is not proper, as Bowen described an intraepithelial carcinoma of the skin.

Microscopically, there is a thickened epithelial area in which the polarity of maturation is lost and is replaced by atypical pleomorphic and mitotic epithelium. There is a distinctively sharp demarcation from the normal to the abnormal epithelium. The basement membrane of the epithelium is intact, and there is no invasion into the subepithelial tissue. Extension onto the cornea is common but the tumor is easily pulled off, leaving Bowman's membrane intact (Fig. 2.68).

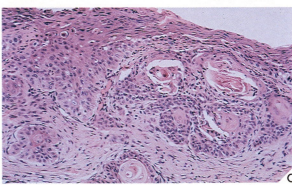

**2.68** | Clinical picture of carcinoma in situ of the conjunctiva. This carcinoma grows with lateral extension in the epithelium without invasion of the underlying layers. Treated with local excisional biopsy, it is easily stripped off Bowman's corneal membrane.

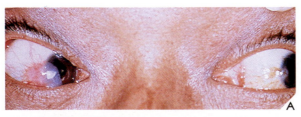

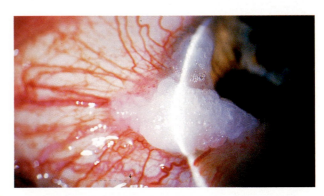

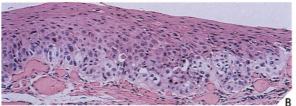

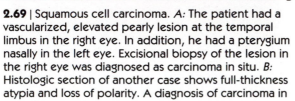

**2.69** | Squamous cell carcinoma. *A:* The patient had a vascularized, elevated pearly lesion at the temporal limbus in the right eye. In addition, he had a pterygium nasally in the left eye. Excisional biopsy of the lesion in the right eye was diagnosed as carcinoma in situ. *B:* Histologic section of another case shows full-thickness atypia and loss of polarity. A diagnosis of carcinoma in situ would be made here. *C:* Other regions show malignant epithelial cells in the substantia propria of the conjunctiva, forming keratin pearls in some areas representing invasive squamous cell carcinoma. (From Yanoff M, Fine BS: *Ocular Pathology. A Color Atlas,* ed 2. New York: Gower Medical Publishing, 1992, 7.14.)

Most squamous cell carcinomas of the conjunctiva start near the limbus on the bulbar surface. Growth is by spread centripetally, with invasion of atypical pleomorphic squamous epithelial cells through the epithelial basement membrane to the substantia propria. Deep invasion is possible to the eyelids or orbit, but most cases are only slightly invasive of conjunctival stroma. Lesions are easily removed with excisional biopsy. Cryoprobe application to the surgery site may reduce the risk of recurrence[80] (Fig. 2.69).

The specimens obtained from these cases show a well-differentiated tumor with acanthosis and commonly some surface keratinization. The stroma exhibits inflammatory cells and areas of atypical epithelial cells with mitotic figures, keratinization, and hyperplasia.

Two variants of squamous cell carcinoma, spindle cell (pseudosarcomatous) and mucoepidermoid carcinoma, are rare. However, these tumors have aggressive growth patterns and invade the eye and orbit. They are also characterized by early recurrence if they are not carefully and totally removed[81] (Fig. 2.70).

Dilatation of preexisting small blood vessels (telangiectasia) can be the result of local irritation or chronic inflammation. In the chronic inflammation of thyroid eye disease, dilated vessels may be seen near the insertions of the rectus muscles.

Hereditary diseases causing telangiectasia can be expressed on the conjunctiva. Examples of these are hemorrhagic telangiectasia [Rendu–Osler–Weber disease with dilated conjunctival blood vessels in a star shape, first seen typically in adolescence (may be present from birth)], ataxia–telangiectasia (Louis–Bar syndrome, with 100% of cases having conjunctival telangiectasia), and encephalotrigeminal angiomatosis (Sturge–Weber syndrome with angiomatous malformations of the bulbar conjunctiva).

A tumor arising from new blood vessel proliferation is a hemangioma. The conjunctiva is an uncommon site.

Palpebral conjunctival involvement is common in eyelid and orbital capillary hemangiomas. These occur early in life, but most regress by 5 years of age.

A granuloma type of capillary proliferation, pyogenic granuloma is associated with areas of prior trauma (such as surgery for strabismus), inflamma-

**Squamous Cell Carcinoma**

## VASCULAR TUMORS

**TELANGIECTASIA**

**HEMANGIOMA**

Capillary Hemangioma

Pyogenic Granuloma

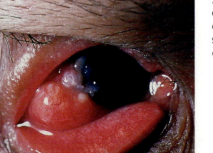

**2.70** | Squamous cell carcinoma of the conjunctiva with invasion into the cornea. Large feeder vessels can be seen, and should make one suspicious of malignancy.

tion (such as a chalazion), or retained foreign body (Fig. 2.71). They are red masses of fibroblasts, proliferating capillaries, lymphocytes, and plasma cells that rapidly enlarge without pain.

### Lymphangiectasia

The clinical appearance of dilated lymphatic channels may be observed in the bulbar or palpebral conjunctiva shortly after birth or in early childhood, denoting a lymphangiectasia. They may also be associated with malformations of the eyelid or orbit (Fig. 2.72).

### Congenital Conjunctival Lymphedema

Also called Nonne–Milroy–Meige disease, this condition is characterized by dilated lymphatic channels in the conjunctiva accompanied by edema, and is thought to be caused by congenital dysplasia of the lymphatics. The condition develops shortly after birth or during childhood. It is usually associated with swelling of the legs.

### Hemorrhagic Lymphangiectasia

In this condition, also called lymphangiectasia hemorrhagica conjunctivae of Leber, there is a connection between blood and lymphatic channels within the bulbar conjunctiva. The affected lymphatics fill with blood and there is some local edema. It can be seen spontaneously, after mild trauma, or with eyelid/parotid gland vascular/lymphatic anomalies. The condition is usually temporary. Persistence of the blood in the lymphatic channels can be treated by excision or by diathermy.[82]

### MELANOTIC TUMORS

Tumors in the conjunctiva of melanocytic origin are in many ways analogous to lesions in uvea or skin. Most researchers believe that melanocytes are

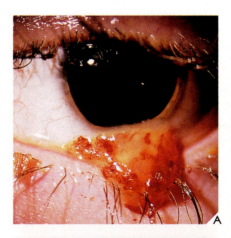
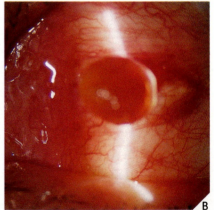

**2.71** | Pyogenic granuloma. A red mass of fibroblasts, lymphocytes, plasma cells and proliferating capillaries enlarges rapidly after prior trauma or inflammation. *A,B:* Two examples of pyogenic granuloma after trauma.

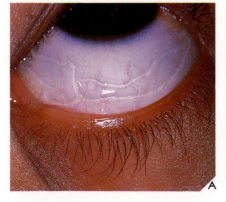
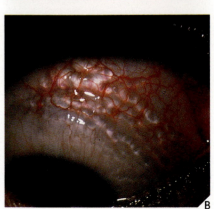

**2.72** | Lymphangiectasia. *A:* This case of congenital lymphangiectasia is seen in a 9-year-old child. The abnormalities are usually stationary once they reach a definite configuration. *B:* Adult with lymphangiectasia.

derived from the neural crest. They may vary in size and abundance of cells and in melanin content, but rarely undergo reactive proliferation. Neoplastic proliferation may occur.

The presence of excessive melanotic pigment is called melanosis. Classification of conjunctival melanosis can be defined by location and time of appearance.

*Melanosis*

A freckle or *ephelis* is a discrete area of melanotic pigment of the basal cell layer of the conjunctival epithelium, present from birth or early childhood. Its clinical appearance is that of a flat brown lesion with irregular borders. It may be present on bulbar or palpebral surfaces, but is most commonly found in the near-limbal conjunctiva. The conjunctival lesion is freely mobile over the sclera. An ephelis has no potential for malignant change. It is more common in darker-skinned races.

*Congenital Epithelial Melanosis*

*Lentigo* is similar to an ephelis, but is slightly larger. Mild melanocytic hyperplasia is seen, in addition to increased pigmentation of the basal cell layer. It is also a freely mobile lesion.

These stationary lesions do not have a true conjunctival location (they consist of increased pigmentation of the uvea, sclera, and episclera), but are often mistaken for conjunctival lesions. The conjunctiva can be moved with no corresponding movement of the lesion. The involved area of the globe of the eye looks blue or slate gray in color, not brownish.

*Congenital Subepithelial Melanosis*

There are two expressions of subepithelial congenital melanosis. Ocular melanocytosis (congenital melanosis oculi) is characterized by an increase in the number and size of pigmented melanocytes of the uvea, with increased numbers of pigmented melanocytes in the episcleral and scleral tissues. It is almost always unilateral and heterochromia of the iris is common. It is very rare in blacks and most common in whites.

When the ocular presentation is combined with same-sided melanosis of the deep dermis of the lids or orbital skin, the condition is called oculodermal melanocytosis or nevus of Ota (Fig. 2.73). This can be a unilateral or a bilateral lesion but exhibits marked asymmetry when bilateral. Asians and blacks have a higher incidence of oculodermal melanocytosis than whites.

Both presentations in white patients have a much higher incidence of uveal malignant melanoma, with few reports of malignant melanoma in nonwhite nevus of Ota patients.[83]

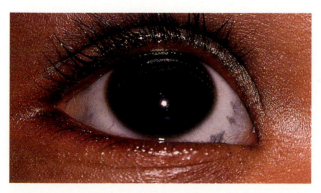

**2.73** | Oculodermal melanocytosis (nevus of Ota). Unilateral or bilateral, the combination of same-sided melanosis of the deep dermis of the lid or orbital skin plus subepithelial melanosis is oculodermal melanocytosis. In white patients this condition is associated with a higher than normal risk for developing choroidal malignant melanoma, with few reports of malignant melanoma in nonwhite nevus of Ota patients. This patient demonstrates the episcleral melanosis plus the increased pigmentation of the lid skin in a unilateral presentation.

*Acquired Melanosis*　　Excessive melanocytic activity of the conjunctival epithelium causes the buildup of melanin within the melanocytes. There is also release of melanin into the substantia propria, where it is gobbled up by histiocytes (melanophages) or connective tissue cells.

*Bilateral acquired melanosis* is related most often to race, with a common finding of acquired melanosis in the conjunctiva of older black patients. There is little chance of cancerous change (Fig. 2.74).

A secondary form of benign acquired melanosis is related to toxic (such as arsenic or thorazine) or metabolic influences (such as Addison's disease or pregnancy) that cause melanin deposition. Melanin cyst or pigment granules can be seen in glaucoma patients on long-term topical epinephrine (Fig. 2.75).

Any source of scarring or cysts of the conjunctiva (e.g., trachoma, vernal conjunctivitis, keratomalacia) may stimulate melanocytes to increased production.

*Unilateral acquired melanosis* is most commonly seen in adult white patients. It consists of a unilateral brownish pigmentation of the conjunctiva that moves freely over the sclera. Progression is highly variable. It can remain benign and enlarge slowly over the years, but there is about a 17% chance that it will become malignant within 5–10 years.[84] Any portion of the conjunctiva may be affected.

Unilateral primary acquired melanosis is classified in two stages. Stage I, benign acquired melanosis, is a precancerous state confined to the epithelium, without invasion of substantia propria. It is subdivided into A and B substages, with a lesion classed as IB when, in addition to melanotic pigmen-

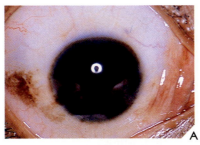

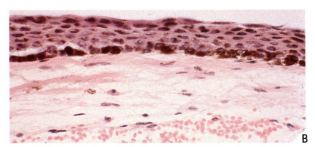

**2.74** | Primary acquired melanosis, benign. *A:* The patient noted the onset of pigmentation of the conjunctiva in adult life. *B:* A histologic section of a biopsy of the lesion shows increased epithelial pigmentation, most marked in the basal layer but also scattered throughout the epithelial layers. Benign acquired melanosis may resemble this or may show benign, pigmented nevus cells in the junctional position. (From Yanoff M, Fine BS: *Ocular Pathology. A Color Atlas*, ed 2. New York: Gower Medical Publishing, 1992, 17.4.)

**2.75** | Adrenochrome pigment caused by epinephrine use. Adrenochrome pigment may develop in the conjunctiva as a result of long-term topical epinephrine use. The epinephrine undergoes oxidation when trapped in conjunctival cysts, forming these pigmented granules, which usually cause no problems.

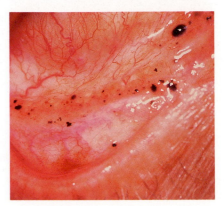

tation, there is atypical melanocytic hyperplasia. In the most worrisome form of stage IB, there is mitotic activity within atypical melanocytes and nests of melanocytes at different levels of the epithelium, but still no invasion of deeper layers. Lesions that have larger epithelioid cells and lesions with atypical melanocytes arranged in nests are highly likely to develop into melanoma.[85]

Stage II, malignant acquired melanosis (cancerous melanosis), is a flat, unilateral onset of pigmentation in adulthood. This invasive malignant melanoma usually arises from a preexisting primary benign acquired melanosis. The cells invading the substantia propria are melanocytes with atypical size, shape, and mitotic activity (Fig. 2.76).

The prognosis for the patient is related to the depth of invasion at the time of excision. This must be measured histologically with a micrometer grid from the surface of the epithelium to the deepest area of invasion of conjunctival stroma. In general, lesions of less than 1.5 mm in depth (Stage IIA) have a better prognosis than those greater than 1.5 mm (Stage IIB). Bulbar cancerous melanosis cases also have a better prognosis. However, even a relatively flat tumor can have early spread if it gains access to lymphatic channels after the epithelial basement membrane is breached.[86]

Cases have been reported of melanocytic hyperplasia without pigment (amelanotic acquired melanosis). Such a case can be difficult to recognize as anything other than nonspecific inflammation of the conjunctiva until it develops into a Stage IIB tumor displaying the histology of a malignant melanoma without melanin.[87]

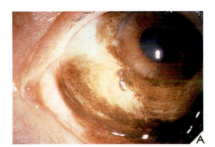
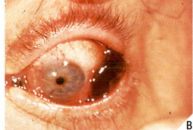
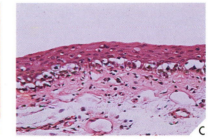
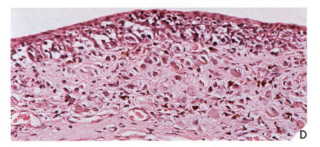
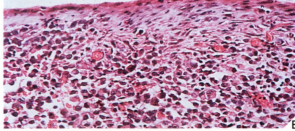

**2.76** | Primary acquired melanosis, cancerous. *A:* The patient developed unilateral onset of conjunctival pigmentation in adult life. The pigmentation was completely flat. As long as the pigmentation was flat, it is unlikely that a melanoma was present. *B:* This patient also had adult-onset increased conjunctival pigmentation. Recently, a mass developed and excisional biopsy was performed. *C:* Some areas of the lesion showed benign acquired melanosis, as represented here by nests of nevus cells in the junctional position. *D:* Other areas showed cancerous melanosis, here at an early stage showing invasion of the superficial subepithelial tissue. *E:* Still other areas showed frank malignant melanoma characterized by deep invasion of the subepithelial tissue. The cells are large and atypical; they show no tendency for maturation or for following the normal cell-size polarity demonstrated in earlier figures. (From Yanoff M, Fine BS: *Ocular Pathology. A Color Atlas,* ed 2. New York: Gower Medical Publishing, 1992, 17.5.)

Nevus

Nevi are well-delineated congenital lesions that may not become pigmented until the second or third decade of life (Fig. 2.77). The nevus is the most common type of conjunctival tumor, and most nevi move with movement of the conjunctiva. This hamartoma is composed mainly of nevus cells, with a mix of epithelial cells in the compound nevi.

Five types exist: (i) intraepithelial (junctional), clusters of nevus cells in the conjunctival epithelium that tend to be flat; (ii) subepithelial, masses of nevus cells in the substantia propria which may elevate the conjunctival surface; (iii) compound, junctional, and subepithelial nevus cells in confluent areas as well as discrete nests in both areas, which may elevate the conjunctival surface (Fig. 2.78); (iv) spindle cell/epithelioid cell (juvenile melanoma or Spitz nevus) which is a rare variety of compound nevus; and (v) blue nevus, heavily pigmented fusiform and dendritic melanocytes crowded in the deep substantia propria with normal overlying epithelium. The subset of cellular blue nevi consists of large spindle-shaped melanocytes in clusters in the conjunctival stroma, but with normal epithelium. Blue and cellular blue nevi do not tend to move with the movement of conjunctiva.

Nevi with growth may become more prominent and more vascular, but they have a very low potential for malignant transformation. Cosmetically, they may detract, and simple excision removes the blemish and eliminates the remote possibility of malignant change. There are cases in which nevi have been present for years without significant change and then give rise to a malignant melanoma. There are also associations of nevi with diffuse atypical melanocytic hyperplasias and malignant melanomas. Therefore, all conjunctival nevi should be carefully observed.

Pigmentation of nevi is variable. Whereas most are dark lesions, the amelanotic ones are difficult to see. As they grow, they may become vascularized and look like an angioma.

Malignant Melanoma

Primary malignant melanomas of the conjunctiva stem from three sources: acquired melanosis, nevi (Fig. 2.79), or de novo. The first two types have been discussed above. De novo appearance of a malignant melanoma occurs in patients with no clinical history of either nevi or melanocytic hyperplasia and represents about 25%–30% of all reported malignant melanomas.

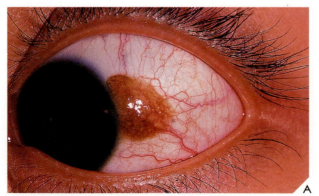
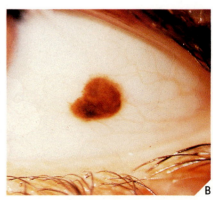

A

B

**2.77** | Benign nevus. *A,B:* Common lesions, usually seen near the limbus, nevi may be present from birth or may wait until adulthood to appear. The pigmented area provides a well-seen counterpoint to the white sclera. Slow growth can be seen, but no treatment (other than photographic documentation) is usually required.

Conjunctival melanomas behave more like cutaneous melanomas than uveal melanomas, by virtue of the fact that they have early access to lymphatic drainage channels to disseminate the cancer. Dissemination is usually to the regional lymph nodes in the preauricular and submandibular areas. Once tumor cells have access to the lymphatics, there is great potential for hematogenous spread. This action does not always foreshadow death from metastases in cases of conjunctival melanoma. Several patients in the AFIP registry have lived more than 10 years after spread to regional lymph nodes from a conjunctival melanoma without the intervention of radiation or chemotherapy.[88]

Like skin melanomas, conjunctival melanomas are not classified according to cell type. There is a loss of normal polarity and the surface and

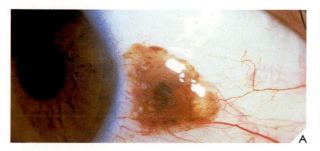
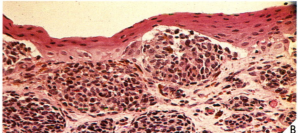

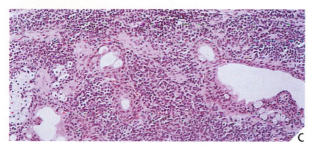

**2.78** | Conjunctival nevus. *A:* The conjunctival nevus near the limbus shows variable pigmentation and small and large cystic structures. *B:* A histologic section of another case shows nevus cells in the junctional region between the epithelial and subepithelial tissues (the substantia propria), producing a junctional nevus. As in the skin, the nevus cells tend to become smaller the deeper they lie in the subepithelial tissue, representing the normal

Junctional nests of nevus cells

Subepithelial nests of nevus cells

polarity of the nevus. *C:* In addition to nevus cells, epithelium-lined cysts are present. These cysts are often found within the nevus and are part of the hamartomatous lesion. The cysts may be noted clinically, as seen in *A.* (From Yanoff M, Fine BS: *Ocular Pathology. A Color Atlas,* ed 2. New York: Gower Medical Publishing, 1992, 17.3.)

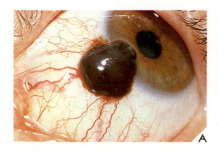
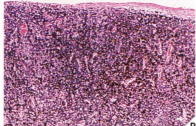
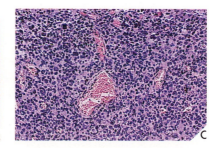

**2.79** | Malignant melanoma. *A:* A pigmented conjunctival lesion near the limbus, present since childhood, had undergone recent rapid growth. *B:* A histologic section of an incomplete excisional biopsy shows a heavily pigmented tumor. *C:* A bleached section shows loss of the normal polarity, i.e., the cells deep in the lesion are of

the same size as those nearer the surface (instead of being smaller). In general, melanomas not thicker than 1.5 mm have an excellent prognosis, whereas those thicker than that tend to be lethal. (From Yanoff M, Fine BS: *Ocular Pathology. A Color Atlas,* ed 2. New York: Gower Medical Publishing, 1992, 17.4.)

deep cells are indistinguishable. The component cells are atypical, with an increase in the nuclear to cytoplasmic ratio and occasional mitoses.

Recurrence of conjunctival melanomas may be seen in conjunctiva, lids, or the orbit. There are several possibilities for recurrence. In cases arising from acquired melanosis, new tumors may occur in other parts of an atypical conjunctiva not adjacent to a resected melanoma. This is due to the potential of the primary acquired melanosis to have multiple areas of malignant change.

Identification of a new primary malignant melanoma is made histologically by demonstration of the atypical melanocytic hyperplasia in the epithelium invading with neoplastic cells into the underlying tissues. Invasion of adjacent tissues is also possible (Fig. 2.80).

Satellite nodules can occur in the conjunctival stroma after excision of a discrete melanoma if it had invaded lymphatic channels before surgery. These nodules are local metastases, as opposed to regional dissemination of tumor. Cell spread during excision is possible, especially with very malignant melanomas, since they have such marked mitotic activity and lack of structure. Malignant cell spread during excision sets the possibility for later local regrowth.

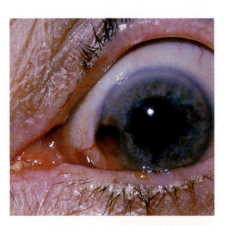

**2.80** | Conjunctival melanoma. Invasion of adjacent tissue by a conjunctival melanoma is possible. This case is an example of a conjunctival melanoma invading the cornea.

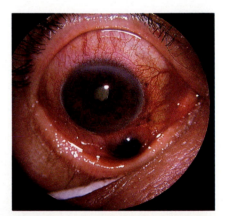

**2.81** | Uveal melanoma. An extension of growth of a uveal melanoma through the sclera can be easily mistaken for a primary conjunctival melanoma that has penetrated deeper structures.

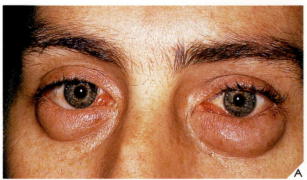

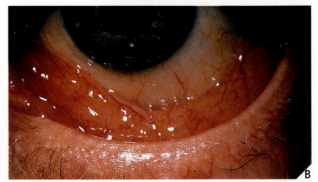

**2.82** | Lymphoma. Lymphomas of the conjunctiva are often just part of a more generalized lesion in the eyelid or the orbit. *A:* Photograph of the eyelids of a patient with lymphoma. *B:* Conjunctival lymphoma in the same patient.

Secondary malignant melanoma of the conjunctiva is a rare event. It is possible to see a conjunctival metastatic melanoma stemming from a distant primary. It is also possible for a uveal melanoma to extend outward through the sclera and to be mistaken for a primary conjunctival melanoma that has invaded deeper structures (Fig. 2.81), and it can be very difficult to distinguish between the two entities.

## STROMAL TUMORS

The connective tissue and vascular channels of the conjunctiva can give rise to the entire spectrum of benign and malignant tumors. Examples of benign lesions include fibroma, myxoma, osteoma, hemangioma, benign lymphoid hyperplasia, neurofibroma, and neurilemmoma.

Sarcoma, angiosarcoma, lymphoma, and malignant schwannoma can also have conjunctival expression. Most of these lesions may exist in the conjunctiva but are rarely confined to it. Often, the more extensive lesion is in the eyelid or orbit (Fig. 2.82).

Metastatic lesions may occur in the conjunctival stroma. An example of leukemia infiltrate presenting in the conjunctiva is shown in Fig. 2.83. It may sometimes present early in the course of the disease.

Rhabdomyosarcoma must be singled out because the conjunctival manifestations may be the initial presentation. Seen in the first decade of life, these tumors may present with a lesion in the superior fornix (or in other quadrants). Rhabdomyosarcoma has the conjunctival manifestation of a swelling of the fornix, extending towards the interpalpebral area. It may look like a nonspecific inflammation of the conjunctiva but it does not shrink with antiinflammatory therapy, and this should alert the physician to the possibility of a neoplasm.

The other conjunctival stromal tumor of note is Kaposi's sarcoma. Reddish-blue vascular macules or nodules develop in the skin of the legs of patients with the classic form of the disease, but patients with acquired immune deficiency syndrome exhibit tumors in the upper body, head, neck, eyelid, and conjunctiva. The conjunctival lesions may be the first clinical signs of AIDS, but the sarcoma usually develops after multiple opportunistic

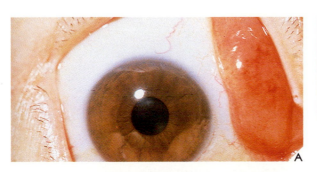
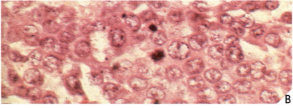

**2.83** | Leukemia. *A:* The patient has a smooth "fishflesh" lesion that had appeared a few weeks previously. The lesion resembles that seen in lymphoid hyperplasia, lymphoma, or amyloidosis. A diagnosis of acute leukemia had recently been made. *B:* Histologic section shows sheets of immature, blastic leukemic cells, many of which exhibit mitotic figures. (From Yanoff M, Fine BS: *Ocular Pathology. A Color Atlas,* ed 2. New York: Gower Medical Publishing, 1992, 7.15.)

infections. It appears as subepithelial nodules or as a diffuse swelling in the fornix or on the palpebral conjunctiva. The histology of this tumor shows spindle-shaped cells with oval nuclei and capillary channels, and biopsy specimens are easily obtained (Fig. 2.84).

## ACKNOWLEDGMENTS

I deeply appreciate the help and suggestions of my editors, Drs. Jack Chandler and Joel Sugar. I thank Jack for the opportunity to write this chapter, and for his aid and counsel. A special thanks to Joel for his prodigious memory, specific additions, and encouraging advice.

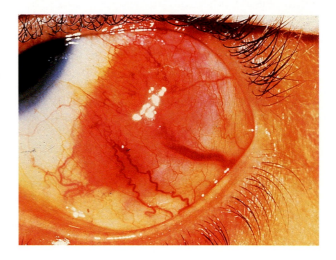

**2.84** | Kaposi's sarcoma. A reddish-blue vascularized nodule in the subepithelium of the conjunctiva is the hallmark of Kaposi's sarcoma. It can be the first clinical sign of AIDS or it can occur after multiple opportunistic infections. The lesions can be on the bulbar conjunctiva, as in this case of an HIV patient, or may represent a diffuse swelling of the fornix or palpebral conjunctiva. (Courtesy of Dr. J Rubenstein)

# LIMBAL TUMORS
## John W. Chandler

The cornea is an unusual site for a neoplasm except for one that arises by extension of a limbal lesion. These tumors typically arise from either squamous epithelial cells or intraepithelial dendritic melanocytes located in the limbal region. In addition, there are congenital lesions located at the limbus that are not neoplastic and involve the peripheral cornea and, in some cases, extend to the central cornea. Chapter 2 details many of these lesions as they arise from or affect the conjunctiva.

## CONGENITAL CORNEAL TUMORS

Most of these are choristomas, which are growths of tissues and structures that do not normally reside in a particular site. A solid dermoid involving the cornea is usually yellow-white and located in the inferotemporal quadrant[1-5] (Fig. 3.1). In most cases they are unilateral. Infrequently, dermoids involve the entire circumference of the limbus, and rarely they cover the entire cornea. Histologic examination reveals a thick collagenous lesion in which any or all of the following may be noted: hair, sweat glands, fat, sebaceous glands, teeth. A dermolipoma is similar, except that fat makes up a larger proportion and other structures are less common. Goldenhar syndrome is characterized by an epibulbar dermoid or dermolipoma associated

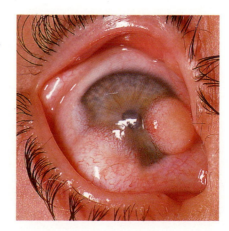

**3.1** | Limbal dermoids. This patient with Goldenhar syndrome had two dermoids. The most elevated led to corneal epithelial drying and irregularities central to it. After removal, vision improved.

with ocular and systemic findings[6,7] (Fig. 3.2). Growth rates in these choristomas parallel those of the rest of the eye. Neoplasia is not common.

The excision of a dermoid or dermolipoma is sometimes difficult. It is frequently difficult to estimate the total size or depth of the lesion. Posteriorly, such lesions may extend into the excretory ducts of the lacrimal gland or around extraocular muscles. In many cases the depth of their extension requires lamellar or penetrating keratoplasty. Because large degrees of corneal astigmatism often accompany these lesions, one of the goals of surgical excision is correction of the astigmatism. Removal of these lesions, however, frequently does not affect the astigmatism.[8]

Another choristoma that may extend from the limbus onto the cornea is an ectopic lacrimal gland, which may also include other tissue elements.[9] These lesions are pinkish and highly vascularized. Ectopic lacrimal gland often extends very deep into the cornea and excision is difficult. Surgical excision usually requires concomitant lamellar keratoplasty. These choristomas have little or no tendency to become malignant. Scleral cysts may occur at the inferotemporal limbus and are discussed in Chapter 13.

## SQUAMOUS EPITHELIAL TUMORS

The palisades of Vogt (Fig. 3.3), reservoirs of corneal epithelial stem cells that are mitotically active, are present along the limbus. This activity may predispose this area to neoplasm. In addition, the exposure of the nasal and temporal limbus to sunlight enhances the risk of neoplasia. Figure 3.4 lists the lesions that may extend from the limbus onto the cornea.[10-12] These represent a spectrum ranging from totally benign to malignant. In all cases, exci-

### Figure 3.2. Findings in Goldenhar Syndrome

| OCULAR | SYSTEMIC |
| --- | --- |
| Epibulbar dermoid or dermolipoma | Preauricular skin tag |
| Lid colobomas | Pretragal fistulas |
| Duane syndrome | Mandibular hypoplasia |
| Microphthalmos | Vertebral abnormalities |
| Iris coloboma | |
| Aniridia | |

**3.3** | Palisades of Vogt. The palisades are pigmented in this patient, highlighting their radial array along the limbus separated by radial vessels.

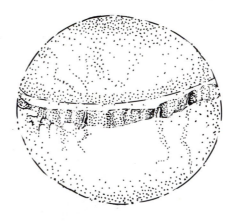
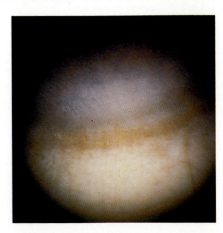

sion and histopathologic examination are indicated. The specimen must be carefully oriented so that the pathologist can provide the surgeon with the most accurate information (Fig. 3.5). Because it is rare for these lesions to invade through Bowman's layer, the extensions onto the cornea can usually be gently scraped off. Some lesions recur and must be re-excised, and may require cryotherapy of the conjunctival sites of involvement. Invasive lesions may occur and prompt more aggressive treatment, including enucleation (Fig. 3.6).

## MELANOCYTIC TUMORS

Melanocytes are widely scattered throughout the conjunctival epithelium. Proliferations and masses composed of these cells cause a number of conjunctival and limbal lesions, some of which involve the cornea[13,14] (Figs. 3.7–3.11). The management of these lesions is discussed in Chapter 2 and in Volume 4 of this series. Limbal pigmentation may increase with age, especially in highly pigmented individuals. The distinction between acquired

### Figure 3.4. Limbal Corneal Lesions Arising from Squamous Epithelium

Benign hereditary dyskeratosis
Benign squamous papilloma
Pseudoepitheliomatous
    hyperplasia
Squamous dysplasia

Carcinoma in situ
Primary corneal epithelial
    dysplasia
Invasive squamous cell carcinoma

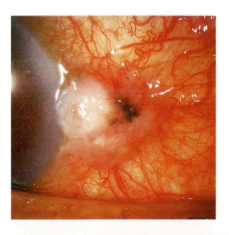

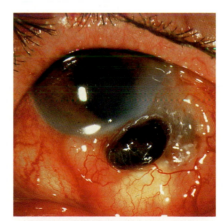

**3.5** | Limbal squamous cell carcinoma. Clinically this lesion is indistinguishable from more benign dysplasia or carcinoma in situ, making excisional biopsy the treatment of choice.

**3.6** | Invasive squamous cell carcinoma with intraocular extension and uveal prolapse. (Courtesy of Dr. A. Sugar.)

### Figure 3.7. Conjunctival Lesions Composed of Melanocytes that May Involve the Cornea

Benign epithelial melanosis
Benign melanocytic nevi
Primary acquired melanosis
Malignant melanoma

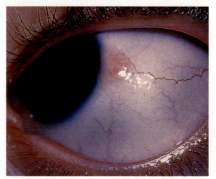

**3.8** | Nonpigmented nevus.

racial conjunctival pigmentation and potentially malignant acquired melanosis is discussed in Chapter 2.

At times, other neoplastic as well as non-neoplastic lesions occur at the limbus (Figs. 3.12–3.14). Excision and histopathologic examination are critical for a definitive diagnosis.

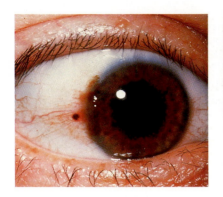

**3.9** | Pigmented nevus.

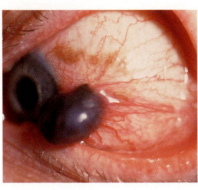

**3.10** | Malignant melanoma arising de novo.

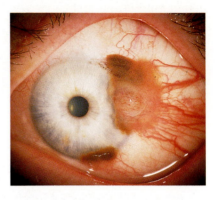

**3.11** | Malignant melanoma arising from primary acquired conjunctival melanosis.

### Figure 3.12. Other Neoplastic and Non-Neoplastic Lesions that May Occur at the Corneal Limbus

| NEOPLASTIC | INFLAMMATORY |
|---|---|
| Lymphoma | Follicles |
| Kaposi's sarcoma | Nodules of limbal vernal keratocon-<br>junctivitis |
| | Phlyctenule |
| | Sarcoid nodule |
| | Conjunctival leproma (leprosy) |
| | Pyogenic granuloma |
| | Keloid |

**3.13** | Limbal granuloma secondary to retained limbal suture.

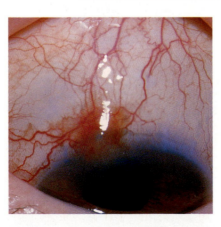

**3.14** | Pyogenic granuloma following pterygium surgery.

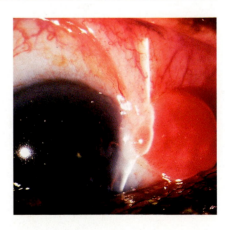

# 4 | THE CORNEAL EPITHELIUM

## Mark L. McDermott

The primary function of the human cornea is image formation, and the corneal epithelium is the most important determinant in achieving this goal. The corneal epithelium is a continuously renewable, transparent surface. Along with the tear matrix components, it forms a superb optical surface that rivals that of any manmade lens. Like all epithelia, it presents a formidable barrier to the external environment. Its intercellular junctions allow the development of microenvironments within its confines and prevent invasion by pathogens. It is a durable, renewable surface well adapted for resisting the daily insults of the external environment.

## EMBRYOLOGY

The human corneal epithelium is derived from ectoderm. In utero, its structure at the 8-week stage (lids fused) consists of two cell layers: a superficial layer, consisting of flat attenuated cells, and an underlying cuboidal basal layer.[1] At 26 weeks of gestation the lids open and the epithelium now consists of four to five cell layers. The basal cells are cuboidal to columnar, with basal nuclei, and rest on a basement membrane. Above this layer are interdigitating wing cells and, most superficially, a layer of flattened epithelial cells.[2] The fetal basement membrane differs substantially from that of a neonate, being less electron-dense and less homogeneous.[3] Early in gestation hemidesmosomes and anchoring fibrils are absent.[1] By 19 weeks of gestation, hemidesmosomes, anchoring fibrils, and a rudimentary Bowman's layer are present.[1] With further development in utero, the number of hemidesmosomes increases, anchoring fibril penetration deepens, and Bowman's layer thickens.[1]

## ADULT ANATOMY

The central epithelium consists of a layer, five to six cells thick, of nonkeratinized stratified epithelium (Fig. 4.1). It is the most regular arrangement of stratified epithelium in the human body. The cells are tightly and orderly arranged without intercellular spaces. This cell layer is modified at its apex to interact with the tear matrix and at its base to adhere to the basal lam-

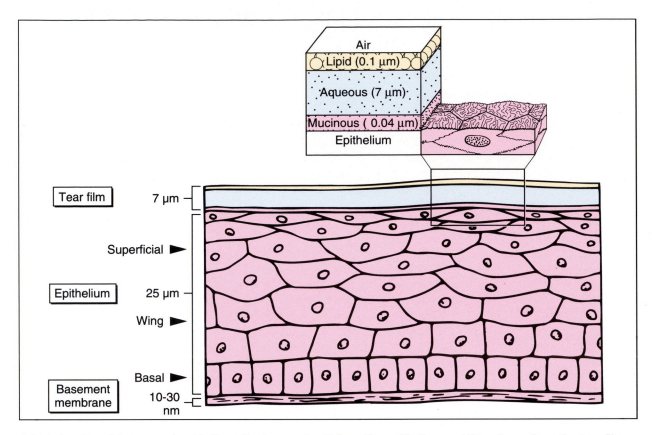

**4.1** | A drawing of the corneal epithelium. Five layers of cells form the epithelium and three layers form the tear film.

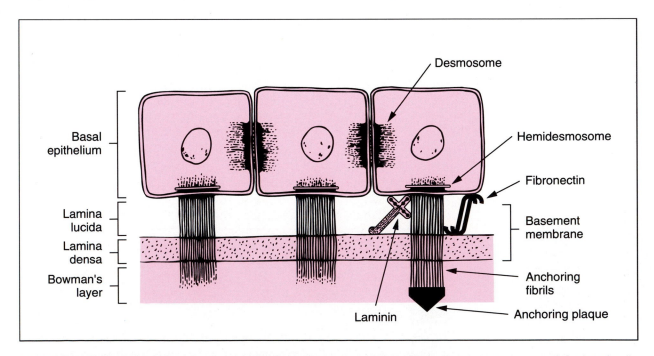

**4.2** | Schematic drawing of human corneal epithelial basement membrane illustrating the attachment of the basal cells of the cornea to Bowman's membrane.

ina. The most superficial layer of the epithelium consists of one to two layers of flattened cells, whose surface is thrown into folds called microplicae. Coating these microplicae is a layer of glycocalyx that interacts with the mucous layer of the tear matrix. The result of this interaction is a smooth, stable optical surface that resists bacterial adherence. Adjacent superficial epithelial cells are joined by zonula occludens, creating a barrier that is relatively impermeable to water. In microelectrode experiments, 60% of total transcorneal resistance to ion flow is provided by the outer membranes and intercellular junctions of the corneal epithelium.[4] The cytosol of these cells is relatively devoid of common organelles but does retain the nucleus. Examination of the superficial epithelial layer in vivo by widefield specular microscopy shows the layer to consist of polygonal cells, usually six-sided, with a variation in shape and size.[5]

Below the surface layer is a layer of polyhedral or wing cells two to three cells thick. There are prominent desmosomal attachments between neighboring wing cells. The cytoplasm contains some organelles as well as cytosolic filaments. A common constituent of these filaments is actin. In proliferating human corneal epithelium, actin has been found to constitute 4%–6% of the total cellular protein.[6] The wing cells are the transitional cell between the basal cylindrical cell and the flattened superficial cells.

The deepest layer of the epithelium, called the basal layer, consists of a single layer of cylindrical cells 18 μm in height, whose cytosol, like that of the wing cells, contains a high concentration of filaments. The basal cells secrete a basal lamina that has two distinct layers when viewed by electron microscopy. A lighter area, the lamina lucida, abuts the basal cell layer, followed by a deeper, more electron-dense layer, the lamina densa. The basal portion of the basal cells is modified to create hemidesmosomes which, along with anchoring fibrils, form the attachment or adhesion complex. Hemidesmosomes have been shown to bind avidly bullous pemphigoid autoantibody. This enables researchers to follow the generation of hemidesmosomes by immunohistochemical methods in research involving wound healing.[7] Anchoring fibrils consist predominantly of type VII collagen dimers and serve to connect the basement membrane to Bowman's layer.

The basement membrane of the corneal epithelium serves several functions. It acts as a structural support for the epithelium, aids in compartmentalization of cells, and functions as a solid-phase modulator of cell attachment, proliferation, and differentiation. The corneal epithelial basement membrane self-assembles from glycoprotein and proteoglycan protomers to create macromolecular arrays. Its two greatest constituents by mass are type IV collagen and laminin.[8]

Type IV collagen, unlike all other collagens, retains terminal carboxyl and amino groups. These groups interact electrostatically to create stable regular arrays. Laminin is an asymmetrical, 850 kilodalton, four-armed glycoprotein constructed of three distinct polypeptide chains. It is a potent modulator of cell spreading, growth, and differentiation. Laminin may self-assemble into polymeric arrays to create a gel-like matrix. Laminin appears to be concentrated in the lamina lucida, whereas type IV collagen is found in larger amounts in the lamina densa. Also present in the lamina lucida are deposits of fibronectin,[9] an extracellular protein that acts as a temporary scaffold for migratory cells and is chemotactic for epithelial cells. The basement membrane of the corneal epithelium changes during life, becoming thicker with age.[3]

The corneal epithelium has a well-developed adhesion complex (Fig. 4.2). It consists of the hemidesmosomes of the basal epithelial cells, the basement membrane, and anchoring fibrils. Together these three components form a remarkably firm attachment for the epithelium. There appears to be a heterogeneity in this complex, however. Hemidesmosomes per basal cell are more numerous in the central cornea than in the peripheral cornea,[10] suggesting that the central epithelium is reinforced to withstand better the shearing force of the eyelids and external trauma.

## PHYSIOLOGY

The epithelium plays several roles in the process of image formation. Its apical cell borders interact with the tear matrix to create an optically smooth surface. The extreme regularity of its cell layers promotes uniform thickness of the epithelium, resulting in a regular surface. Corneal smoothness is evaluated with a Placido disc (Figs. 4.3, 4.4). Moreover, the tight packing of the individual epithelial cells leaves only minimal intercellular spaces, thereby causing only minor variation in the refractive index between and within these cells. This dense packing, maintained by the many desmosomes between adjacent cells, results in minimal scattering of light by the epithelium, as well as extreme clarity. Processes that lead to an increase in the variation of the refractive index within the epithelium cause increased light scattering and reduced clarity.[11] Corneal edema is a common cause of reduced epithelial clarity and can be the result of either intraepithelial cell edema or intercellular edema. Variation in refractive index is the cause of the reduced clarity. A common cause of intraepithelial cell edema is epithelial hypoxia resulting from contact lens overwear. Intercellular edema may result when high intraocular pressure, such as in acute angle-closure glaucoma, forces aqueous humor across the endothelial barrier and stroma into the corneal epithelium, where it collects in the intercellular spaces.

In both health and disease the corneal epithelium has a strong tendency to smooth over underlying irregularities. An everyday example is the epithelial facet. This plug of epithelium fills in focal defects in Bowman's layers, bringing them up to surface grade much the way an asphalt patch does on a roadway. This smoothing tendency is also active to some degree in areas undergoing excimer photoablation. In this case, the epithelium's tendency

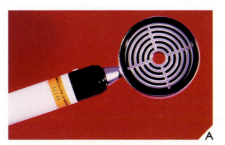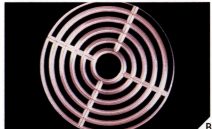

**4.3** | *A:* Placido disc to evaluate spherical nature of corneal surface. *B:* Enlarged view.

**4.4** | Placido disc mires showing irregular astigmatism.

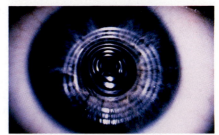

to bring the underlying areas back up to grade may mitigate the refractive effect of the ablation.[12]

The physiology of epithelial cell turnover is an area of active research (Fig. 4.5). It is widely accepted that the basal corneal epithelial cells undergo mitosis, but there is evidence to suggest a difference in the mitotic potential of central, peripheral, and juxtalimbal basal epithelial cells. In cell culture experiments comparing the mitotic rate of human limbal, peripheral, and central corneal epithelium, limbal epithelium had the highest mitotic rate. Peripheral corneal epithelium was intermediate, and the central epithelium had the lowest mitotic rate.[13,14]

These data provide supporting evidence for the X, Y, Z hypothesis (Fig. 4.6) of centripetal corneal epithelial movement proposed by Thoft and Friend.[15] In this theory, at steady state the rate of desquamation of apical cells (Z) equals the sum of cells dividing (X) and superficial and wing cells migrating from the periphery centripetally (Y). Lemp and Mathers have suggested that this centripetal movement of epithelial cells is not uniform and is responsive to local areas of both increased and decreased rates of desquamation.[16]

As a corollary to this theory, several authors have discussed the existence of a multipotent stem cell believed to exist in the paralimbal area.[17,18]

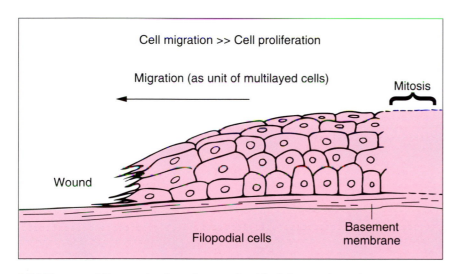

**4.5** | Diagram of the mechanism of corneal epithelial wound repair.

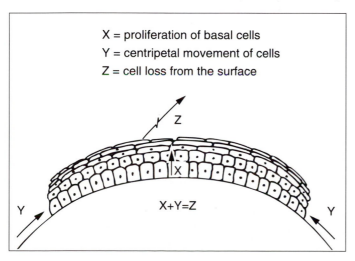

**4.6** | The X,Y,Z hypothesis of corneal epithelial maintenance. Loss of cells from the surface of the cornea (Z) is balanced by basal cell proliferation (X) and centripetal movement of cells from the periphery (Y). (From Thoft RA, Friend J: The X,Y,Z hypothesis of corneal epithelial maintenance. *Invest Ophthalmol Vis Sci 1983;24:1442–1443.*)

This stem cell is thought to be the source of the corneal epithelial cells that arise to replace large reductions in epithelial cell mass.

## BIOCHEMISTRY

The biochemical pathways in corneal epithelium are well described. The primary energy source is glucose, which is metabolized by both anaerobic (glycolysis) and aerobic (tricarboxylic acid cycle) pathways (Fig. 4.7). In aerobic metabolism the source of oxygen is primarily from the atmosphere, with small contributions from dissolved oxygen in the tears and oxygen in the limbal vasculature. Other metabolic pathways in corneal epithelium include an inducible polyol pathway that is unresponsive to the effects of insulin. Other

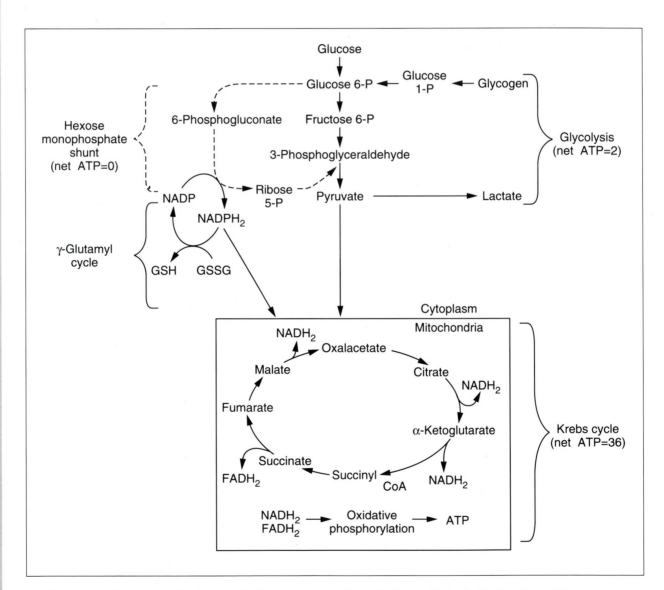

**4.7** | Schematic of corneal epithelial metabolism, cytoplasmic glycolysis, hexose monophosphate shunt, and γ-glutamyl cycle, as well as mitochondrial Krebs cycle.

(From Anderson RE (ed): *Biochemistry of the Eye.* San Francisco: American Academy of Ophthalmology, 1983, 25.)

enzyme systems are present that regulate electrolyte balance in the epithelium. There is an Na,K-ATPase-dependent active transport system for Na⁺. There are also active transport systems for Cl⁻ ions which are regulated by a β-adrenergic receptor/adenylate cyclase complex[19] (Fig. 4.8).

The cornea also contains enzyme systems for detoxification and drug metabolism. Catalase, glutathione peroxidase, and superoxide dismutase have been shown to be present in corneal epithelium.[20,21] These enzyme systems scavenge the oxygen free radical superoxide as well as hydrogen peroxide to provide a protective function. Also present in human corneal epithe-

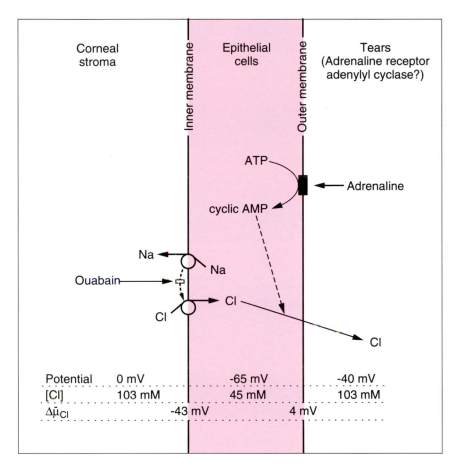

**4.8** | Model for action of epinephrine in the stimulation of epithelial Cl⁻ transport. (From Klyce SD, Wong RKS: Site and mode of adrenaline action on chloride transport across the rabbit corneal epithelium. *J Physiol 1977;266:777.*)

lium are high levels of heme oxygenase and NADPH cytochrome P-450 reductase.[22] The existence of these enzyme systems supports the role of the epithelium in drug metabolism. Moreover, this enzyme system may be important in the production of prostaglandins as part of the inflammatory response.

## INNERVATION

Innervation of the human cornea is complex (Fig. 4.9). There is evidence for both sensory and sympathetic innervation. Moreover, there is growing acceptance of the efferent role of innervation in normal corneal epithelial functioning.[23] Immunohistochemical studies have shown that the nerve supply to the human cornea contains both peptidergic and catecholaminergic components.[24] Electron microscopy of corneal nerves allows them to be divided into large dense-core vesicle fibers and small dense-core fibers.[24] The large dense-core vesicle fibers may be sensory, whereas the small dense-core fibers appear to be catecholaminergic.

## IMMUNOLOGY

Class I HLA antigens are present on the membranes of all corneal epithelial cells, with increased density of expression on cells closer to the limbus.[25,26] The presence of Class II (DR) antigens on central corneal epithelial cells is controversial. However, these antigens are present on the Langerhans cells near the corneal limbus.[27] As in other parts of the body, the Langerhans cells in the corneal epithelium may play an important role as inflammatory mediators.[27]

## DIAGNOSTIC TESTS

Diagnostic tests for the corneal epithelium are centered on tests for optical smoothness and tests for intactness of the cell layer. Tests for optical smoothness are designed to assess the ability of the corneal surface to act as a mirror. If the surface is irregular the quality of the mirror is low, as will be the quality of the cornea as a refractive surface. Tests for epithelial smoothness include quality of the corneal light reflex and quality of the reflected mires from the ophthalmometer or Placido disc (see Figs. 4.3, 4.4). Distortion of these reflections indicates an irregular surface that may in part be responsible for a patient's decreased vision. There are a variety of tests for intactness of the

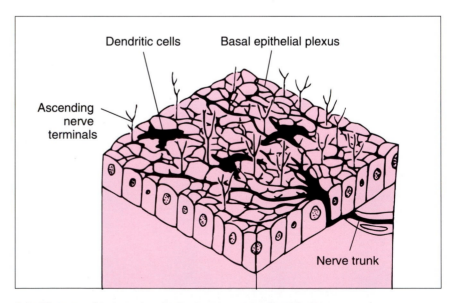

**4.9** | Diagram of innervation in the human corneal epithelium.

epithelial cell layer. Some of these rely on the intactness of the tight junctions between cells. Both electrical conductance studies and fluorophotometry[28] allow characterization of the "tightness" of the intercellular junctions. Both of these techniques, however, are research oriented and are not widely used in clinical practice. On a larger scale, the presence or absence of epithelial cell layers can be seen with specular microscopy. The advantage of this technique is that it allows repeated, atraumatic in vivo observation of the epithelium in a variety of disorders.[5,29]

Instillation of the dyes fluorescein (Fig. 4.10) or rose bengal (Figs. 4.11 and 4.12) provides gross evidence of epithelial discontinuity. Fluorescein dye adheres to areas at which epithelial cells have desquamated; it does not adhere to dying cells. Rose bengal, on the other hand, stains dead and dying epithelial cells as well as areas of the cornea denuded of epithelium.

When areas of epithelial discontinuity are diagnosed, several additional tests can assist in determining the etiology. These include corneal sensation determination, Schirmer testing, adnexal and eyelid exam, tear break-up time, conjunctival impression cytology, microbiologic cultures, and quantitation of blink frequency.

An understanding of epithelial physiology is essential to evaluation and treatment of epithelial defects. In examining patients with epithelial defects it is important to hypothesize a mechanism for the defect. From the patient's history, medical illnesses, and exam one can usually determine if the defect is secondary to increased rate of desquamation of epithelial cells, poor migration of epithelial cells, or a possible stem cell defect.

An extreme example of a clinical situation characterized by an increased rate of desquamation is the traumatic corneal epithelial abrasion. In this injury, full-thickness corneal epithelium is lost but the underlying basement membrane and anchoring fibrils are intact. The initial event, like in any wound, is an exudation of plasma proteins, including fibrinogen and fibronectin, which coat the denuded area. The wing cells in the epithelium surrounding the defect lyse their desmosomes, flatten, and assume amoebic

## CLINICAL ASPECTS

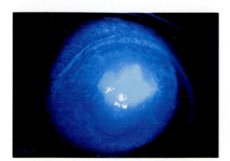

**4.10** | Fluorescein staining of an epithelial defect.

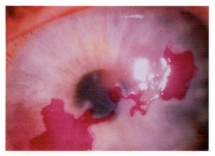

**4.11** | Rose bengal in patient with *Herpes simplex* virus epithelial dendritic ulcer.

characteristics and begin to migrate into the fibronectin-rich defect. In cell culture experiments these migrating cells have been shown to send out filapodia rich in actin fibers and vinculin.[6] It appears that actin fibers are essential for this migration process.[30] In addition, with the exposure of the lamina lucida, laminin and fibronectin in the basement membrane are able to assist in the mobilization and adhesion of these migrating epithelial cells to cover the defect as a single cell layer.[31] Closure of small defects by a single layer of epithelium occurs rapidly, usually within 24 to 48 hours. With a slower-onset proliferative response the epithelium regains its usual thickness. The rapidity of the proliferative response is, however, dependent on the location of the defect. Defects that are closest to the limbus have the potential for greater proliferative response than defects present centrally.[13] Using Thoft and Friend's hypothesis[15] to characterize an abrasion, a large increase in Z (cell loss from the surface) is initially counterbalanced by an increased centripetal movement of cells (Y) and a later increase in proliferation of basal cells (X). This centripetal movement follows a predictable pattern. At the wound periphery, three to six distinct areas of cells form convex migrating fronts. These fronts move centrally, and as the sides of adjacent fronts contact each other a variety of polygonal figures are formed.[32] With complete closure of the defect a contact line shaped like a "Y" or like two "Ys" placed end to end is formed[32] (Figs. 4.13–4.15).

The rapid closure of traumatic epithelial defects is in part due to the relatively intact underlying basement membrane. Damage to the underlying

**4.12** | Rose bengal in superior limbic keratoconjunctivitis.

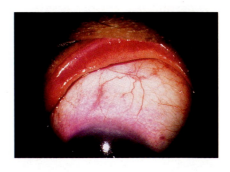

**4.13** | Corneal epithelial healing following corneal abrasion (From Dua HS, Forrester JV: Clinical patterns of corneal epithelial wound healing. *Am J Ophthalmol 1987;104:481–489.*)

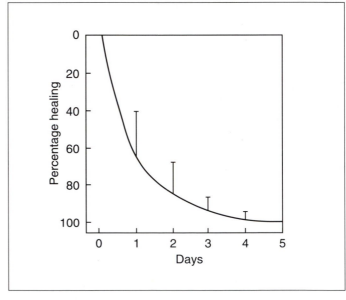

basement membrane caused by trauma, inflammation, infection, or excimer laser[12] may result in less efficient epithelial migration, leading to slower closure of the defect.[31] Once closed, the area may spontaneously erode owing to poor restoration of the adhesion complex. One common systemic disease associated with defects in epithelial adhesion complexes is diabetes mellitus, in which there is decreased penetration of the anchoring fibrils into the corneal stroma.[33] This explains the tendency of the diabetic corneal epithelium to desquamate as a large sheet with the thickened basement membrane adherent to the epithelium, thus leaving bare stroma exposed.[34]

Alterations in the proliferative response of the basal cells may also affect epithelial healing and physiology. The use of systemic chemotherapeutic agents can reduce the proliferative response of the corneal epithelium, resulting in epithelial defects. These agents include cytosine arabinoside, 5-fluorouracil, and chlorambucil.[35] Epithelial defects have been recognized as complications of local 5-fluorouracil injections to maintain patent fistulas after trabeculectomy.[36] It is likely that the local concentration of 5-fluo-

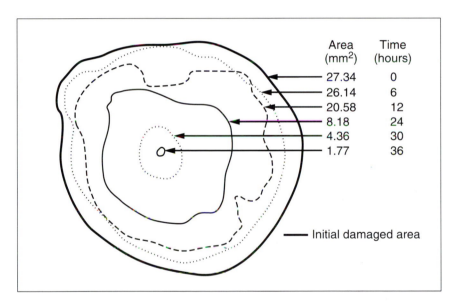

| Area (mm²) | Time (hours) |
|---|---|
| 27.34 | 0 |
| 26.14 | 6 |
| 20.58 | 12 |
| 8.18 | 24 |
| 4.36 | 30 |
| 1.77 | 36 |

—— Initial damaged area

**4.14** | Measurement of corneal re-epithelialization after mechanical epithelial debridement (rabbit).

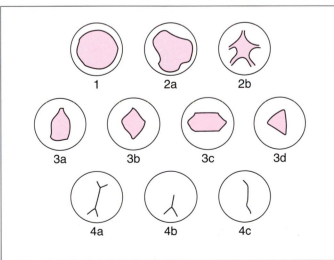

**4.15** | Diagrammatic representation of the sequence of patterns that develop during the resurfacing of corneal epithelial defects: (1) large cornea abrasion, (2) formation of convex leading fronts, (3) geometric shapes, (4) contact line (shaded area, epithelial defect; clear area, surface covered by epithelium). (From Dua HS, Forrester JV: Clinical patterns of corneal epithelial wound healing. *Am J Ophthalmol 1987;104:481–489.*)

rouracil is high enough to reduce basal cell proliferation, leading to disorganization of epithelial physiology and thus to punctate keratitis and frank epithelial defects. In cell culture studies of corneal epithelium, certain growth factors appear to stimulate epithelial mitosis. These growth factors include epidermal growth factors, fibroblast growth factor, and mesodermal growth factor.[37] The most widely investigated is epidermal growth factor, but data on clinical efficacy are incomplete.[37,38] This is in part due to differences between the activity of epithelial cells in culture and in intact corneal epithelium.

Many other drugs may affect the epithelium via preservatives present in the medication's vehicle. The preservatives benzalkonium chloride and chlorhexidine have been shown to significantly increase human corneal epithelial permeability to fluorescein.[39] There is a synergistic effect on corneal epithelial permeability when these two preservatives are combined with the local anesthetics tetracaine or oxybruprocaine.[39]

In addition to drugs, contact lens use has also been shown to alter corneal permeability. Both daily wear soft and rigid gas-permeable lenses reduce human corneal epithelial permeability to fluorescein.[40] It is hypothesized that contact lens wear causes a reduction in epithelial desquamation, resulting in an increase in epithelial cells. The increased number of epithelial cells is then responsible for the reduction in permeability. If epithelial cells are being shed at a slower rate, one would expect the cells on average to be larger. In fact, this has been observed in patients using extended-wear lenses. Lemp and Gold[41] performed widefield specular microscopy on 12 patients wearing extended-wear soft contact lenses. They observed a shift of the surface cells towards larger cells, suggesting that a reduced rate of desquamation probably occurs.[41]

# 5

# THE MOLECULAR STRUCTURE OF THE CORNEAL STROMA IN HEALTH AND DISEASE

## Charles Cintron

The cornea, basically composed of three discrete tissue layers (epithelium, stroma, and endothelium), contributes to the outer coat of the eyeball, and is continuous with the sclera and conjunctiva. In addition to serving as a mechanical barrier, the cornea is the major refractive organ of the optic system. These optic and mechanical properties are a direct consequence of the stromal macromolecular components and their arrangement in the tissue.

Several ocular tissues are required by the stroma to maintain its optic and structural properties. By regulating fluid transport through the cornea, the endothelium maintains stromal deturgescence and carries nutrients and waste products to and from the stroma. An extensive innervation, working in conjunction with the tears and the eyelid, protects the cornea from damage and infection at the corneal epithelial surface. The tear layer and epithelium, in turn, serve as an optically clear and smooth surface to ensure distortion-free refraction, and act as a barrier to help maintain proper hydration of the stroma. As in other connective tissues, the major portion of the stroma is composed of extracellular matrix macromolecules which are responsible for the strength and transparency of this tissue. Alteration in one or more of these macromolecules often results in the loss of some stromal function with accompanying clinical symptoms. Therefore, differences in stromal macromolecules from normal and diseased corneas provide us with a greater understanding of their functions in these tissues.

## STROMAL COMPONENTS

The stroma can be divided into four extracellular matrix components: the basal lamina of the epithelium, Bowman's layer (membrane), lamellar stroma, and Descemet's membrane, each of which is morphologically and biochemically distinct from the others (Fig. 5.1).

The basal lamina of the corneal epithelium consists of a lamina lucida and a lamina densa. The lamina lucida contains

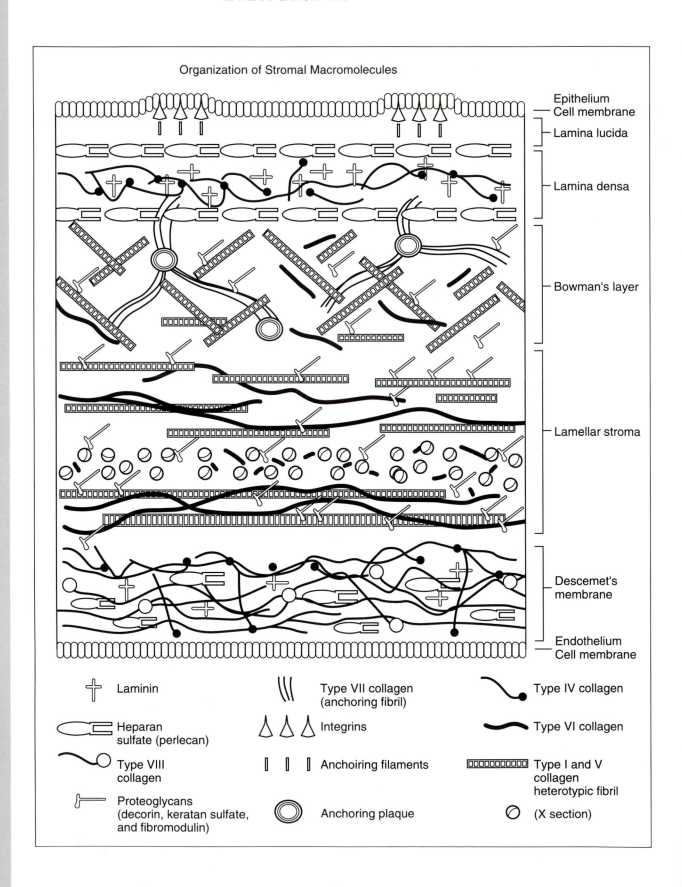

Organization of Stromal Macromolecules

Epithelium
Cell membrane

Lamina lucida

Lamina densa

Bowman's layer

Lamellar stroma

Descemet's
membrane

Endothelium
Cell membrane

Laminin

Heparan
sulfate (perlecan)

Type VIII
collagen

Proteoglycans
(decorin, keratan sulfate,
and fibromodulin)

Type VII collagen
(anchoring fibril)

Integrins

Anchoiring filaments

Anchoring plaque

Type IV collagen

Type VI collagen

Type I and V
collagen
heterotypic fibril

(X section)

fine filaments that are believed to bridge the gap between integrin components within the hemidesmosome and the lamina densa.[1]

Cell substrate adhesion occurs when the extracellular matrix molecules are bound by cell surface receptors, as it happens with a family of membrane glycoproteins called integrins (Fig. 5.2). The integrins consist of noncovalently associated α and β polypeptide subunits. Of the 20 α–β combinations known, adult rabbit and chicken corneal epithelial cells express α6β4 in the basal cell surfaces in contact with basement membrane.[2-4] These integrins may be linked to the actin-containing cytoskeleton via α actinin and talin. In addition, integrins may transduce biochemical signals from the extracellular matrix (ECM) to the cell interior. The basal cell surface of corneal epithelium is reinforced by hemidesmosomes. These structures contain an electron-dense cytoplasmic plaque to which intermediate filaments associate. In addition to bullous pemphigoid antigens and proteins having some homology to desmoplakins, the hemidesmosome is associated with the specific integrin heterodimer α6β4. Although the ligand for this integrin has not been determined, kalinin[5,6] is a candidate. Kalinin, a possible component of the anchoring filaments in the lamina lucida, links the hemidesmosome complex to the lamina densa. The lamina densa is composed of heparan sulfate proteoglycan (HSPG), laminin, and perhaps type IV collagen (see Fig. 5.1). Cyto- and immunocytochemical evidence indicates that HSPG may have a specific orientation with respect to the basal lamina cell–matrix interfaces.[7,8] Embedded in and extending from the lower surface of this lamina densa are the anchoring fibrils composed of type VII collagen. All these macromolecules are believed to be synthesized by the corneal epithelium and they function to adhere the epithelium to the stroma.

Bowman's layer, composed mainly of randomly organized collagen fibrils, is an acellular region of the stroma immediately under the basal lamina of the epithelium (see Fig. 5.1). Anchoring fibrils extend from the basal lamina into this layer and insert into patches of electron-dense structures termed "anchoring plaques," which contain the globular domain of type VII collagen and some basal lamina components such as laminin. The collagen fibrils are uniform in thickness and measure about two thirds that of the fibrils in stromal lamellae. Immunoelectron microscopic analyses of Bowman's layer in chicken indicate the presence of types I, V, and VI collagen (personal communication, John Fitch, Tufts University, Boston, MA). Fibrils are composed of types I and V collagen, whereas the interfibrillar spaces are probably filled

**5.1** I (OPPOSITE PAGE) In this representation of the major macromolecules in the extracellular matrix of the cornea, the integrins, associated with hemidesmosomes of the basal surface of the epithelium, interact with anchoring filaments that bridge the space between the cell and the lamina densa. The lamina densa is composed of several macromolecules, including heparan sulfate, laminin, and perhaps type IV collagen. Extending from the lamina densa into Bowman's layer, are the anchoring fibrils, composed of type VII collagen. Although the fibrillar collagens in this layer are randomly arranged, a fairly sharp transition to a lamellar arrangement is seen in the deeper portions of the stroma. The fibrils are parallel to each other within bundles (lamellae). Intertwining the fibrils are filaments of type VI collagen. Proteoglycans associate with both fibrillar and filamentous collagens. In humans, the collagen fibrils and lamellae of the deeper portions of the stroma are thicker and more orthogonal. Descemet's membrane, a product of the underlying endothelium, is a modified basement membrane composed of type IV, type VIII, and possibly type III collagen. As in other basal laminae, this membrane also contains heparan sulfate and laminin.

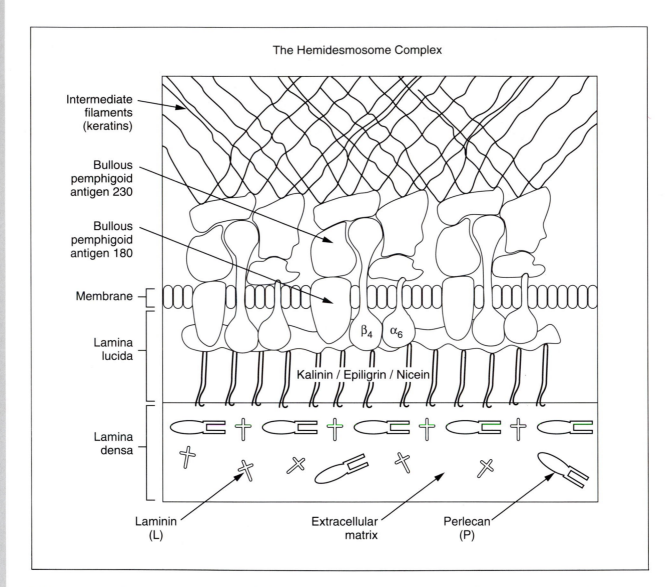

## The Hemidesmosome Complex

Intermediate filaments (keratins)

Bullous pemphigoid antigen 230

Bullous pemphigoid antigen 180

Membrane

Lamina lucida

$\beta_4$  $\alpha_6$

Kalinin / Epiligrin / Nicein

Lamina densa

Laminin (L)

Extracellular matrix

Perlecan (P)

**5.2** | Integrins and other proteins, such as the bullous pemphigoid antigens, are embedded in the cell membrane, associate with hemidesmosome components, and communicate with both intracellular and extracellular matrix components. The anchoring filaments in the lamina lucida contain a protein known as kalinin, epiligrin, or nicein. Kalinin is embedded in the lamina densa to unknown components. $\beta_4\alpha_6$ = integrins. BPA = bullous pemphigoid antigen. Kalinin/Epiligrin/Nicein = anchoring filaments. Membrane = basal membrane of epithelium.

with type VI collagen filaments and proteoglycans such as keratan sulfate (personal communication, James Funderburgh, Kansas State University, Manhattan, KS). At the posterior surface of Bowman's layer the collagen fibrils appear to organize into bundles of fibrils that are continuous with the anterior lamellar stroma.

The "lamellar stroma" forms the bulk of the tissue and can be morphologically and physiologically divided into an anterior and a posterior lamellar stroma (see Fig. 5.1). Bundles of parallel collagen fibrils in the anterior lamellar stroma appear as short narrow sheets (lamellae) with extensive interweaving, whereas the lamellae in the posterior stroma are long, wide, and thick (about 2 μm) structures with minimal interweaving among layers. Stromal cells (keratocytes) are dispersed between the lamellae and occupy 3%–5% of the stromal volume. Collagen fibrils in both regions of the stroma are fine, uniform structures composed of types I and V collagen. The diameter of the fibrils is increased slightly in the posterior stroma. As in Bowman's layer, the interstices of the fibrils are filled with type VI collagen and proteoglycans, keratan sulfate, decorin, and fibromodulin.

Descemet's membrane is a specialized basement membrane sandwiched between the posterior stroma and the endothelium from which it is derived. The deeper stromal lamellae merge with Descemet's membrane. This membrane is composed of very regularly arranged stratified layers of filamentous material, forming a lattice with nodes at intersecting filaments. The nodes constitute the corners of equilateral triangles along a plane tangential to the surface and in register to successive layers to form a linear pattern in meridional sections. Types IV, III, and VIII collagen and HSPG have been identified in Descemet's membrane, but their relationship to the filamentous lattice structure is not known.[9,10] Monoclonal antibodies that label various domains of the hexagonal lattice of Descemet's membrane also recognize a fragment of a protein postulated to be derived from type VIII collagen.[11]

## THE COLLAGENOUS MATRIX

Ten different collagen types have been characterized in stroma from fetal, adult, and diseased corneas of various animal species (Fig. 5.3). At least two distinct classes of collagens are now recognized: those that are present in the fibrillar form and those that are nonfibrillar or filamentous.

In corneal stroma the collagen fibrils contain two or more distinct types of collagen and therefore are heterotypic.[12] It has been demonstrated in the chick cornea that collagen types I and V interact as heterotypic fibrils and that this interaction is at least partially responsible for regulation of collagen fibril diameter.[13] The corneal stroma contains a large amount of type V collagen compared with other type I-containing connective tissues. Changes in the proportion of types I/V collagen have been observed in scar tissue and may be related to the altered physical properties of the scar.[14] It has also been demonstrated that in the primary stroma of the chick heterotypic types I/II-containing fibrils are present,[12] whereas in the human fetal cornea types I/III collagen fibrils are present.[15] These interactions of different collagen types may provide a mechanism whereby fibril architecture can be regulated.

A variety of nonfibrillar collagens including types IV, VII, and VI have been studied in the cornea. Type IV collagen present in basal laminae has important structural properties as well as the ability to mediate specific cell–matrix interactions. Corneal epithelial cell interactions with either the intact basal lamina or matrix components produce changes in cell shape and organization as well as in rates of synthesis.[16] Specific receptors have been shown to mediate these interactions.[17] Type VII collagen of the anchoring fibrils has been studied in the cornea during development and wound repair.[18,19] Type VI collagen is a filamentous collagen which forms networks in most soft connective tissues. Appearing in the electron microscope as beaded filaments with a characteristic periodicity of 100 nm, type VI collagen has been detected in many organs and is very abundant in the corneal stroma located between collagen fibrils.[20-22] Although its function is unknown, recent studies have suggested that it plays a role in restricting movement of collagen fibrils relative to each other. The alteration in the proportions of type VI to other collagens in corneal scar tissue and its interactions with proteoglycans are indicative of a function in maintaining the interfibrillar structure important for transparency.[21] Type VIII collagen, a major component of Descemet's membrane, has been localized and its protein and genomic structure have been partially characterized.[23]

**5.3** | At least ten genetically distinct collagens have been described in the corneas from different animal species, ages, and pathology. Type I, II, III, and V collagens are present as fibrils in tissues. Types IV, VI, VII, and VIII form filamentous structures. Types IX and XII are fibril-associated collagens. The sizes of the collagens are not to scale, and their polypeptide constituents and association into macromolecular structures are not completely known. Type II collagen is found only in embryonic chick collagen associated with the primary stroma. Type III collagen is found in Descemet's membrane and in scar tissue. Types I and V form the heterotypic fibrils of the lamellar stroma. Type VII has been identified with the anchoring fibrils, and type VIII collagen is present only in Descemet's membrane. Type IX collagen, associated with type II fibrils in the primary stroma, and type XII collagen, associated with type I/V fibrils, are part of a family of fibril-associated collagens with interrupted triple helices. Both type IX and XII are covalently-associated with a chondroitin sulfate chain.

| Heterogeneity of Collagens in the Cornea | | | |
| --- | --- | --- | --- |
| Type | Polypeptides | Monomer | Polymer |
| I | $[\alpha 1(I)]_2\alpha 2(I)$ | | |
| II | $[\alpha 1(II)]_3$ | | |
| III | $[\alpha 1(III)]_3$ | | |
| IV | $[\alpha 1(IV)]_2\alpha 2(IV)$ | | |
| V | $[\alpha 1(V)]_2\alpha 2(V)$ | | |
| VI | $\alpha 1(VI)\alpha 2(VI)\alpha 3(VI)$ | | |
| VII | $\alpha 1(VII)_3$? | | |
| VIII | $[\alpha 1(VIII)]_2\alpha 2(VIII)$? | | |
| IX | $\alpha 1(IX)\alpha 2(IX)\alpha 3(IX)$ | | |
| XII | $\alpha 1(XII)_3$ | | |

Collagen fibrils form three-dimensional structures in the extracellular matrices of tissues and organs. Because similar fibrillar types vary in their organization from one tissue to another, these patterns may be dependent on molecular interactions with other molecules between the fibrillar collagens. Matrix components that bind to fibril surfaces are good candidates for such pattern-generating interactions. Among these are proteins belonging to the class of FACIT collagens (Fibril-Associated Collagens with Interrupted Triple helices) such as collagens IX, XII, and XIV. Type IX collagen is a fibril-associated collagen containing a glycosaminoglycan side chain. It is found in cartilage and vitreous, where it is associated with type II fibrils, and has been found in the chick primary corneal stroma, which also contains collagen type I/II fibrils. The form of this collagen located in the corneal stroma is missing a large terminal domain present in the cartilage form.[24] This collagen is present in a very narrow developmental window and may have an important regulatory function in stromal morphogenesis.[25]

Type XII has recently been cloned and localized in adult mammalian and chick corneas.[26,27] Type XII appears associated with the surface of type I-containing fibrils. Type XII contains three 60 nm fingers and a 75 nm-long collagen tail extending from a central globular region. It has been suggested that the collagen tail binds to the surface of collagen fibrils while the noncollagenous fingers project into the perifibrillar matrix.

Adult, fetal, and diseased stroma contain all or in part four types of proteoglycans (PGs) and hyaluranan (Fig 5.4). Hyaluranan, present in developing

## PROTEOGLYCAN MATRIX

| Heterogeneity of Proteoglycans in the Cornea | | | |
|---|---|---|---|
| Type | Core Protein Mol Wt (kDa) | Glycosamino-glycans | Structure |
| Dermatan sulfate (decorin) | 37 | CS/DS | |
| Keratan sulfate (lumican) | 37&25 | KS | |
| Fibromodulin | 41 | KS | |
| Heparan sulfate | 400 | HS | |
| Hyaluranan | --- | HA | |
| Biglycan | 37 | CS/DS | |
| Core protein | | Glycosaminoglycan | |

**5.4** I The major proteoglycans in the cornea are decorin and lumican. These are part of a family of small proteoglycans that includes biglycan and fibromodulin. All four proteoglycans contain genetically distinct core proteins and are covalently associated with one or more long glycosaminoglycans. In addition to lumican, the cornea has at least two additional keratan sulfate proteoglycans differing in the protein and glycosaminoglycan moieties. Only small quantities of fibromodulin have been identified in the cornea. This proteoglycan is distinguished by its sulfate group on the N-terminal tyrosine. Hyaluranan, not covalently bound to a protein, is present only in fetal and healing corneas. Biglycan, detected by immunohistchemistry, may be a component of the scar tissue. Heparan sulfate, present in the basal lamina of the epithelium and Descemet's membrane, has not been characterized. CS/DS=condroitin sulfate/dermatan sulfate. KS=keratan sulfate. HS=heparan sulfate. HA=hyaluranan.

and healing corneas, is not detected in normal adult stroma.[28] HSPG is present in the lamina densa of the epithelium, in Descemet's membrane, and perhaps associated with corneal nerves. The predominant PGs in the cornea reside in the lamellar stroma and have been characterized as keratan sulfate, decorin, and minor quantities of chondroitin and fibromodulin.[29-34]

Proteoglycans are highly acidic macromolecules that possess at least one sulfated glycosaminoglycan (GAG) chain covalently bound to a peptide core. The two major types of GAGs in corneal stroma are keratan sulfate (KS) and chondroitin/dermatan sulfate (CS/DS) (see Fig. 5.4). Each GAG is a polymer of a disaccharide, which in KS consists of N-acetylglucosamine and galactose and in DS consists of N-acetylgalactosamine and glucuronic or iduronic acid. Sugars in GAGs are sulfated to various degrees, and the GAG chain is covalently linked to a core protein. Corneal PGs are part of a family of small PGs with a core protein similar in molecular weight and amino acid composition and sequence.[35] There are three different KSPGs in bovine cornea, each with a different core protein and unique pattern of glycosylation.[35,36] The KSPGs contain 1-3 chains of keratan sulfate N-linked to the core through a mannose-containing linkage oligosaccharide similar to those in complex glycoproteins.[37] Extensive studies of the KS GAG structure, its peptide linkage region, and the immunologic similarity of corneal KSPG to others in many tissues have indicated that the core protein of cornea KSPG is related to other glycoproteins.[35] Although the core proteins may be derived from different gene products,[38] they all may be closely related to the proteins of decorin, fibromodulin, and biglycan.[34] One of the isoforms of KSPG has been cloned and called lumican.[39]

The chondroitin/dermatan sulfate proteoglycans isolated from chick cornea have been cloned and identified as decorin.[40] This PG contains one chondroitin/dermatan sulfate side chain and one to three N-linked oligosaccharides.[41] The high degree of homology between bovine bone, human fibroblast, and chick cornea core proteins strongly supports the idea of an evolutionarily conserved single-copy gene for the decorin core protein. Comparative analyses of proteoglycans from rabbit, bovine, cat, and human indicate marked similarities among species.[33]

## ROLE OF PGS IN CORNEAL TRANSPARENCY AND HYDRATION

The functions of PGs within the corneal stroma are related to their hydrophilic properties, their location between collagen fibrils, and their interactions with other macromolecules. These macromolecules are important to the generation and maintenance of a precise pattern of hydration in normal cornea. When this pattern is disturbed by endothelial damage or contact lens hypoxia, corneal transparency is compromised. Because the space between collagen fibrils is occupied by PGs, these polyanions may play an important role in maintaining small, uniform spaces between stromal collagen fibrils, necessary for transparency. The transparency and rigidity of the corneal stroma depend on PG types, their molecular properties, distribution, organization, and interactions with other macromolecules.

The major PGs in fetal rabbit cornea are CS/DSPGs, which have a higher charge density than the KSPG in this tissue.[42] The charge density and relative quantity of these PGs are the reverse of those in the adult. Scar tissue has smaller PGs than normal cornea, except for a population of CS/DSPGs markedly larger than normal.[43,44] Although there is no direct evidence, the appearance of the large CS/DSPGs during early stages of wound healing may indicate the presence of biglycan.[45] As in developing cornea, KSPG in scar is low-sulfated, and its proportion to other PGs in scar is markedly lower than in normal adult cornea. The unusually large CS/DSPG molecule and low-sulfated KSPG in these tissues may play a fundamental role in determining collagen fibril spacing.

Proteoglycans are important to corneal hydration. The water content of the cornea and its capacity for water absorption increase across the cornea from the anterior to the posterior stroma.[46] The total-water gradient has been correlated with the distribution of nonfreezable water and stromal PGs. Considering that KSPGs from adult corneas have more swelling ability but less water-retentive power than DSPGs, the differences in distribution of these PGs in cornea may function in the establishment of water gradients across this organ. The distribution of PGs in neonatal cornea is the reverse of that in adult cornea. Chemical analyses of these PGs, however, indicate that their water-sorptive properties may differ from those in the adult.[42] In corneal scars, the high charge density and size of some fractions of CS/DSPGs and the synthesis of chondroitin-6-sulfate correlate with the high water content in this tissue.

The temporal and topographic distribution of PGs in the cornea may be important for development and maintenance of proper hydration in this tissue. Proteoglycans may not be uniformly distributed throughout the corneal stroma. Analyses of bovine corneas have indicated an increasing ratio of KSPGs to CS/DSPGs from the anterior to the posterior stroma.[46] Chondroitin sulfate-like GAGs are deposited first in posterior stroma and subsequently in anterior stroma in developing rabbit cornea.[47] Immunologic evidence indicates that KS is present early in corneal development,[48] and there are at least two immunologically distinct species of KS, based on their distinctive temporal and topographic distribution in fetal cornea. At birth the PGs are distributed throughout the stroma, with most of the KSPG in anterior regions and CS/DSPG concentrated in posterior stroma. Although early studies failed to show KSPG in rabbit corneal scar tissue, a low-sulfated KSPG is indeed synthesized during the early stages of scar formation.[49] In addition, there are distinct differences between the quantity and quality of GAGs synthesized in the anterior and posterior regions of the young scars.[28,50]

The mechanism by which these PGs are differentially distributed in cornea is unknown. The hypothetical role of oxygen in GAG synthesis[51] and the nonuniform distribution of oxygen in cornea suggest an explanation for PG distribution in this organ. Moderate restrictions on the atmospheric source of oxygen result in activation of the Pasteur effect, with increased levels of lactate in the stroma. It is primarily the osmotic effect of increased lactate that causes corneal edema due to contact lens wear. Extended or recurrent periods of low oxygen concentrations, as in contact lens wear, may have longer-lasting and potentially more serious effects, such as increased endothelial cell polymegathism[52] and possible changes in PG synthesis in the stroma as well.[53]

Severe pathologic conditions that affect the corneal stroma result in edema and reduction of corneal transparency. Edema is often due to damage or abnormal development of endothelium. Although the endothelial junctional complexes, dependent on calcium for their integrity, do not constitute a barrier against the penetration of small molecules from the anterior chamber to the stroma, these structures maintain a small intercellular space and limit the flow of water. In the normal endothelium, the leak rate equals the metabolic pump rate so that the endothelium maintains a constant stromal water content. This biochemical pump mechanism, which normally keeps the stroma in a relatively dehydrated state, counteracts the osmotic properties of the hydrophilic stromal PGs. The final state of the cornea depends on the severity of the pathology and the healing rate. In rabbit cornea, transient stromal edema due to surgical damage of the endothelium is accompanied by changes in corneal GAGs. These changes are characterized by the loss of KSPG and CS/DSPG, approaching 50% of the total GAG before regeneration of the endothelium and return of the PGs to their normal level.[54] Perfusion of rabbit cornea with calcium-free medium damages junctions between endothelial cells, swells the tissue and causes ultrastructural changes consistent with the loss of PGs.[55,56] Marked loss of PGs is paralleled by alterations in the collagen fibrils, pointing to the importance of PGs in maintaining the structure of the stroma necessary for corneal transparency and rigidity.[55] Thus, the ultrastructural association and hydrophilic properties of corneal PGs are factors in the stromal hydration as well as in the regular arrangement of collagen fibrils. The distribution and types of corneal PGs lost and regenerated during endothelial wound healing are indicative of interactions between PGs and collagen matrix as well as the rapid turnover of PGs in vivo.

## MOLECULAR INTERACTIONS BETWEEN PGS AND COLLAGEN

The interactions between PGs and other macromolecules in the extracellular space are generally assumed to contribute to the functional properties of the tissues. PGs interact with many molecules through ionic interactions.[57] Although size is an important factor, the strength of GAG interactions with other extracellular matrix (ECM) proteins is related to GAG charge density and usually lacks specificity. Core protein has also been shown to bind to collagen and other ECM components.[58,59] The core protein of decorin binds to collagen,[60,61] and inhibits collagen fibrillogenesis.[62,63] Decorin, as its name implies, "decorates" the outer surface of collagen fibrils in a periodic fashion. The core protein is mostly composed of a repeat of a 24 amino acid unit characterized by an arrangement of conserved leucine residues.[40,64,65]

These repeats have been implicated as a basic protein-binding domain. Decorin exhibits growth regulatory effects, in part because of its ability to bind transforming growth factor-$\beta$.[66] Decorin binds to collagen at specific sites separated by the 67-nm repeat distance of the fibrils.[57] CS/DSPGs in tendon and sclera have been localized to the "d" bands of collagen fibrils with a periodicity of 62 nm.[67,68]

In cornea, the situation is more complicated because of the presence of at least two types of PGs, lumican and decorin. Cytochemical evidence indicates that KSPG interacts with corneal collagen fibrils.[69] In these studies, two groups of PGs located orthogonally to the corneal collagen fibrils at either the periodic collagen banding pattern "a" or "c" or bands "d" or "e" were shown to be KSPGs or DSPGs, respectively, by enzyme sensitivity. Low-angle x-ray diffraction techniques have confirmed the location of PGs on the collagen fibril.[70] The precise arrangement of the corneal PGs presumably reflects specific intermolecular interactions with collagen.

Type VI collagen is located abundantly between collagen fibrils as fine, filamentous structures containing beads with a periodicity of 100 nm in corneal stroma and other tissues.[20,22,71] These periodic beads represent the globular domains of this filamentous collagen (see *The Collagen Matrix* above). The interaction between PGs and type VI collagen is suggested cytochemically and immunocytochemically,[72–75] and biochemically.[76] Because the PGs are associated immunocytochemically with the globular domains of type VI collagen, the spacing of collagen fibrils in cornea may be dependent on the proper association of PGs with type VI collagen.

# MATRIX DEGRADATION AND TURNOVER

The stroma is maintained by a balance between processes that lead to extracellular matrix deposition and degradation. Corneal ulceration can be considered as a disorder of tissue maintenance. Its physical manifestation, loss of the structural components of the corneal stroma, is due to an excess of specific, extracellular matrix degrading activities within the cornea. The best characterized of the degradative proteinases found in cornea during ulceration is collagenase, the only known enzyme that can cleave the native type I collagen helix at neutral pH. Type V collagen is degraded not by collagenase but by a gelatinase called type V collagenase. We have seen that the corneal stroma contains a variety of collagen types that change during development and repair. In animal models, the epithelial basement membrane disappears just before the onset of stromal ulceration. Enzymes must exist that can degrade the collagenous component of this structure.

The matrix metalloproteinases (MMPs) operative within the corneal stroma are important to normal matrix turnover as well as to matrix repair and abnormal degradation in various pathobiologic conditions. Members of this family have closely related structures, a requirement for zinc as a co-factor and calcium for stability, and exhibit optimal activity at the neutral pH of the extracellular space.[77] Each enzyme is secreted as an inactive species, and in vitro activation usually results in a decrease in molecular weight owing to proteolytic cleavage from the N-terminal of the protein. Similar activation mechanisms may occur in vivo within the extracellular space. The MMPs can be grouped into three subfamilies on the basis of their substrate specificity. Collagenases degrade native types I, II, and III collagen; stromelysins can specifically cleave proteoglycans, fibronectin, and laminin;[78] and gelatinases hydrolyze denatured collagen molecules (gelatin) as well as native types IV, V, and VII collagens.[79] Two different gelatinase species have been characterized: a lower molecular weight species (72 kD) called type IV collagenase and a higher molecular weight form (90–100 kD) called type V collagenase.[80] Sequencing studies have established that the two gelatinase species are products of separate genes.[81] Corneal epithelial cells produce predominantly the 92 kD form of progelatinase, whereas stromal fibroblasts synthesize mostly the 72 kD progelatinase. The 72 kD progelatinase can be extracted from the stroma without culturing, whereas 92 kD progelatinase expression appears to be stimulated in organ or cell culture.

Although controlled expression or activation of gelatinase might facilitate homeostatic processes, overexpression or inappropriate activation of these enzymes could have detrimental effects. A gelatin-degrading activity also was observed in cultures established from ulcerating corneas. Persistent or recurrent epithelial defects almost always precede stromal ulceration.[82] Adhesion of the corneal epithelium to the stromal layer is mediated by components of the basement membrane. When epithelial defects are present, stromal ulceration usually does not occur until after the basement membrane disappears. Therefore, gelatinases may play an important role during the development of the epithelial defect that leads to corneal ulceration. Keratectomized corneas synthesize and secrete both pro-collagenase and pro-stromelysin. Collagenase, synthesized by stromal cells, continues to be produced for over nine months after keratectomy, which is indicative of scar tissue remodeling. A gradient of collagenase expression exists across the radius of the keratectomized cornea, with the highest in the wound area, suggesting communication between stromal cells. The factors that control expression as well as activation of the MMPS by corneal epithelial cells and stromal fibroblasts will be important to determine.

## CORNEAL DYSTROPHIES

The corneal dystrophies are a heterogeneous group of relatively uncommon disorders, usually inherited. They may begin early in life or become manifest during aging. The exact causes of dystrophic disorders of the cornea are not well understood. Some are thought to result in part from abnormalities in corneal stromal cell function. Corneal stromal cells synthesize and degrade matrix materials during corneal morphogenesis and wound healing, and proper metabolism of such materials is essential for maintaining corneal transparency. An understanding of normal stromal cell metabolism is essential to defining abnormal conditions in corneal disorders and dystrophies, particularly in disorders that recur in grafts after penetrating keratoplasty.

Keratoconus is a progressive disease that involves thinning and scarring of the central cornea. A variety of morphologic and biochemical abnormalities have been detected in corneas with keratoconus, but these observations have not been consistent and there is no general agreement concerning their significance. Moreover, some abnormalities have not been confirmed by independent investigators. Part of the confusion stems from the fact that keratoconus has been linked to several different diseases, including atopic dermatitis and Down syndrome, and might therefore have a genetic component. Characterization of keratoconus has been difficult because corneal tissues have been obtained from patients of different ages and at different stages of the disease, often with associated complications such as corneal scarring or edema. Studies have shown that corneas obtained from patients with keratoconus contain significantly less total protein per milligram of dry weight than those of normal controls.[83,84] Moreover, stromal thinning may involve modification of stromal extracellular matrix metabolism.[85] These results have led to the hypothesis that degradation of macromolecules, including proteins, may be one of the mechanisms affected in keratoconus. In support of this hypothesis, cells derived from keratoconus corneas display enhanced collagenase[86] and gelatinase activities.[87] Immunohistochemical evidence indicates that keratoconus corneas have less keratan sulfate than normal.[88] In addition, lysosomal acid hydrolase levels are elevated in keratoconus cornea.[89] Finally, the levels of α-1-proteinase inhibitor in keratoconus were shown to be significantly lower than in normal corneas.[90] The exact mechanism underlying the α-1-proteinase inhibitor defect in keratoconus remains to be disclosed.

Macular corneal dystrophy is an inherited disorder in which a diffuse clouding of the cornea is accompanied by the appearance of small, ill-defined stromal opacities. The cornea synthesizes an abnormal KSPG which has an immunologically normal protein core. Until recently, the keratan chains in this variety of proteoglycan were thought to be normally elongated but never sulfated. However, immunohistochemical evidence has shown that sulfated keratan sulfate is present in the cornea of some individuals with macular dystrophy.[91] To differentiate between these two forms of the disease, patients are now classified as having type I (no sulfated KS in the cornea or the serum) or type II (detectable sulfated KS in the cornea and the serum) macular corneal dystrophy. This heterogeneity has been related to the collagen interfibrillar spacing in the stroma.[92,93]

## STROMAL HEALING OF EXCIMER LASER ABLATION WOUNDS

The use of lasers as a surgical tool in ophthalmology has demonstrated the importance of healing to obtain the desired outcome. Because the basic response of a wounded tissue is to repair the defect, the surgeon is then confronted with wound and healing phenomena that unpredictably alter the biochemistry, morphology, and tissue function. Clearly, understanding these phenomena is of utmost importance.

Several studies have shown that the 193-nm argon fluoride excimer laser discretely removes corneal tissue by photoablation without thermal damage to surrounding tissue.[94–97] Ultrastructural analysis of the walls of the ablated areas shows that damage to the adjacent structures is confined to a 60- to 200-nm wide zone.[95] Nonpenetrating incisions reaching within 40 μm of Descemet's membrane result in endothelial cell loss beneath the line of the irradiation.[95–97] Corneal ridging, epithelial cell damage, stromal swelling, and difficulty in making incisions to predictable depths argue for caution in human application.[97] Standard ultrastructural analyses indicate that each laser pulse removes discrete quantities of tissue, leaving clean-cut collagen fibrils. However, no information is available on the effect of ablation on quantities of proteoglycans and interfibrillar type VI collagen, macromolecular stromal components that may be important for transparency and strength.[21,22,43]

The tissue healing response after excimer laser photoablation appears to be dependent on the nature of the damage.[98] Photoablation under conditions that result in undulating stroma and uneven cutting results in poor epithelial healing with irregular basal lamina and hemidesmosome formation, and elicits extensive stromal cell invasion. On the other hand, smooth ablation of the tissue results in rapid regeneration of epithelial components and minimal cellular response from the stroma. In rabbits, the endothelial response to anterior stromal ablation leads to the appearance of electron opaque material in Descemet's membrane and immunohistochemical evidence of basement membrane components in the posterior stroma.[98,99] The major response to rabbit corneal ablation is the deposition of new connective tissue under the epithelium.[100]

Rabbit corneas are known to respond vigorously to wounds by synthesizing scar tissue. However, higher vertebrates, such as humans and monkeys, are more sluggish in healing. Nevertheless, monkeys respond to photorefractive ablation of anterior cornea by depositing an extracellular matrix[101] (Sundar Raj et al, personal communication), suggesting that humans may respond similarly. Recent studies have shown that photorefractive keratectomy in monkeys results in deposition of scar tissue with subsequent tissue clearing within months after treatment.[102,103] This rapid change in scar opacity may be due to the minimal quantities of tissue removed, the uniform surface of the stroma, and the rapid epithelial movement over the denuded area, offering an environment in which invading stromal cells are guided into the defect to deposit extracellular matrix without complications. Because the healing process partially recapitulates some morphologic and biochemical events seen in normal corneal morphogenesis,[104] scar tissue undergoes remodeling to become less opaque.[28] However, the unpredictability in the final refraction after photorefractive keratectomy may be related to the biological variability in scar remodeling.[103] The addition of new matrix to replace the ablated region does not completely fill in the defect and the extent of replacement is as yet unpredictable.

Corneal stromal wounds are repaired by the deposition of scar tissue by fibroblasts. Understanding the mechanisms by which fibroblasts contribute to wound healing is important for the development of pharmacologic agents that alter the healing process. Various stages of scar formation, such as activation and migration of stromal cells, cell proliferation and orientation, and synthesis of extracellular matrix proteins and the remodeling process, have been targeted for pharmacologic manipulation to alter the repair of tissue.[105] However, these attempts have been crude and largely ineffective. The use of steroids to discourage fibroblast invasion of the wound may nevertheless be useful. It is possible that delay of stromal cell invasion may allow the epithelium time to cover the defect and to deposit its basal lamina components and anchoring fibrils. Subsequent release of stromal cells from steroid inhibition results in minimal migration, if any, owing to the absence of tissue discontinuity.

Excimer laser ablation of corneal tissue appears to be an efficient method to remove tissue with minimal damage to adjacent areas. Subsequent tissue healing does not seem to be impaired or altered. However, laser ablation of the tissue does not always heal to form a mechanically strong and transparent tissue. In addition, in every instance the extent of deposition of new tissue remains unpredictable. A deeper understanding of scar formation is needed to predict and subsequently to alter the healing process to a desired end.

# THE CORNEAL ENDOTHELIUM

## H. F. Edelhauser

The main physiologic functions of the corneal endothelium are: to maintain an effective barrier from the aqueous humor; to maintain a metabolic pump; and, ultimately, to maintain corneal transparency. The anatomic and physiologic aspects of the corneal endothelium are illustrated in Figure 6.1. Endothelial cell size, shape, and number are indications of age and degree of stress.[1] For example, a high cell density with uniform

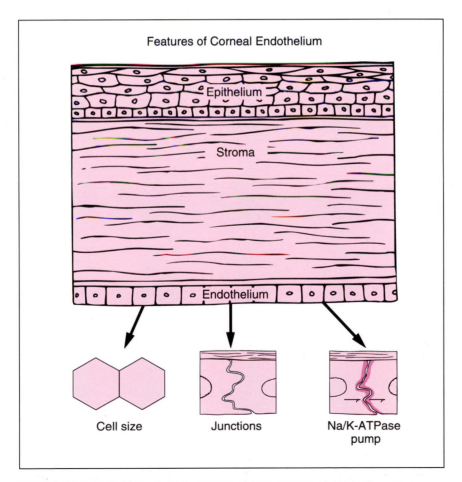

**Features of Corneal Endothelium**

Epithelium

Stroma

Endothelium

Cell size

Junctions

Na/K-ATPase pump

**6.1** | The three important features of the corneal endothelium are the cell shape and size, the junctions between the cells (barrier), and the Na,K-ATPase (metabolic pump).

hexagonal cells and a low coefficient of variation is the normal state; however, a low cell density, with few hexagonal cells and a high coefficient of variation, is indicative of a stressed endothelium.[2] The integrity of the endothelial cell junction establishes the barrier and is of the utmost importance in controlling the endothelial metabolic pump, which is located on the lateral membranes of the endothelial cells.

Clinically, if the endothelial pump function balances the leak rate, the corneal stromal water content will be 78% and the corneal thickness (0.52 mm) will be maintained (Fig. 6.2). Therefore, a compromise in either cell number, barrier function, or metabolic pump function can lead to corneal edema.

## THE ENDOTHELIAL BARRIER

The basis of barrier function is the existence of tight junctions and gap junctions between endothelial cells (Fig. 6.3). With maturation of the developing corneal endothelium and wound healing, the tight junction becomes more complex.[3] Laboratory studies have shown the tight junctions to be very sensitive to calcium (exposure to $Ca^{++}$-free solution causes the junctions to break down) and to the level of glutathione within the endothelial cell (Fig. 6.4). Surgically, trauma to the endothelium (e.g., from intraocular lens insertion) can break the endothelial cell junctions and lead to corneal edema. Once the tight junction is reestablished, the barrier function of the corneal endothelium is restored. The tight junctional complex is also regulated by the cytoskeleton (F-actin) of the endothelial cells.[4] Factors and agents that cause endothelial cell swelling and corneal edema do not appear to compromise the tight junction but do result in the loss of gap junctions.[5] Ouabain is a

**6.2** | A balance exists between the endothelial leakage and the metabolic pump, thus maintaining corneal thickness.

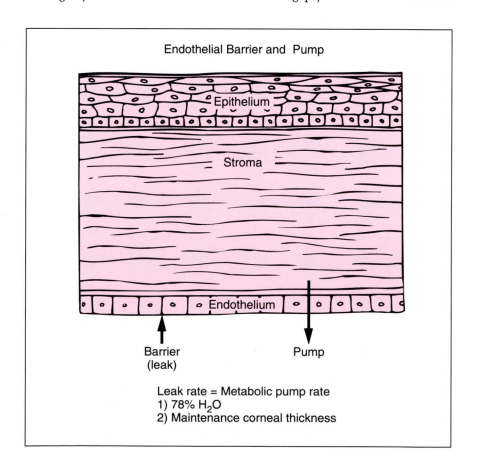

Endothelial Barrier and Pump

Epithelium

Stroma

Endothelium

Barrier (leak)

Pump

Leak rate = Metabolic pump rate
1) 78% $H_2O$
2) Maintenance corneal thickness

good example of such an agent. Inhibition of the endothelial Na,K-ATPase causes endothelial and stromal edema; as the endothelial cells swell the gap junctions break down but the tight junctions are maintained.

The metabolic pump of the corneal endothelium is controlled by the Na,K-ATPase located in the lateral membranes.[3] The location of the enzyme has been shown histochemically to be in the lateral membranes,[6] and the number of pump sites has been quantified with [3H]-ouabain.[7] These studies

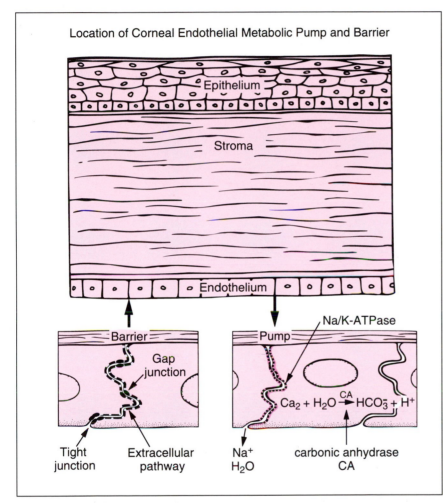

Location of Corneal Endothelial Metabolic Pump and Barrier

**6.3** | The function of corneal endothelial barrier is provided by the endothelial tight junctions and the gap junctions. The metabolic pump is maintained by the activity of Na,K-ATPase in the lateral membrane, which pumps Na+ from stroma to aqueous humor, and by a high concentration of intracellular carbonic anhydrase (CA), which forms $HCO_3^-$.

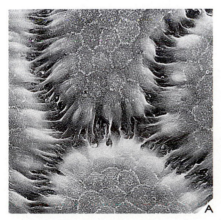
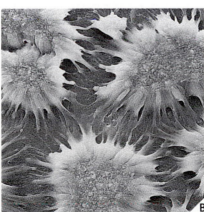

**6.4** | Oxidation of corneal endothelial cell glutathione to the GSSG form with diamide causes breakdown of the endothelial cell junctions and loss of endothelial barrier function. Breakdown of the junctions is shown at 15 *(A)* and 30 *(B)* minutes of diamide perfusion to the endothelium.

have shown that there are three million pump sites per endothelial cell and that they can be adequately contained in the lateral cell membranes. Studies have also demonstrated an active $HCO_3^-$ pump and/or $HCO_3^-$ secretion across the endothelium.[8] There is, however, a question as to whether this is active $HCO_3^-$ secretion controlled by the enzyme carbonic anhydrase or simply the diffusion of bicarbonate down its concentration gradient from the cytoplasm of the endothelial cell to the aqueous humor. It is important to point out that $HCO_3^-$ always moves in association with $Na^+$ and water then follows the active movement of the ions.

Figure 6.5 illustrates the permeability of the human cornea endothelium as a function of age (note that with the continued loss of endothelial cells that occurs with age there is no increase in permeability). When the endothelium is removed (Fig. 6.6), the permeability increases sixfold, from 2.26 to 12.85 ($10^{-4}$ cm/min).[9] Because the corneal endothelial permeability is a key factor in maintaining corneal transparency, the wound repair process and junctional integrity is of great importance. Recently, studies by Stiemke et al[3] on the developing rabbit corneal endothelium have shown that as the cornea matures and tight junctions are formed the endothelial permeability decreases.[3] The density of pump sites in corneal endothelial cells increases and the cornea becomes dehydrated.[10]

**6.5** | Human corneal endothelial permeability vs. age. Without a corneal endothelium, the permeability can increase sixfold.

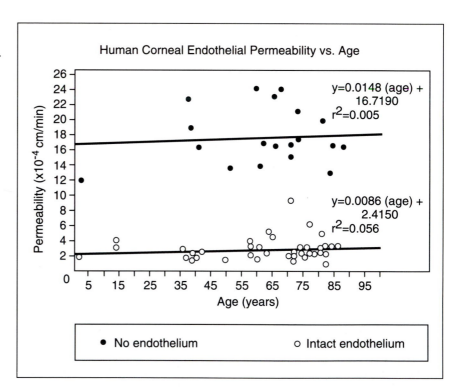

The major role of the wound repair process in corneal endothelium is to restore the barrier function. The mechanism of endothelial wound repair is by cell migration, with a limited degree of mitosis (Fig. 6.7). A number of studies have shown that wound repair of the corneal endothelium in the rabbit is by both mitosis and migration, whereas cell proliferation in the primate and human cornea is minimal. Watsky et al[9] have shown that when the permeability of the corneal endothelium is measured in human corneas

## CORNEAL ENDOTHELIAL WOUND REPAIR

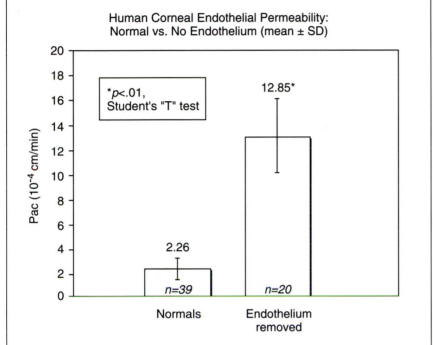

**6.6** | Human corneal permeability with and without endothelium.

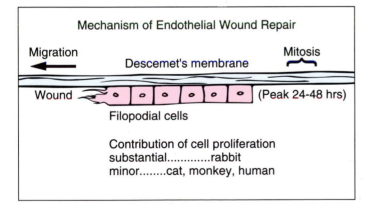

**6.7** | Mechanism of corneal endothelial wound repair. All wound repair occurs by migration and sliding in the human cornea.

obtained from the eye bank that have previously had cataract surgery, the endothelium is compromised and the permeability is increased (Fig. 6.8). The results of this study suggest that even though wound repair occurs after the trauma of cataract surgery, the endothelial barrier function does not return to normal. After cataract surgery, corneas return to normal thickness and are transparent; therefore, the metabolic pump may function at a higher level to compensate for the increased permeability.

## CORNEAL ENDOTHELIAL METABOLIC PUMP

A diagram of the metabolic pump is shown in Figure 6.9. The corneal stroma has a total $Na^+$ concentration (bound and unbound) of 179 mEq/L, with $Na^+$ activity of 134.4 mEq/L (the remaining 44.6 mEq/L is bound to the stromal proteoglycans). The aqueous humor contains only unbound $Na^+$ with an activity of 142.9 mEq/L. Therefore, a sodium gradient exists by which the stromal water can diffuse from the stroma to the aqueous humor. The diffusion of water from the stroma is regulated by the active metabolic pumping of sodium from the endothelial cells to the extracellular space by the Na,K-ATPase ($3 Na^+/2 K^+$) in exchange for a $K^+$. The corneal endothelial cells also contain a high concentration of carbonic anhydrase, which forms bicarbonate from metabolic $CO_2^-$. The $HCO_3^-$ will also diffuse down its concentration gradient into the extracellular space or across the membrane associated with the $Na^+/HCO_3^-$ exchanger. To maintain the osmotic flux of water across the endothelium to control the water content of the stroma, the tight junction maintains the extracellular space between endothelial cells, and water from the stroma can diffuse through the junction.

This point is further demonstrated in Figure 6.10, which diagrams the osmotic force and subsequent movement of water generated by the difference in sodium activity between the corneal stroma and aqueous humor. The

**6.8** | Effect of cataract surgery on permeability of the corneal endothelium. Note that aphakic eyes and eyes with either a posterior chamber (PC) lens or an anterior chamber (AC) lens have increased endothelial permeability.

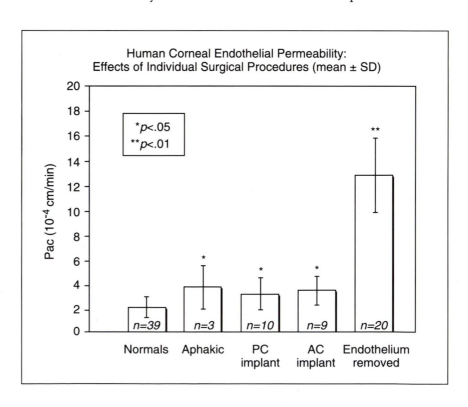

Human Corneal Endothelial Permeability: Effects of Individual Surgical Procedures (mean ± SD)

$*p<.05$
$**p<.01$

Pac ($10^{-4}$ cm/min)

Normals (n=39), Aphakic (n=3), PC implant (n=10), AC implant (n=9), Endothelium removed (n=20)

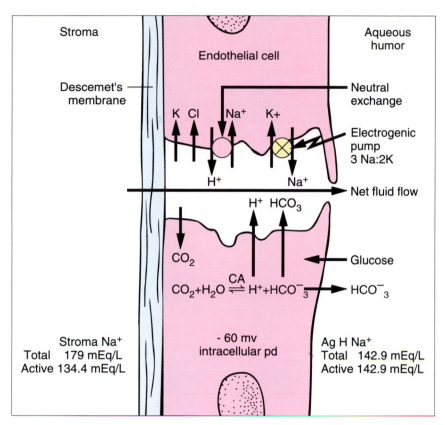

**6.9** | Diagram of the corneal endothelial pump mechanism.

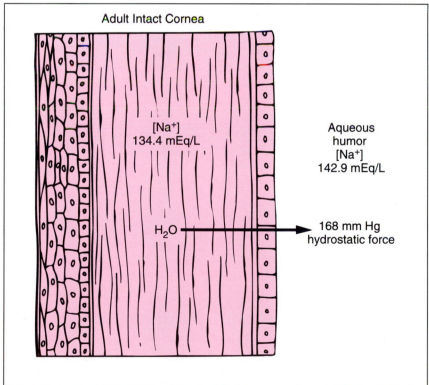

**6.10** | Sodium activity gradients across the normal endothelium.

Na$^+$ activity within the aqueous humor is greater than within the stroma (142.9 vs. 134.4 mEq/L). Assuming the reflection coefficient of the endothelium to be 0.6, an osmotic force of 98.5 mm Hg is established from stroma to aqueous humor to draw water from the stroma. In reality, the osmotic force of 30.4 mm Hg (Fig. 6.11) exists across the endothelium when the chloride activity and the stromal inhibition pressure are accounted for, both of which oppose the hydrostatic force established by the sodium ion activity. The metabolic pump aids the direction of water diffusion with the net flux of sodium from the stroma to the aqueous humor (i.e., water osmotically follows the Na$^+$ movement).

In cases of corneal endothelial dysfunction in which the corneal edema results from loss of endothelial cells (Fig. 6.12), the sodium ion activity within the stroma is greater than that of the aqueous humor (149.8 vs. 142.3 mEq/L). Therefore, aqueous water diffuses into the stroma owing to the loss of the corneal endothelial barrier and pump function. The increased sodium ion concentration within the stroma is the result of the unopposed diffusion of aqueous humor sodium to the stroma and the increase of stromal sodium activity from the amount bound in the stromal proteoglycan (i.e., as the hydration of the corneal stroma increases there is a decrease in the bound sodium). For transparency to be restored and the cornea to return to normal, the endothelial barrier function must be reestablished.

**6.11** | Net hydrostatic force across the corneal endothelium. Sodium ion activity of the aqueous humor is the major driving force that osmotically maintains the corneal stroma in the deturgescent state.

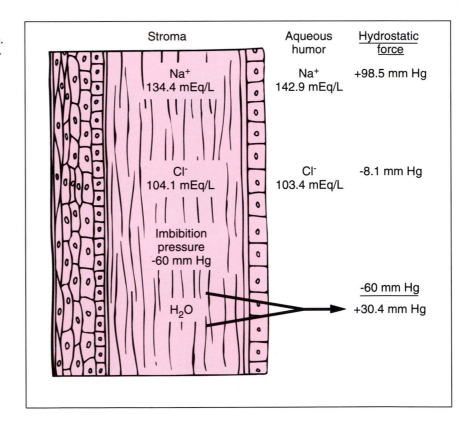

Studies by Geroski and Edelhauser[7] have shown the pump site density of the human cornea to be $4.4 \times 10^9$ sites/mm and Burns et al[11] have demonstrated the fluorescein permeability of the corneal endothelium to be 2.89 mm/min $\times 10^3$ (Fig. 6.13A). In a series of patients with endothelial guttata,

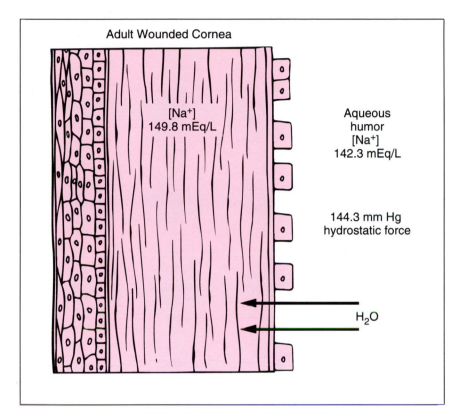

Adult Wounded Cornea

[Na$^+$]
149.8 mEq/L

Aqueous humor
[Na$^+$]
142.3 mEq/L

144.3 mm Hg
hydrostatic force

H$_2$O

**6.12** | Sodium activity gradients across the wounded corneal endothelium. The endothelial barrier is lost and the hydrostatic force is 144.3 mm Hg at the stroma, resulting in corneal hydration.

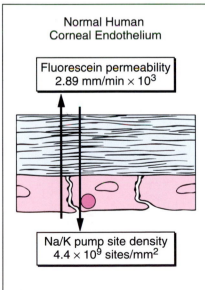

Normal Human
Corneal Endothelium

Fluorescein permeability
2.89 mm/min $\times 10^3$

Na/K pump site density
$4.4 \times 10^9$ sites/mm$^2$

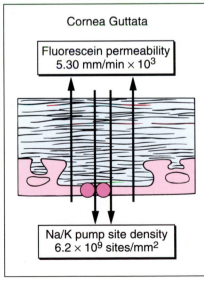

Cornea Guttata

Fluorescein permeability
5.30 mm/min $\times 10^3$

Na/K pump site density
$6.2 \times 10^9$ sites/mm$^2$

**6.13** | *A:* Normal corneal endothelial cell permeability to fluorescein and normal pump site density. *B:* In corneal guttata the permeability increases twofold and the leak is balanced by a doubling of the pump site density. The cornea remains transparent.

Burns et al reported that the permeability increased to 5.30 mm/min x $10^3$.[11] These corneas have an endothelium that has become progressively leaky; however, they have a normal corneal thickness of 0.52 mm and are transparent. Geroski and Edelhauser[7] showed that in the case of early guttata (1,700 cells/mm$^2$) the density of the Na/K pump sites increased to 6.2 x $10^9$ sites/mm$^2$ (Fig. 6.13B). Even though the corneal endothelial cells do not undergo mitosis, a physiologic adaptation can occur that balances the endothelial leak, i.e., the production of more pump sites.

## BARRIER AND PUMP FUNCTION WITH LOW CELL DENSITY

The following is a summary of the changes in the barrier and pump function of the corneal endothelial cell that can take place as the cell number decreases and corneal decompensation occurs (Fig. 6.14). In corneal endothelium, if there are no junctions between the cells, there can be no barrier or metabolic pump function. In the normal human cornea with 2,000–3,000 cells/mm$^2$, with tight junctions for the barrier and Na,K-ATPase for the metabolic pump, the pump can balance the leak of aqueous humor into the stroma and the Na$^+$ activity will be greater in the aqueous humor than in the stroma, so that the hydrostatic movement of the water would be in the direction of stroma to aqueous. In the case of a stressed corneal endothelium with a decreased cell number (i.e., between 800–1,500 cells/mm$^2$), the corneal endothelium can adapt to the increased leakage and balance the increased permeability by producing more pump sites on the lateral membranes. (A similar phenomenon occurs in the cells of the proximal tubule of the kidney to adjust for an increased salt load.) The point at which corneal decompensation occurs results from a progressive loss of endothelial cells to below the critical level of less than 500 cells/mm$^2$. At this low cell number, the permeability has greatly increased and the endothelial cells are spread so thin that there is not enough room on the lateral cell membrane for the metabolic pump sites. Therefore, the metabolic pump cannot balance the leak and corneal edema results.

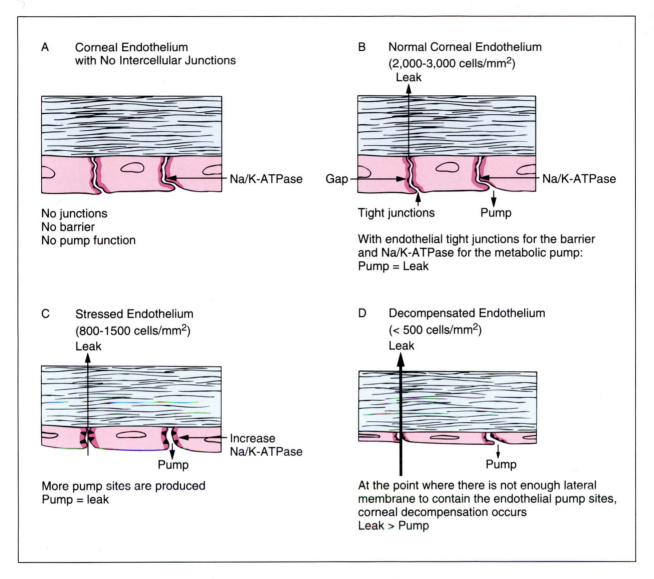

A   Corneal Endothelium
with No Intercellular Junctions

Na/K-ATPase

No junctions
No barrier
No pump function

B   Normal Corneal Endothelium
(2,000-3,000 cells/mm$^2$)
Leak

Gap

Na/K-ATPase

Tight junctions     Pump

With endothelial tight junctions for the barrier
and Na/K-ATPase for the metabolic pump:
Pump = Leak

C   Stressed Endothelium
(800-1500 cells/mm$^2$)
Leak

Increase
Na/K-ATPase

Pump

More pump sites are produced
Pump = leak

D   Decompensated Endothelium
(< 500 cells/mm$^2$)
Leak

Pump

At the point where there is not enough lateral
membrane to contain the endothelial pump sites,
corneal decompensation occurs
Leak > Pump

**6.14** | *A:* A corneal endothelium with no intercellular junctions. There is no barrier and no pump function. *B:* A normal corneal endothelium with 2,000–3,000 cells/mm², with endothelial cell tight junctions for the barrier and Na,K-ATPase for the metabolic pump. There is a balance, and the cornea maintains its transparency. *C:* In a stressed endothelium with 800–1,500 cells/mm², the endothelial barrier becomes leaky; however, the endothelial cells can produce more pump sites, the metabolic pump can balance the leakage, and the cornea remains transparent. *D:* When the corneal endothelium has fewer than 500 cells/mm², the cells are spread so thinly that there is not enough membrane for the Na,K-ATPase pump sites. At this point, corneal endothelial decompensation occurs.

# 7 | WIDEFIELD CLINICAL SPECULAR MICROSCOPY AND COMPUTERIZED MORPHOMETRIC ANALYSIS

## Richard W. Yee

The corneal endothelium is essential for the maintenance of normal cornea hydration, thickness, and transparency.[1,2] The first direct visualization of this monolayer of cells was demonstrated by Vogt in 1918.[3] With the slit-lamp microscope, Vogt showed that the endothelial mosaic could be visualized in the axis of a reflected light beam. Unfortunately, fine continuous eye movements, limited magnification, and annoying light reflexes precluded the routine systematic study of the endothelium. In 1968, David Maurice modified metallurgical microscopes and, using the principle of reflective light microscopes, he obtained specular reflections from the endothelial surface of excised corneas through a fluid medium at high magnification.[4] Modifications of this laboratory specular microscope were made by Laing et al,[5] and later by Bourne and Kaufman,[6] allowing routine clinical examination and photography of the corneal endothelium. These early specular microscopes were narrow-field scopes and provided a field of view of only 0.04 mm[2]. These microscopes were commercially available as the Syber (known later as the Heyer Schulte specular microscope) and the Bio-Optics specular microscope. The optic principles of the clinical specular microscope are well documented[7,8] (see Vol. 1 of *Textbook of Ophthalmology*, Chapter 19).

Current specular microscopes have multiple advantages. They have a wider field of view and utilize optic improvements to minimize annoying reflections from incident light.[9,10] Widefield specular microscopes offer a full-field view providing better examination of the endothelial mosaic. The addition of highly sensitive video cameras and recording systems,[11] as well as a variety of optic improvements such as the scanning-mirror system introduced by Koester[12] and modification of the applanating objective cone for the contact specular microscope,[13] have improved the resolution of the endothelium and increased the field of view to as much as 1 mm[2]. Current specular scopes are marketed by Alcon, Bio-Optics, and Keeler. Eyebank specular microscopes are available by Alcon and Bio-Optics.

## PATIENT SET-UP

Commercially available contact widefield specular microscopes are easy to use with minimal discomfort to the patient. The procedure is first explained to the patient to relieve any anxiety. Typically, there is no pain involved and patients are told that the procedure is very similar to that of Goldmann applanation tonometry. It is important to explain to patients that they will see a flash of light and hear the whirring of the motor drive so that they will not be frightened and move during the actual procedure. The positioning of the head and the patient's comfort are extremely important to minimize movement and allow optimal photographs of the endothelium.

One or two drops of proparacaine anesthetic should be used before the eye is contacted. Once the corneas are contacted with the dipping cone, a few epithelial irregularities may be seen; however, these usually disappear within a few hours. If necessary, an assistant can hold the patient's head and separate the eyelids so that optimal photographs can be obtained. Positioning the eye in a straight-ahead position is best achieved with a fixation light. If there is significant eye movement, additional pressure of the applanation cone on the cornea is sometimes helpful. At times, it is simply better to stop for a rest if the patient is getting anxious.

Optimal photographs are obtained when the cornea is relatively thin, clear with minimal scarring or edema, and has an intact epithelium. Light reflexes from the iris can obscure the endothelial mosaic and are best eliminated by dilating the pupil. Kodak TMAX fine-grain black-and-white film pushed to ASA 1600 will give excellent resolution. To ensure adequate exposure, bracketing the exposures can be performed using different flash intensities. TMAX film developed in Kodak D-19 film developer for 5 minutes at 70°F yields high border contrast.

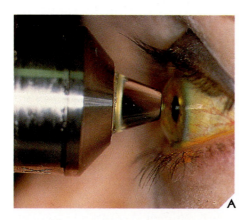

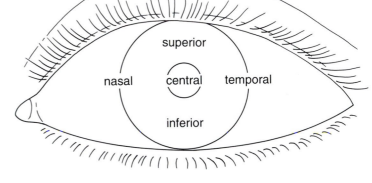

**7.1 |** *A:* The applanation cone should be placed centrally with the light shining through the pupil. *B:* The cornea should be systematically scanned to ensure complete evaluation of the endothelial mosaic, centrally, superiorly, inferiorly, nasally, and temporally.

A standard approach to examining the corneal endothelium is very important. The beam of light is directed through the pupil to ensure the placement of the cone on the most central portion of the cornea (Fig. 7.1A). Systematically scanning superiorly, inferiorly, nasally, and temporally will ensure a thorough evaluation of the monolayer (Fig. 7.1B). These regions can be individually photodocumented with a video camera or a 35-mm camera. If an area greater than 1 mm$^2$ needs to be photodocumented, a photographic montage of the entire area can be made by taking multiple photographs with overlapping fields (Fig. 7.2). Specific endothelial regions can be relocated with certainty using a combination of the widefield capability, montage photographic technique, and artifacts induced by the contact applanation cone known as posterior corneal rings.[14] This scanning method using widefield specular scopes offers a more complete qualitative and quantitative evaluation of the corneal endothelium.

Analyzing specular micrographs can be done qualitatively by looking at the morphology and giving an interpretation, or quantitatively by counting cell density and doing morphometric analysis. Interpretation requires knowledge of normal endothelium mosaic appearance (Fig. 7.3). The normal specular micrograph should demonstrate a regular endothelial mosaic with cell sizes

# REGIONAL SPECULAR MICROSCOPY

## QUALITATIVE ANALYSIS

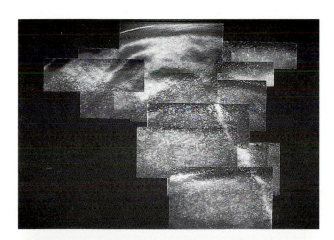

**7.2** | Photographic montage (representing approximately 4 mm of the cornea) in a patient with ICE (Chandler) syndrome. Note the superior portion of the cornea with relatively normal corneal endothelium surrounded by abnormal endothelial cells demonstrating a typical "reversal pattern" appearance.

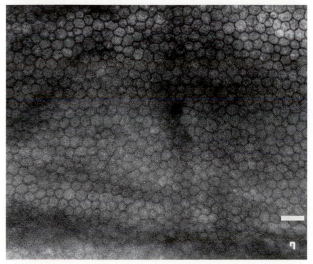

**7.3** | Widefield specular micrograph of the human corneal endothelium in a 69-year-old normal subject has a cell density of 2,201 cells/mm$^2$, a coefficient of variation of 0.27, and 66% hexagonal cells. (Bar = 50 µm.)

**7.4** | *A:* Classification by Laing describing morphologic structures seen frequently on specular microscopy. (Adapted from Laing RA: Specular microscopy of the cornea. *Curr Top Eye Res 1980;3:157–219.*)

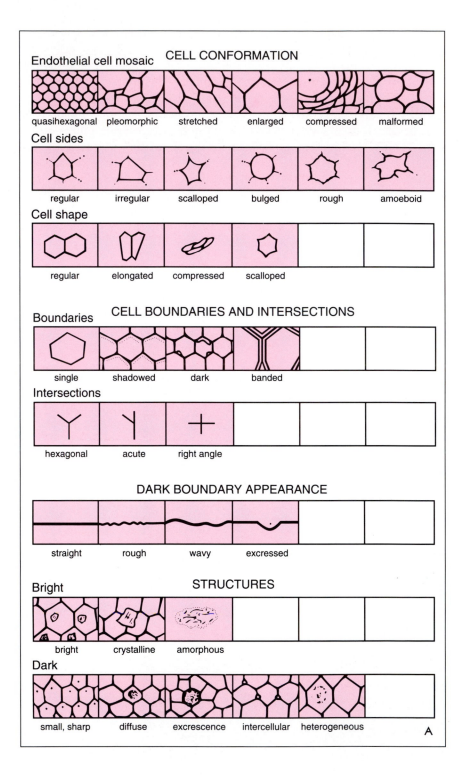

between 200 and 400 $\mu m^2$, depending on the patient's age. The presence of bizarre cell shapes, intracellular vacuoles, irregular blurring of endothelial cell borders, or additional components such as cornea guttata, inflammatory cells, or pigmented keratic precipitates is considered abnormal. Many times the clustering of cells or other specific characteristics will provide the diagnosis. A classification of these morphologic structures has been described by Laing[15] (Fig. 7.4A). Although this classification system has not been standardized, these morphologic structures are helpful in describing the appearance of structural changes in the monolayer (Fig. 7.4B).

The most common quantitative analysis of specular micrographs consists of cell counting and cell area measurements. Cell area is typically given as mean cell area ($\mu m^2$/cell) which is equal to $10^6$/cell density (cells/$mm^2$) or as cell density (cells/$mm^2$) which is equal to $10^6$/mean cell area ($\mu m^2$/cell). Cell counting methods exist for determining these two parameters. These include a *comparison* cell analysis in which the endothelial cell mosaic is visualized and compared with a cell pattern of known size,[16–18] *fixed-frame* cell analysis in which the number of cells within a constant area is counted, and *variable-frame* cell analysis in which the number of cells counted is constant and thus the area varies. The cell density is calculated by dividing the number of cells

## QUANTITATIVE ANALYSIS

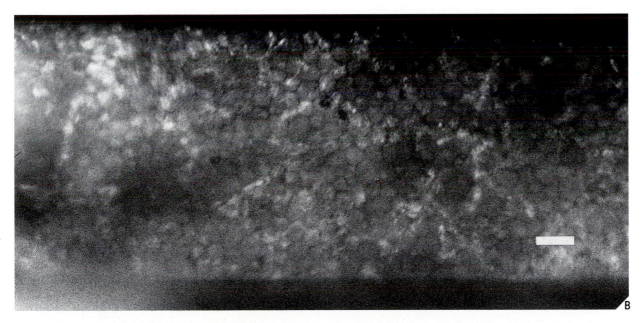

B

**7.4 | (Continued.)** *B:* Specular micrograph demonstrating a variety of morphologic structures in a patient with HIV-positive serology and CMV retinitis. Note pleomorphic and enlarged malformed cells and a variety of bulging and rough-shaped borders. Cell shapes are regular and elongated, and cell boundaries and intersections vary. A number of bright and amorphous areas overlie the endothelial mosaic. Many dark intracellular and intercellular changes are present. (Bar = 50 $\mu m$.)

by the area of that frame.[19] Although these methods are commonly used in clinical practice, there are inherent sampling errors as well as inaccuracies in the assessment of the cell densities.[19] However, these errors are usually within 10% of the actual cell density and are sufficient for routine preoperative clinical evaluations.[20,21] *Individual* cell analysis of each cell in a cluster can be used to determine cell density or average cell area, either manually or semiautomatically. This analysis provides much more information about the individual cells and is probably the most accurate for the determination of cell density.[15] With additional computation, other morphometric parameters, such as the perimeter and the coefficient of variation of the mean cell area (polymegathism) and/or cell shapes (pleomorphism) can be documented.

## COMPUTERIZED MORPHOMETRIC ANALYSIS

Information obtained from specular microscopy has been based primarily on cell density measurements and morphologic appearance. Little correlation has been seen between cell density and the functional capacity of the endothelial mosaic. In addition, there is no direct correlation between cell density and endothelial function as indicated by corneal thickness measurements.[1] Several investigators have suggested that the variation in the individ-

## Figure 7.5. Morphometric Baselines of Normal Endothelium

### ENDOTHELIAL SIZE PARAMETERS IN A NORMAL POPULATION (MEAN ± SEM)

| AGE | EYES | PERIMETER (μ) | MEAN CELL AREA (μM²) | COEFFICIENT OF VARIATION | CELL DENSITY (CELLS/MM²) |
|---|---|---|---|---|---|
| 10–19 | 3 | 64.2 ± 0.5 | 293.8 ± 3.5 | 0.22 ± 0.015 | 3404 ± 40 |
| 20–29 | 11 | 69.3 ± 1.4 | 345.2 ± 13.4 | 0.27 ± 0.016 | 2942 ± 116 |
| 30–39 | 6 | 70.9 ± 0.8 | 359.5 ± 7.8 | 0.27 ± 0.017 | 2787 ± 58 |
| 40–49 | 6 | 73.2 ± 1.9 | 383.7 ± 20.0 | 0.28 ± 0.016 | 2640 ± 133 |
| 50–59 | 7 | 72.3 ± 1.3 | 375.1 ± 12.9 | 0.29 ± 0.008 | 2685 ± 94 |
| 60–69 | 9 | 72.6 ± 1.7 | 375.2 ± 18.0 | 0.30 ± 0.016 | 2711 ± 121 |
| 70–79 | 9 | 72.9 ± 0.8 | 381.7 ± 8.5 | 0.29 ± 0.013 | 2630 ± 60 |
| 80–89 | 9 | 80.9 ± 3.2 | 449.0 ± 30.8 | 0.29 ± 0.012 | 2316 ± 154 |

### ENDOTHELIAL SHAPE PARAMETERS IN A NORMAL POPULATION (MEAN ± SEM)

| AGE | RELATIVE FREQUENCY (%) OF CELL SHAPES NUMBER OF SIDES | | | | | |
|---|---|---|---|---|---|---|
| | 4 | 5 | 6 | 7 | 8 | 9 |
| 10–19 | 0.3 ± 0.3 | 12.7 ± 1.8 | 75.3 ± 1.8 | 11.7 ± 0.3 | 0 | 0 |
| 20–29 | 0.3 ± 0.2 | 13.9 ± 1.1 | 72.6 ± 2.0 | 12.7 ± 1.1 | 0.7 ± 0.2 | 0 |
| 30–39 | 0.7 ± 0.2 | 16.2 ± 0.8 | 67.2 ± 2.8 | 14.5 ± 2.7 | 1.5 ± 1.4 | 0 |
| 40–49 | 0 | 18.7 ± 1.4 | 64.2 ± 2.0 | 16.0 ± 0.7 | 0.8 ± 0.4 | 0 |
| 50–59 | 0 | 18.3 ± 1.4 | 63.9 ± 3.0 | 16.3 ± 1.6 | 1.6 ± 0.5 | 0 |
| 60–69 | 1.0 ± 0.4 | 16.6 ± 1.0 | 64.3 ± 2.3 | 16.4 ± 1.4 | 1.7 ± 0.6 | 0 |
| 70–79 | 0.2 ± 0.1 | 19.1 ± 0.7 | 60.6 ± 1.4 | 18.7 ± 1.1 | 1.0 ± 0.7 | 0.2 ± 0.1 |
| 80–89 | 0.6 ± 0.3 | 18.2 ± 0.6 | 61.4 ± 1.0 | 18.6 ± 0.5 | 1.2 ± 0.4 | 0 |

(Modified from Yee RW, Matsuda M, Schultz RO, Edelhauser HF: Changes in the normal corneal endothelial cellular pattern as a function of age. *Curr Eye Res* 1985;4:671–687. By permission of Oxford University Press.)

ual cell area (polymegathism) as well as cell shape, i.e., cells with different number of sides (pleomorphism), may better reflect endothelial cell integrity and function.[22,23] Schultz et al[24] have shown that detailed descriptions of cellular polymegathism and pleomorphism are more sensitive than cell density measurements alone for detecting early endothelial changes.[5] Normal morphometric baselines for proper comparison in evaluation of the endothelium when pathologic states are compared have been previously reported[25–27] (Fig. 7.5). Several investigators have demonstrated a gradual reduction of cell density with age in the normal human corneal endothelium.[6,28,29] Similarly, there is a definite increase in cellular polymegathism and polymorphism and decrease in the number of cells with age.[26] Along with these age-related changes is the loss of the regular hexagonal pattern. There are no apparent regional disparities or differences between paired human corneas in cellular polymegathism or polymorphism by specular microscopy.

Many published studies have demonstrated the sensitivity of morphometric analysis for detecting abnormalities of the endothelial monolayer. Morphometric analysis has been used to describe changes seen in diabetic cornea,[24] unilateral keratoconus,[30] donor corneal endothelium,[31] long-term hard and soft contact lens wearers,[32–35] unilateral ptosis,[36] after penetrating keratoplasty[37] and cataract extraction,[38,39] with anterior chamber intraocular lenses,[40] in a number of animal laboratory experiments evaluating the toxicity of irrigating solutions[41] in diabetic dogs,[42] rats,[43] wound healing,[44,45] and inflammatory mechanisms.[46]

The methodology for morphometric analysis has been previously published.[24] Briefly, a specular photograph is chosen on the basis of cell boundary clarity and is enlarged to 400 times the original magnification. Before the specular photograph is printed, a calibration negative of a micrometer scale is taken with the same specular camera and placed in an enlarger to ensure accurate cornea-to-print magnification. A hundred individual cells are outlined with a fine-point felt-tipped pen and are numbered consecutively to minimize sampling and analysis error (Fig. 7.6A). Individual cells are digitized by marking each cell apex with a graphics tablet pen.

The coordinates are entered into a digitizing tablet and analyzed by endothelial analysis software that has been previously developed[47] (Fig. 7.6B). Cell density measurements are obtained as previously mentioned. The coefficient of variation (polymegathism) is calculated by dividing the standard deviation of the cell area by the mean cell area. The coefficient of

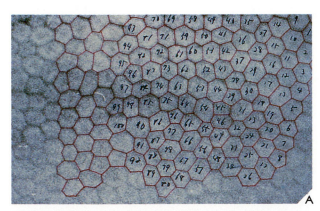

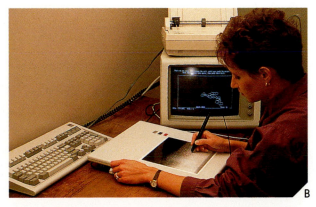

**7.6** | *A:* Specular photograph outlined with a fine-tipped pen and numbered consecutively before digitization.

*B:* Coordinates are manually entered into a digitizing tablet to obtain morphometric parameters.

variation is a dimensionless index independent of cell size and provides quantitative measurement of cell variation.[48] Cell shapes are described by the number of apices of each cell, and the variation is analyzed automatically by digitizing the apex of each cell (pleomorphism). The quantitative description of these additional cellular patterns is complementary to cell density measurements and is descriptive in defining the endothelial population and possibly its functional status.[22,23,49] It has been suggested that these shape changes may also reflect compensatory mechanisms of the endothelium to accommodate stress[50] (Fig. 7.7).

The increased sensitivity of morphometric analysis in detecting abnormalities of the endothelial monolayer can be reasonably explained by considering endothelial wound healing.[51-53] Depending on the severity of the injury, endothelial cell loss may not be reflected by a decrease in cell density or an increase in mean cell area. For example, if only one cell is lost in a cluster of 100 cells, the mean cell area would increase maximally by 1%, a statistically nondetectable increase.[54] On the other hand, if a six-sided cell is lost in the cluster of 100 cells, at least two cells (2%) or possibly a maximum of six cells (6%) will show significant changes in cell pattern as adjacent cells stretch, slide, or even fuse together to cover the cell-free or traumatized area. This process can result in an increase in cellular polymegathism. Therefore, cell loss that is not detectable by cell density measurements alone may be detectable by quantitation of cellular polymegathism and pleomorphism.

Further studies are in progress to describe better the relationship between anatomic form and functional capability.[50,55-57]

# CLINICAL INDICATIONS FOR SPECULAR MICROSCOPY
## PREOPERATIVE EVALUATION

Clinical specular microscopy is a practical tool not only for the cornea subspecialist in evaluating donor corneas and corneal dystrophies but also for the ophthalmic surgeon in identifying subtle changes in the cornea when the slit-lamp examination is normal. A clear cornea with a normal pachymetry reading is no assurance of a normal endothelial morphology or cell density. Because of the increased sensitivity of morphometric analysis, it is important to assess not only cell density but also polymegathism and polymorphism. The cell density threshold for the development of corneal edema

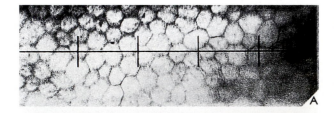

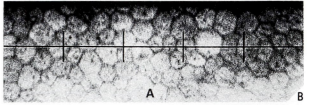

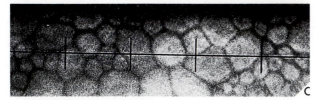

**7.7 |** Specular photomicrographs of the endothelium. *A:* A 60-year-old normal subject with a cell density of 2,702 cells/mm² and a coefficient of variation of 0.32 with 61% hexagonal cells. *B:* A 61-year-old patient with significantly less pleomorphism and polymegathism has a cell density of 2,464 cells/mm² and a coefficient of variation of 0.38 with 45% hexagonal cells. *C:* A 61-year-old patient demonstrating pleomorphism and polymegathism secondary to type II diabetes. Cell density is 2,983 cells/ mm² and a coefficient of variation is 0.88 with 45% hexagonal cells. (Bars = 50 µm.) (Modified from Schultz RO, Matsuda M, Yee RW, et al: Corneal endothelial changes in type I and type II diabetes mellitus. *Am J Ophthalmol* 1984;98:401–410. Copyright by The Ophthalmic Publishing Company.).

and bullous keratopathy has been estimated to be between 400 and 700 cells/mm$^2$,[1,58] which requires a patient to have at least 1,000 to 1,200 cells/mm$^2$ before most anterior segment surgery (assuming that cell loss is in the range of 0%–30%). Moreover, when the cell density approaches this cell count, it behooves the surgeon to make certain that the patient understands the increased risk of developing postoperative corneal edema and subsequent corneal decompensation. Because there is a large range of variation in cell densities in all age groups, age cannot be used to predict endothelial cell count. Most patients, including those over the age of 70, should have a cell count of at least 2,000 cells/mm$^2$. Typically, there should be no significant cell density differences or morphologic differences between pairs of eyes. It has been noted that the cell density between a pair of eyes must be greater than 280 cells/mm$^2$ to be meaningful.[59]

Because there is evidence that a polymegathic and pleomorphic corneal endothelium does not tolerate intraocular surgery as well as a more uniform endothelium, a monolayer with a coefficient variation of greater than 0.40 or with less than 50% hexagonal cells should be considered abnormal and possibly at greater risk for postoperative edema. As in cell density measurements, there is a range of variation of polymegathism and pleomorphism in all age groups; therefore, age cannot be used to predict the endothelial morphologic appearance. Presumably the difference in cell polymegathism and pleomorphism between a pair of eyes should be greater than 15%–20% to be meaningful.

Clinical use of the specular microscope includes preoperative evaluation of the endothelial monolayer whenever an endothelial abnormality is noted by slit-lamp examination.[60] Slit-lamp abnormalities include corneal guttata, keratic precipitates, pigmented and inflammatory cells, endothelial surface or Descemet's membrane irregularities, and increased corneal thickness. A history of possible endothelial involvement, i.e., family history of corneal dystrophy,[61] trauma,[62] acute narrow-angle[63–66] or chronic open-angle glaucoma, uveitis,[67–70] keratitis, graft rejection,[71] previous ocular surgery,[72,73] secondary intraocular implantation,[40] or corneal transplantation[74] may affect the surgical outcome. It is important again to reemphasize the use of widefield regional scanning of the monolayer for a more accurate assessment of the entire endothelial layer. This is particularly important in evaluating postoperative corneas, because a regional disparity in cell density and morphology has been reported.[38–40]

## DONOR CORNEAS

Specular microscopy has been suggested as a useful and reliable method of screening tissue for keratoplasty. Evaluation of corneal tissue can be performed on whole globes[31,75] as well as on corneas stored in tissue culture medium.[76–78] At present, most eye banks rely only on historical and slit-lamp information as criteria for accepting or rejecting corneal tissue. Unfortunately, this allows donors with undetectable endothelial abnormalities such as guttata to be transplanted,[79] as well as exclusion of donors rejected simply because of age restrictions.[78]

Cell counts required for transplant surgery should be at least 2,000 to 2,500 cells/mm$^2$. Survival of the graft depends on this initial cell count as well as on the degree of endothelial trauma during the intraoperative and postoperative course. Cell loss after routine penetrating keratoplasty will range from 30%–60%, with stabilization of the endothelial monolayer in 3 to 4 years.[37,80]

## ENDOTHELIAL DYSTROPHIES

Specular microscopy has been a useful tool for helping to confirm the diagnosis of certain endothelial dystrophies. The morphologic changes of the corneal guttata in Fuchs endothelial dystrophy have been characterized by Laing and others[81,82] (Figs. 7.8A and 7.8B). With widefield regional specular microscopy, assessment of a cornea with Fuchs dystrophy before an intraocular procedure can be performed and evaluated with greater certainty with regard to the prognosis for postoperative corneal clarity. This regional specular evaluation, in addition to the clinical history of frequent fluctuating vision, abnormal pachymetry readings, and formation of microcytic bullae (as indicated by the subepithelial fibrosis), can aid in deciding whether penetrating keratoplasty is necessary at the time of cataract surgery. If there are a significant number of peripheral cells and the guttata are primarily located centrally, there is a decreased likelihood that corneal transplantation is necessary (Fig. 7.9A). On the other hand, if there is complete confluence of guttata even in the peripheral cornea, one might consider a combined procedure (Fig. 7.9B).

Sometimes deep corneal opacities seen on slit-lamp examination are due to posterior polymorphous dystrophy, especially early in the disease process. This can be confused with changes caused by other corneal conditions such as Fuchs dystrophy, iridocorneal endothelial syndromes, interstitial keratitis, and even keratoconus.[82] In old Descemet's membrane tears, a rail-track border is characteristically seen with specular microscopy and differs from

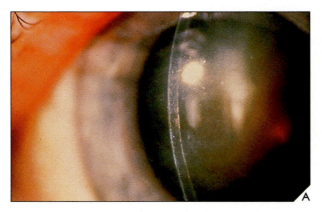

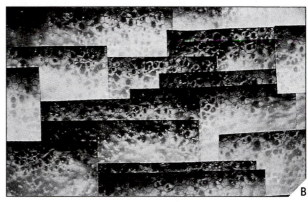

**7.8** | *A:* Slit-lamp appearance in Fuchs dystrophy shows endothelial irregularities and subepithelial fibrosis.

*B:* Photographic montage of the guttata in Fuchs dystrophy.

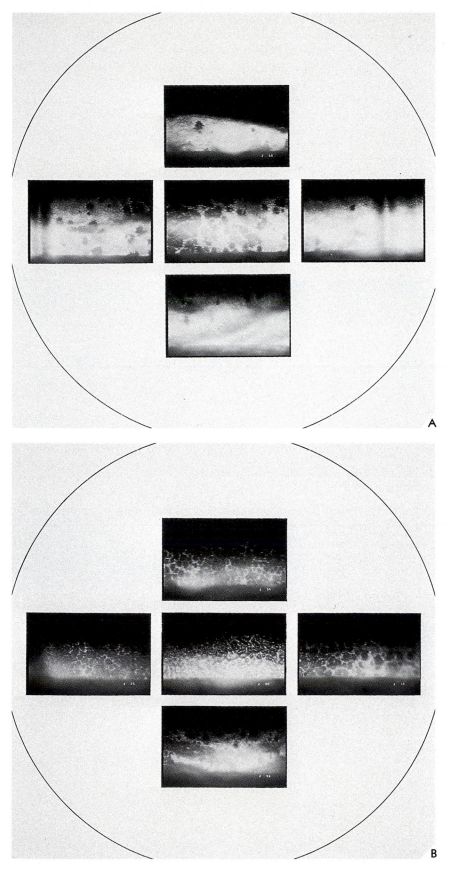

**7.9** | *A:* Widefield regional specular examination in a patient with moderate Fuchs dystrophy. Note the confluent guttata centrally, and relatively normal appearing cells in the midperiphery of the cornea. *B:* Widefield regional specular examination in a patient with severe Fuchs dystrophy. Note the confluent guttata centrally and throughout the midperiphery of the cornea.

the characteristic rounded, vesicular, band-shaped lesions circumscribed by areas of morphologically abnormal cell shapes seen in posterior polymorphous dystrophy[83–85] (Figs. 7.10A and 7.10B).

The iridocorneal endothelial (ICE) syndrome also demonstrates a characteristic specular microscopy appearance.[86,87] Although the early form of these endothelial abnormalities may be confused with cornea guttata, the corneal clarity and thickness typically are within normal limits. In addition, patients often have unilateral involvement but the other eye may also be involved.[88] Early in the disease there is rounding of the endothelial cells with loss of cell border clarity, increase in granularity of the intercellular details, and the appearance of small, dark areas which may enlarge and become completely blacked-out areas within the cell. As the disease progresses, the endothelial monolayer is no longer recognizable as a mosaic of cells and there may be a "reversal appearance" with black central areas and white borders as the cells overlap each other[86,87] (Figs. 7.2, 7.11A and 7.11B).

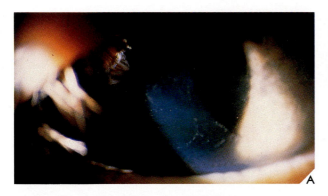 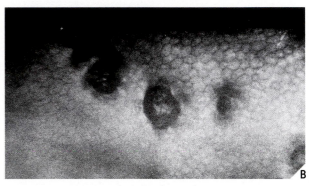

**7.10** | *A:* Slit-lamp appearance of posterior polymorphous dystrophy. *B:* Specular micrograph demonstrates round vesicles circumscribed by elongated abnormal cells.

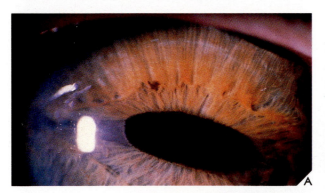 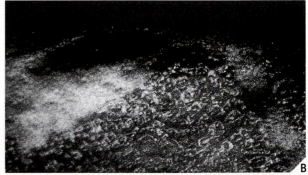

**7.11** | *A:* Slit-lamp appearance of ICE (Chandler) syndrome. *B:* Specular micrograph shows loss of cell border clarity, increased granularity, and blacked-out areas.

# 8 | PATHOPHYSIOLOGY OF CORNEAL ENDOTHELIAL DYSFUNCTION

## David B. Glasser

Maintenance of barrier and pump function is essential to the continued normal functioning of the corneal endothelium and ultimately to maintenance of corneal clarity. Endothelial dysfunction associated with medical and/or surgical problems occurs because of disruption of the endothelial barrier and pump via one of several mechanisms. Mechanical trauma, cell toxicity of therapeutic agents or their vehicles and preservatives, inflammation, and toxic byproducts of epithelial or endothelial metabolism are discussed in this chapter. Primary and secondary endotheliopathies associated with degenerations, dystrophies, and infectious processes are discussed elsewhere.

## TRAUMA

Mechanical trauma is the greatest single source of endothelial damage during intraocular surgery, assuming that no toxic solutions are placed inside the eye. The principal sources of mechanical trauma are endothelial contact with surgical instruments, the lens, the iris, or an intraocular lens implant. During phacoemulsification, lens fragments and air bubbles are ejected from the ultrasonic tip at high speeds and can damage the endothelium (Fig. 8.1). Ultrasonic energy itself is not harmful to

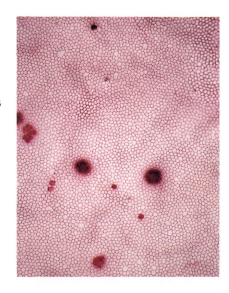

**8.1** | Vital-dye staining of rabbit cornea immediately after phacoemulsification shows areas of endothelial damage suggestive of impact craters from flying lens fragments or air bubbles ejected at high speed from the phacoemulsification tip.

the endothelium,[1,2] but warming from an inadequately cooled phacoemulsification tip can destroy endothelial cells and denature stromal proteins.

The denuded areas of Descemet's membrane that result from mechanical trauma have no endothelial pump or barrier function until wound healing occurs (Fig. 8.2). Healing begins with elongation and sliding of adjacent endothelial cells into the wounded area. Mitosis plays only a small role in human endothelial wound healing. A monolayer covering Descemet's membrane is reestablished within 3 days, at which time the endothelial barrier begins to function and corneal swelling begins to reverse. Pump sites are regenerated over the next 3 to 4 days, and corneal thickness returns to normal. Endothelial remodeling occurs and cell morphology normalizes, consisting of mostly hexagonal cells of fairly uniform size by 2 to 3 months.[3–5]

Remodeling may be delayed by prolonged inflammation or by iris-supported or closed-loop anterior chamber intraocular lens implants. These

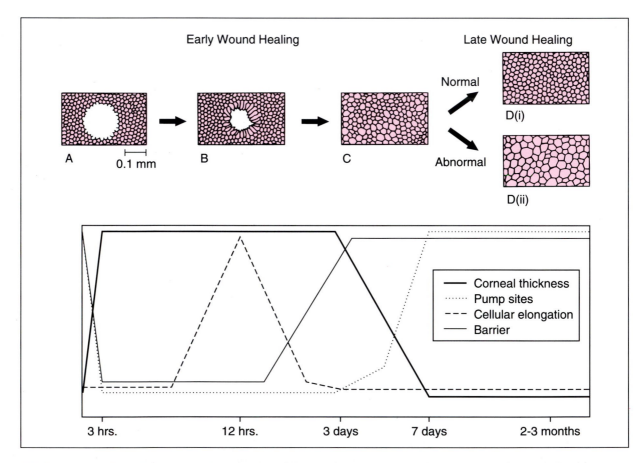

**8.2** | Schematic of events in early and late endothelial wound healing. *A:* Absence of cells immediately after injury. The endothelial pump and barrier functions are interrupted, and corneal thickness increases. *B:* Elongation and sliding of cells to cover the adjacent defect begins within 12 hours after injury. *C:* By 3 to 4 days the defect is covered and the endothelial monolayer is reestablished. Barrier function returns first, followed by an increase in pump sites. Corneal thickness and cellular elongation return to normal by 1 week. Variability in cell size (polymegathism) and shape (pleomorphism) persist until late wound healing occurs. *D.i:* Normal late wound healing consists of endothelial remodeling, resulting in cells of fairly uniform size and shape. Cell density is lower than before injury. The monolayer is stable but continues to lose cells slowly with age. *D.ii:* Abnormal late wound healing occurs if the endothelium continues to be stressed, as with chronic inflammation or an improperly fixated intraocular lens. Polymegathism and pleomorphism persist, and cell loss continues at an accelerated rate. If the underlying stress is not alleviated, corneal decompensation eventually will occur.

lenses may cause chronic inflammation or may act as a sink for the continued loss of endothelial cells at the lens footplates. Endothelial morphology remains abnormal and accelerated cell loss can occur in these instances. Cell loss continues throughout life, and the cornea remains clear by virtue of the tremendous cell reserve present from birth. Any surgical or nonsurgical insult shifts the cell loss curve towards decompensation[6] (Fig. 8.3). Even a slight increase in the rate of cell loss can significantly reduce the number of years before corneal decompensation occurs as the result of endothelial failure (Fig. 8.4). Unless the underlying source of endothelial stress is removed, the endothelial pump eventually will be unable to balance the increased leak through a damaged endothelial barrier. Patients with low cell densities or morphologic abnormalities of the endothelium (e.g., diabetics) are more susceptible to surgical trauma[7-10] and other stresses, such as contact lens wear,[11] which might result in corneal decompensation. Diabetics are also more likely to require cataract surgery or vitrectomy, and may require multiple procedures. It is particularly important to minimize trauma and other endothelial stresses in these patients.

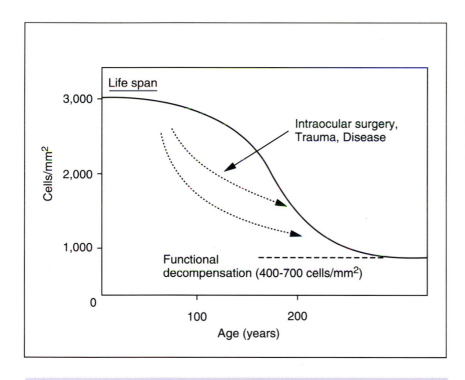

**8.3** | Endothelial cell density at birth is over 3,000 cells/mm², and declines at a constant rate thereafter. Corneal decompensation occurs at about 500 cells/mm², giving the cornea a useful life span of about 200 years. Any insult to the corneal endothelium will shorten the period of time before corneal decompensation occurs.

## Figure 8.4. Corneal Longevity

| Percentage of Cell Loss/Year | Longevity (Years) |
| --- | --- |
| 0.5 (Normal) | 200 |
| 1.0 | 100 |
| 2.0 | 50 |
| 3.0 | 33 |

## TOXICITY

All therapeutic agents, including their vehicles and preservatives, have the potential to injure the corneal endothelium. This potential for injury is much greater when an agent is used inside the eye than when it is applied externally because the concentrations to which the endothelium is exposed are much higher. A variety of surgical solutions are used to facilitate intraocular surgery. They include irrigating solutions, viscoelastics, mydriatics, miotics, glucose, tissue plasminogen activator (tPA), and thrombin. Endothelial toxicity can result from exposure to hyper- or hypotonic solutions and to alkaline or acidic pH. The corneal endothelium can tolerate osmolalities between 200 and 400 mOsm[12] and pH values between 6.8 and 8.2.[13] A lack of essential ions or metabolic substrates may interfere with intercellular junctional complexes and metabolism. Lack of calcium causes loss of the tight junctions between the endothelial cells and therefore leads to loss of the barrier function.[14,15] Glutathione is also needed for maintenance of cell junctions and plays a role in endothelial fluid transport.[16,17] The reduced form of glutathione protects endothelial cells from oxidative damage. Glucose is an essential energy source for maintenance of aerobic metabolism, with production of ATP for the $Na^+,K^+$ pump and NADPH to reduce glutathione.[18] Preservatives and detergents, although not deliberately added to surgical solutions, may also adversely affect the endothelium, usually by destroying cell junctions or by direct damage to the cell membrane.

Glucose, tPA, thrombin, antibiotics, steroids, and a host of other drugs have been suggested as useful intraocular agents or as additives to irrigating solutions. It must be emphasized that almost all drugs formulated for extraocular use contain vehicles, preservatives, antioxidants, and solubilizers that are not intended for intraocular use. The potential, therefore, exists for direct toxicity from the drug itself, its vehicle, preservatives, or any number of interactions that might alter the electrolyte balance, pH, or osmolality of the irrigation solution. The surgeon must be aware that such additives render the solution's formulation, stability, and toxicity unknown, and that use of such a solution constitutes an in-vivo human experiment. Accordingly, additives should be used only for specific indications, never "routinely."

## IRRIGATION SOLUTIONS

An essential component in most intraocular surgical procedures is the irrigation solution. The irrigant keeps the globe inflated and maintains normal pressure–volume relationships during surgery. The potential for damage to the corneal endothelium is related to the chemical composition, pH, and osmolality of the solution that bathes those tissues and to the endothelial contact time. As intraocular manipulations have become more complex, the duration and volume of irrigation have increased.[19] Despite a lack of controlled clinical studies, longer irrigation times, higher flow rates, and larger volumes are probably more traumatic to the corneal endothelium.[20] In addition, contact time between the endothelium and the irrigating solution is often underestimated, especially for short procedures. A solution may be in use for less than 30 minutes during cataract surgery. However, given the aqueous volume after cataract surgery with lens implantation, and assuming normal aqueous flow, McDermott et al[19] calculated that it takes over 4 hours for aqueous to replace the fluid left in the anterior chamber at the end of surgery. If surgery and postoperative medications (beta blockers, carbonic anhydrase inhibitors) reduce aqueous flow by 50%, it may take over 8 hours for the aqueous to turn over.

Normal saline was the predominant irrigant until Merrill, Fleming, and Girard[21] showed that its acidic pH of 6.8 and incomplete electrolyte balance were toxic to intraocular tissues.[21] The balanced salt solution (BSS) developed by Merrill and associates in 1960 has a stable but nonphysiologic citrate-acetate buffer, a pH of 7.5 to 8.2, and contains potassium, calcium, and magnesium chloride in addition to sodium chloride. This composition began to approximate that of aqueous humor (Fig. 8.5), but was still unable to maintain normal endothelial function and structure.[22] In 1972, Dikstein and Maurice[23] used in vitro perfusion techniques to show that a modified bicarbonate Ringer's solution containing glutathione, glucose, and adenosine (GBR) could preserve corneal endothelial function and ultrastructure. Edelhauser and associates,[24,25] using the same in vitro perfusion techniques, compared GBR to four other commonly used irrigants (normal saline, Plasma-lyte 148®, lactated Ringer's, and BSS). In each case GBR was superior at maintaining corneal endothelial function (as measured by corneal swelling rates) and ultrastructure. However, commercial formulation of a stable GBR solution was difficult because of the instability of reduced glutathione, adenosine, and bicarbonate. To circumvent these problems, BSS Plus® (Alcon Laboratories, Fort Worth, TX) was formulated to be as similar to GBR and aqueous humor as possible (see Fig. 8.5) while maintaining pharmacologic stability. BSS Plus is a two-component, bicarbonate-buffered electrolyte solution containing oxidized glutathione and glucose but no adenosine. Once reconstituted, the solution maintains a physiologic pH for 6 to 24 hours.[19,26]

## Figure 8.5. Chemical Composition* of Human Aqueous Humor, BSS Plus, BSS, and SMA$_2$

| | HUMAN AQUEOUS HUMOR | BSS PLUS | BSS | SMA$_2$ |
|---|---|---|---|---|
| Sodium | 162.9 | 160.0 | 155.7 | 145.7 |
| Potassium | 2.2–3.9 | 5.0 | 10.1 | 4.8 |
| Calcium | 1.8 | 1.0 | 3.3 | 1.2 |
| Magnesium | 1.1 | 1.0 | 1.5 | — |
| Chloride | 131.6 | 130.0 | 128.9 | 120.1 |
| Bicarbonate | 20.15 | 25.0 | — | 25.0 |
| Phosphate | 0.62 | 3.0 | — | — |
| Lactate | 2.5 | — | — | — |
| Glucose | 2.7–3.7 | 5.0 | — | 8.3 |
| Ascorbate | 1.06 | — | — | — |
| Glutathione | 0.0019 | 0.3 | — | — |
| Citrate | 0.12 | — | 5.8 | 3.4 |
| Acetate | — | — | 28.6 | 4.4 |
| pH | 7.38 | 7.4 | 7.6 | 7.3 |
| Osmolality (mOsm) | 304 | 305 | 298 | 290 |

*All concentrations are in millimoles or milliequivalents/liter.

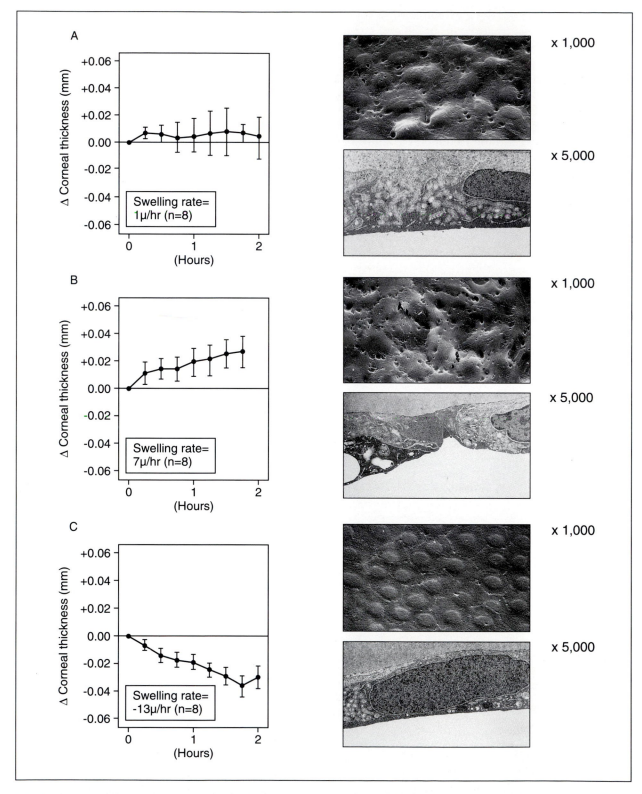

**8.6** | Corneal swelling and scanning and transmission electron micrographs of corneal endothelial cells after in vitro perfusion of human donor corneas at 37°C. *A:* BSS: Corneas swell at 1 μ/hr. Electron micrographs show endothelial swelling, clarified cytoplasm, and dilated intercellular spaces. *B:* SMA₂: Corneas swell at 7 μ/hr. Electron micrographs show disruption of intercellular junctions, rounding up of endothelial cells, and cytoplasmic vacuoles. *C:* BSS Plus: Corneas deswell at 13 μ/hr due to the temperature reversal effect, demonstrating normal endothelial function. Electron micrographs show normal regular hexagonal cells with normal junctional complexes and normal intracellular organelles.

BSS Plus maintains normal endothelial structure and function during in-vitro perfusions of human donor corneas (Fig. 8.6), whereas BSS and SMA$_2$® (Senju Pharmaceutical Co., Osaka, Japan) do not.[22,27] In vivo anterior chamber irrigations in cats and monkeys confirm that BSS and SMA$_2$ can reversibly stress the endothelium, inducing corneal swelling after 1 hour and abnormal cell morphology after as little as 15 minutes of irrigation.[20,22] BSS Plus prevents changes in cell morphology and corneal swelling after irrigations lasting 2 hours. These differing effects are probably related to the different buffers used in the solutions. Bicarbonate (in BSS Plus) is the major buffer present in aqueous and is effective in the physiologic pH range of 6.0 to 8.0. Citrate-acetate (in BSS and SMA$_2$) buffers most effectively between pH 3.6 and 6.2. Citrate may also chelate calcium, thereby disrupting cell junctions and barrier function.[14,15] Araie[28] has shown that endothelial permeability is substantially increased after perfusion with SMA$_2$. This suggests that the corneal swelling seen in SMA$_2$ perfused corneas (see Fig. 8.6) is due in part to compromised endothelial barrier function. Increased permeability is consistent with the disruption of intercellular junctions seen in scanning and transmission electron micrographs of corneal endothelium after perfusion with SMA$_2$ and BSS (see Fig. 8.6). The paucity of lateral cell membrane area (where the Na$^+$,K$^+$-ATPase pump is located) and the presence of abnormal mitochondria in these corneas suggest a decrease in endothelial pumping capacity as well. Other chemical differences between the solutions (see Fig. 8.5) that may play a role include the presence of glutathione and glucose in BSS Plus. In 1988, McDermott et al[19] summarized the requirements for a state-of-the-art irrigating solution as follows: pH of 7.4, osmolality between 300 and 310 mOsm, bicarbonate buffer, glucose, glutathione, and pertinent electrolytes.

Many studies have been published evaluating the effects of irrigating solutions on rabbit corneal endothelium, but few clinical studies have compared BSS with BSS Plus in humans. The rabbit eye is young, presumed free of disease, has the capacity for endothelial cell regeneration, and can withstand great metabolic stresses. Conclusions about rabbit tissue may not reflect the behavior of human tissue 60 to 70 years old. Therefore, use of drugs or solutions shown to be safe for rabbit endothelium may still result in damage to some human patients. Kline and associates[29] found significantly less endothelial cell loss with BSS Plus (15.4%) than with BSS (22.7%) in 100 patients after extracapsular cataract surgery and posterior chamber lens implantation performed without viscoelastic. However, the use of narrow-field specular microscopy (with its inherent high sampling error) to calculate endothelial cell density (ECD) and the relatively high mean cell loss compared to other reports (8% after similar surgical procedures)[30] make it difficult to generalize these results. Rosenfeld and associates[31] were unable to demonstrate any difference in cell loss between use of BSS and BSS Plus use during vitrectomy. Part of the difficulty in demonstrating significant differences in cell loss in clinical studies that compare BSS and BSS Plus is related to the large sampling errors inherent in the use of small patient groups and small numbers of cells to determine cell density.[32,33] In addition, follow-up times for most clinical studies may be too short to detect significant changes in ECD. Cell loss associated with the mechanical trauma of surgery is probably too great to allow more subtle changes associated with an irrigating solution to be detected during the early postoperative period.

Another area of concern is the proper temperature of the irrigation solution. Although 37°C is physiologic, the risk of overheating the irrigant presents a substantial danger to intraocular tissues. Accelerated metabolic activity with increased glucose and oxygen consumption, and even denaturation of some proteins, might occur at temperatures just a few degrees above 37°C. Cooling irrigation solutions to reduce inflammation and metabolic effects has also been proposed. Although probably safer than heating, cooling of these solutions has not been shown to be of benefit. Until in-line temperature sensors and control systems are developed to regulate strictly solution temperature, room temperature irrigants present less risk.

A final source of endothelial toxicity from irrigation solutions comes from formulation errors, packaging problems, and contamination. Filamentous fungi, yeasts, and anaerobic bacteria have been isolated from various irrigation solutions and corneal storage media in recent years.[34-37] Container failures and manufacturing errors have been implicated as sources of contamination. An epidemic of *Candida parapsilosis* endophthalmitis demonstrated that a single lot of contaminated irrigation solution may cause widely dispersed cases of postoperative endophthalmitis, many of which may be delayed in onset or difficult to diagnose.[36,37] It is, therefore, advisable to inspect visually the irrigation solution before surgery to ensure clarity and container integrity. Reuse of irrigation solutions significantly increases the risk of contamination. Irrigation solutions contain no preservatives and are designed to be used immediately after opening. Reuse contradicts all standard infection control principles and increases the chance for error in the operating room. The reliability, safety, and resistance to breakage of filters and devices designed to allow the use of a single bottle of solution on several patients are unknown. Poor packaging led to the recall in 1983 of 500-ml bottles of BSS after reports of corneal decompensation linked to its use. Analysis of the solution revealed a pH of 9.1.[38] Irreversible endothelial damage occurs with exposure to solutions outside a pH range of 6.5 and 8.5.[13] The glass used to package the solution reacted with the irrigant, resulting in an alkaline pH shift during storage. Improper formulation and variations in quality control resulted in intraoperative endothelial cell edema and temporary corneal clouding during use of another brand of BSS in 1988. Samples of the solution were shown to induce reversible endothelial cell edema in rabbit and human donor corneas in the laboratory.[19] The osmolality of the solution ranged from 217 to 402 mOsm/L, and the pH ranged from 6.3 to 7.2.[19,39] Although endothelial cells might survive exposure to osmolalities and pH values in this range,[12,13] the status of the endothelium at the time it is exposed to such a solution can determine the extent of the damage. A normal cornea may respond to a hypotonic solution with reversible endothelial cell edema, whereas a cornea with a low cell count will develop stromal edema due to junctional breakdown (Fig. 8.7).

## VISCOELASTIC SOLUTIONS

Viscoelastics are used for protection of the corneal endothelium and for manipulation of tissues during anterior segment surgery. They were initially developed as vitreous substitutes, but have been supplanted by the use of intraocular gases and silicone oil in vitrectomy surgery. Wide clinical experience with these solutions suggests that they are effective and well tolerated in anterior segment surgery. Sodium hyaluronate (Healon®, Kabi Pharmacia, Piscataway, NJ; Amvisc®, Med-Chem Products, Woburn, MA), chondroitin sulfate/sodium hyaluronate (Viscoat®, Alcon Laboratories, Fort Worth, TX), and hydroxypropyl methylcellulose-based viscous solutions are nontoxic to cat endothelial cells under conditions analogous to cataract surgery in humans.[40] These solutions do not significantly bind drugs commonly used in the perioperative period.[41] Problems associated with viscous solutions have been related to increased intraocular pressure (IOP), formulation problems, and intraocular inflammation.

All viscoelastics have the potential to raise IOP to dangerous levels.[42–47] The peak pressure usually occurs within 6 to 8 hours after surgery, so studies using measurements 24 hours after surgery may miss the pressure rise.[40,46–49] The mechanism responsible for the increase in IOP is probably related to a decrease in outflow facility. Sodium hyaluronate (and probably other viscous solutions) is eliminated from the anterior chamber primarily through the trabecular meshwork.[50,51] Berson and associates[50] found a 65% decrease in aqueous outflow facility after anterior chamber injection of 1% sodium hyaluronate into enucleated human eyes. Anterior chamber washout does not eliminate the decrease in outflow facility,[50] but it does decrease the level and

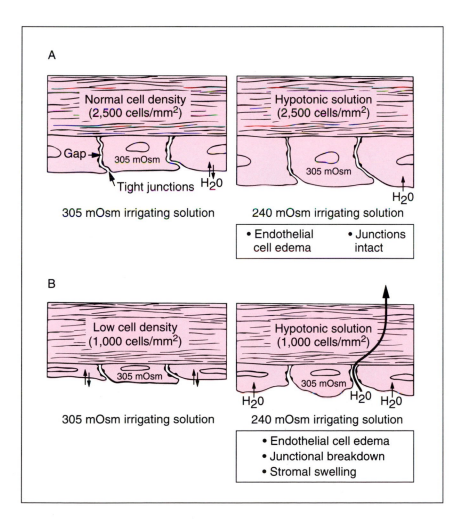

**8.7** | *A:* Normal corneal endothelium exposed to hypotonic irrigation solution will develop intracellular edema without junctional breakdown. If the osmotic stress is not too great (i.e., osmolality between 200 and 400 mOsm), the cell will volume-regulate and resume normal functioning within minutes. *B:* Endothelium with a low cell density exposed to hypotonic irrigation solution may develop junctional breakdown because the cell is thin, with little lateral cell membrane to begin with. Stromal edema results. (Adapted from McDermott ML, Edelhauser HF, Hack HM, Langston RHS: Ophthalmic irrigants: A current review and update. *Ophthalmic Surg 1988;19:724–733.*)

duration of the postoperative pressure rise (Fig. 8.8).[40] Therefore, viscous solutions should be washed out or aspirated at the end of surgery in all cases. Viscoat requires more meticulous aspiration (in all quadrants of the anterior chamber) than other viscous solutions. Removal of the viscous solution will not prevent the intraocular pressure rise in all cases,[47] so the use of intraocular carbachol, topical apraclonidine, or a systemic carbonic anhydrase inhibitor is also recommended for IOP control during the first 24 hours after surgery. We have been less impressed with the ability of topical beta blockers to prevent postoperative pressure rises. A study by West and associates[52] suggests that topical levobunolol may be more effective than timolol or betaxolol given immediately after surgery. However, possible technical differences between the three participating surgeons in this study were not analyzed.

Several cases of severe IOP elevation occuring days to weeks after the use of a polyacrylamide viscoelastic (Orcolon®) led to the recall of the product in 1991. According to the manufacturer, the mechanism of pressure elevation in these cases was the formation of microgels during preparation and delivery of the product. Changes in the preparation of the product are being considered to eliminate the formation of microgels.

The ionic composition of the vehicle used to formulate a viscous solution is an important determinant of endothelial toxicity in tissue culture.[53] Currently available viscous solutions are formulated in phosphate-buffered saline (Healon), physiologic saline (Amvisc), phosphate-buffered water (Viscoat), and balanced salt solution (Occucoat®, Storz Ophthalmics, St. Louis, MO). They all are nontoxic to the endothelium when injected into the anterior chamber in vivo.[40] An early formulation of Viscoat did result in several cases of calcific deposits in the corneal stroma and Bowman's membrane after cataract surgery.[54,55] Calcium precipitation was attributed to excessive

**8.8** | Intraocular pressure after anterior chamber injection of viscoelastics in the cat. Upper four curves, no washout of viscoelastic. Lower four curves, viscoelastic washed out. Note that the pressure rise is less pronounced and of shorter duration if the viscoelastic is washed out. (From Glasser DB, Matsuda M, Edelhauser HF: A comparison of the efficacy and toxicity of the intraocular pressure response to viscous solutions in the anterior chamber. *Arch Ophthalmol* 1986;104:1819–1824. Copyright 1986, American Medical Association.)

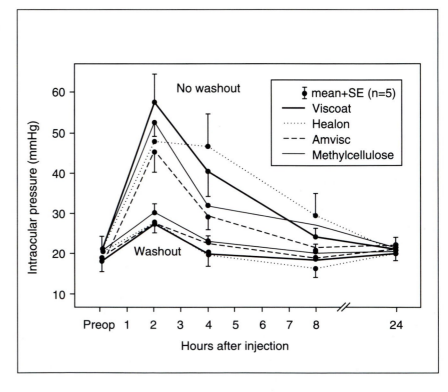

phosphate concentration (93 mM) in the Viscoat vehicle. Reformulated Viscoat contains less phosphate (18 mM), and there have been no further reports of calcium deposition.

Human donor corneas covered with Healon demonstrated significant cell death after 30 minutes, and almost complete cell death after 2 hours. Hyndiuk and Slack,[56] therefore, recommend the use of corneal preservation medium rather than viscoelastic material to cover the endothelial surface of trephined donor corneas while the host bed is prepared. The cause of cell damage is not known, but may be due to transmission of shearing forces to cell membranes or to inability of nutrients to diffuse through the viscoelastic to the endothelial cells.

Commercially available highly purified viscoelastics are nonantigenic according to the manufacturers and to studies by Richter and associates.[57,58] However, intrastromal injection of Healon, Amvisc, or Viscoat induces a mild acute inflammatory reaction in rabbit corneas.[59,60] Injection of sodium hyaluronate into the vitreous of owl monkeys produces inflammation that varies with the batch of viscoelastic used and which is independent of concentration or source of the material.[61] Clinical inflammatory reactions related to the use of viscous solutions are uncommon. They can occur because of impurities or deficiencies in formulation. As early as 1959, Fleming et al[62] reported that a 0.5% solution of methylcellulose in balanced salt produces no inflammatory or foreign-body reaction after injection into the anterior chamber of rabbit eyes, whereas 0.5% methylcellulose in physiologic saline produces iridocyclitis. Clinical reports of severe intraocular inflammation after cataract surgery with Viscoat led to a recall in 1987.[63] The inflammation was probably caused by the presence of endotoxins or other protein impurities present in the viscoelastic, despite the fact that the lots involved met standards for purity. A tightening of standards corrected the problem. This episode highlights the difficulty manufacturers may have in detecting and eliminating impurities in long-chain, high molecular weight proteins from biological sources. Another potential source of inflammation is the reuse of cannulas that have been used to inject viscoelastics. These cannulas may retain toxic detergents, as discussed below.

A host of new viscous solutions based on sodium hyaluronate, chondroitin sulfate, HPMC, polyacrylamide, and collagen are being developed. An ideal viscoelastic should effectively protect and manipulate tissues. It should be uniform from one lot to the next, inexpensive, and easy to manufacture and purify. It should contain no antigenic proteins. Its viscosity should decrease within 1 hour through dissolution or metabolism into components that do not impede aqueous outflow or raise IOP. It should be formulated in a balanced salt solution that mimics as closely as possible the composition of aqueous humor.

## MYDRIATICS

Repeated application of topical phenylephrine was used to maintain pupillary dilatation in the early 1970s during lengthy vitrectomy procedures. This was abandoned because of corneal clouding and endothelial toxicity of commercial preparations containing a nonphysiologic buffered vehicle and benzalkonium chloride.[64–66]

Intraocular epinephrine has been the mydriatic of choice for most ophthalmologists for over a decade. In 1972 and 1982, reports of corneal edema after its use led to studies of the effects of commercially available epinephrine preparations on the corneal endothelium.[67,68] Toxicity of 1:1,000 and 1:10,000 solutions formulated for intravascular or intracardiac use was determined to be due to the presence of sodium bisulfite (a preservative–antioxidant), acidic pH of 3–4, and a nonphysiologic buffer (citrate) with high buffering capacity. Addition of 1 ml of 1:1,000 (not 1:10,000) epinephrine to at least 5 to 15 ml of BSS or BSS Plus to dilute the preservative and buffer was recommended. Buffer capacity, and therefore resistance to neutralization of pH, varied considerably from one manufacturer's preparation to the next. McDermott and associates[19] demonstrated that 1:1,000 epinephrine from certain manufacturers (Parke-Davis, Morris Plains, NJ; Elkins-Sinn, Cherry Hill, NJ) diluted to a final concentration of 1:500,000 in BSS Plus is nontoxic and maintains normal endothelial function during 3 hour perfusions of isolated human corneas. Slack and colleagues[69] showed that a preservative-free, sulfite-free brand of 1:1,000 epinephrine (American Regent Laboratories, Shirley, New York) was able to maintain normal endothelial pumping function and ultrastructure during perfusion after dilution to a final concentration of 1:250,000. We recommend 0.5 ml of 1:1,000 epinephrine from one of the above manufacturers added to 500 ml of BSS Plus. The resulting concentration of epinephrine (1:1,000,000) will dilate the pupil within 1 minute without compromising endothelial function.

## MIOTICS

Coles[70] has shown that pilocarpine is toxic to the endothelium, and that its intraocular use should be avoided. Sympatholytic agents such as thymoxamine and dapiprazole have been recommended for intracameral use in selected cases.[71,72] However, these agents are not commercially available and have not yet undergone the type of rigorous toxicity testing, including perfusions of human donor corneas, used to evaluate other intraocular solutions. Currently available intraocular miotics include Miochol® (Iolab Pharmaceuticals, Claremont, CA) and Miostat® (Alcon Laboratories, Fort Worth, TX). In their current formulations, Miochol is a 1% solution of acetylcholine in mannitol and water, and Miostat is a 0.01% solution of carbachol in BSS (Fig. 8.9).[73–75] Yee and Edelhauser[76] found corneal swelling and ultrastructural endothelial changes during perfusion of human corneas with Miochol, whereas Miostat prevented corneal swelling and endothelial toxicity. They attributed this difference to the more physiologic vehicle used to formulate Miostat. In contrast, Birnbaum et al[77] did find reversible corneal swelling without ultrastructural changes during perfusion with Miostat. However, this study used rabbit rather than human tissue, and no comparison with the current formulation of Miochol was made. There are no clinical reports of endothelial toxicity related to current formulations of either Miochol or Miostat. The choice of miotic should be based primarily on the desired clinical

## Figure 8.9. Intraocular Miotics

|  | **MIOCHOL** | **MIOSTAT** |
| --- | --- | --- |
| Miotic | 1.0% acetylcholine | 0.01% carbachol |
| Vehicle | 3.0% mannitol/water | Balanced salt solution |
| pH/osmolality | Physiologic | Physiologic |
| Onset of miosis | Under 1 minute | 2 minutes |
| Duration of miosis | 10–20 minutes | 2–24 hours |
| Pressure lowering | 1–6 hours | 1–3 days |

effects (see Fig. 8.9). If endothelial toxicity is of particular concern, the formulation and laboratory evidence suggest that Miostat is more physiologic.

Intraocular use of drugs originally intended for extraocular use should be avoided whenever possible. Almost all drugs formulated for topical, intravenous, intracardiac, or intratracheal use contain preservatives and other chemicals that are toxic to the endothelium or may adversely affect the physiologic balance of the ocular irrigant.

Sodium bisulfite, a preservative/antioxidant, was the endothelial toxin responsible for cases of corneal edema associated with epinephrine use discussed above.[67,68] Other preservatives present in drugs include propyl- and methylparabens, benzalkonium chloride, cetylpiridium chloride, benzyl alcohol, chlorhexidine, and thimerosal. All have been shown to affect adversely endothelial structure and function, particularly benzalkonium chloride.[78–84] Preserved solutions should not be used within the eye. Experimental studies have demonstrated endothelial damage after subconjunctival injections[83] and topical drops[79] due to toxicity of the preservatives benzalkonium chloride, sodium bisulfite, and methyl- and propylparabens. Lemp and Zimmerman[84] have reported a case of endothelial decompensation due to chronic topical use of benzalkonium chloride-preserved artificial tears. Corneal decompensation associated with the placement of collagen shields soaked in undiluted tobramycin and steroid at the conclusion of cataract surgery has also been reported.[85] Increased penetration of the therapeutic agents and their preservatives due to the presence of the collagen shield may have resulted in endothelial damage. Detergents are also highly toxic to the corneal endothelium. Benzalkonium chloride, a preservative and cationic detergent, is toxic at concentrations of only 0.0001%.[82] Nuyts and associates[86] demonstrated loss of endothelial barrier function in human donor corneas after exposure to concentrations of a nonionic detergent used for instrument cleaning as low as 0.06%. At higher concentrations, detergents can cause cell membrane lysis and fusion (Fig 8.10).

Another potential source of preservative and detergent toxicity is reuse of instruments and irrigation tubing. Human corneal endothelium can withstand exposure to levels of ethylene oxide and its reaction products, ethylene glycol and ethylene chlorohydrin, that are 25 times higher than those recommended for ophthalmics by the Food and Drug Administration. However,

## PRESERVATIVES AND DETERGENTS

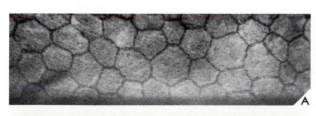
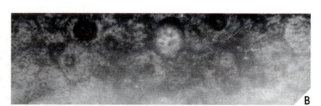
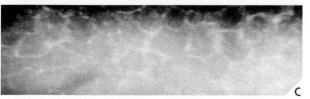

**8.10** | Specular microscopy of human donor endothelium after perfusion with 1.0% detergent for 3 minutes. *A:* Normal endothelium at beginning of exposure. *B:* Eleven minutes after exposure; endothelial cell edema has developed. *C:* Thirty minutes after exposure; total destruction of the endothelial mosaic has occurred. (From Nuyts MMA, Edelhauser HF, Pels E, Breebaart AC: Toxic effects of detergents on the corneal endothelium. *Arch Ophthalmol 1998;108:1158.* Copyright 1990, American Medical Association.)

ethylene oxide gas sterilization of plastic irrigation tubing may cause release of complex compounds (plasticizers, clarifiers, monomers, polymers) that can combine with sterilant residues, resulting in toxicity[87] or inflammation.[88] Kim[89] reported three cases of iritis and corneal decompensation after cataract surgery due to toxicity from thimerosal residues in reused viscoelastic cannulas. Breebaart and associates[90] reported 18 cases of severe postoperative corneal edema caused by a nonionic ethoxylated fatty acid detergent residue in reused irrigation cannulas. These reports suggest that reuse of instruments and cannulas should be avoided when possible, and that particular care must be taken in cleaning and rinsing reusable instruments.

Toxicity of scrub solutions is also related to the presence of a detergent, as well as to inherent toxicity of the antiseptic itself, to concentration, and to contact time. Reports of keratitis resulting from accidental exposure to Hibiclens® (Stuart Pharmaceuticals, Wilmington, DE) highlight the potential for toxicity if the scrub solution is allowed to enter the conjunctival sac.[91-94] Phinney and associates[92] reported five patients accidentally exposed to Hibiclens who presented with symptoms of pain and decreased vision. A large corneal epithelial defect was usually present, although punctate keratitis was described in one patient. Stromal edema and vascularization developed and progressed over a period of 2 to 10 weeks. Intrastromal hemorrhages occurred in areas of stromal neovascularization in one patient. Two patients developed irreversible bullous keratopathy and required penetrating keratoplasty. The edema cleared within 6 to 7 months in the remaining three patients, leaving reduced endothelial cell density and mild stromal scarring. Two of five patients had decreased corneal sensation. Hamed and associates[91] reported stromal thinning and ectasia in two cases with persistent epithelial defects treated with steroids. Dense irreversible corneal scarring occurred in both cases. In contrast, Shore[94] reported two cases of accidental Hibiclens exposure which were limited to epithelial involvement and which recovered without sequellae within 5 days. The benign course was attributed to routine irrigation of the conjunctival sac with balanced salt solution after the skin preparation. It is noteworthy that eight of the nine reported cases of severe keratitis occurred in association with nonocular surgery performed by nonophthalmologists. The paucity of cases related to ophthalmic procedures may be related to the tendency of many ophthalmologists to irrigate the conjunctival sac at the end of the preparation.[95] Irrigation reduces contact time and the potential for toxicity.

Hibiclens contains chlorhexidine gluconate 4% in a detergent vehicle and has bactericidal activity against a wide range of gram-positive and gram-negative bacteria. Chlorhexidine itself is toxic to corneal epithelium and endothelium, and penetration may be enhanced by the detergent present in Hibiclens.[78,91] Chlorhexidine also binds to stromal proteins and is slowly released, which may explain the progressive course of stromal edema and vascularization noted in the clinical reports.[78] MacRae and associates[96] studied the ocular toxicity of a number of antiseptics and found marked corneal deepithelialization, conjunctival chemosis, and anterior stromal edema in rabbits treated with Hibiclens, tincture of iodine, 3% hexachlorophene with detergent (pHisoHex®, Winthrop-Breon, New York, NY), 70% ethanol and 7.5% povidone-iodine with detergent (Betadine Surgical Scrub®, Purdue Frederick, Norwalk, CT). Only 10% povidone-iodine *without detergent* (Betadine Solution®) prevented the severe toxic reactions seen with the other antiseptics in this study.

Corneal toxicity from antiseptic solutions is a potentially blinding complication. Because the potential for corneal exposure to the scrub solution cannot be completely eliminated, we recommend the use of a nontoxic antiseptic: 10% povidone-iodine *without detergent* (Betadine *Solution*). This solution is germicidal against a broad range of gram-positive and gram-negative bacteria, fungi, yeasts, viruses, and protozoa. Apt and associates[97] placed half-strength (5%) povidone-iodine without detergent directly into the conjunctival sac before ocular surgery in 30 patients. They found no significant toxicity and a 91% reduction in colonies cultured. This solution is now available commercially (Escalon Ophthalmics, Skillman, NJ). In addition, we recommend irrigation of the conjunctival sac after completion of the skin prep if the antiseptic used is potentially toxic or contains a detergent.

## GLUCOSE

In diabetic patients, intraoperative posterior subcapsular opacification can be prevented by adding glucose to the BSS Plus used during vitrectomy.[98,99] Addition of 3 ml of 50% dextrose (in sterile water with no preservatives) to a 500-ml bottle of BSS Plus increases its osmolality to 330 mOsm. This maintains osmotic equilibrium between the solution and the lens and prevents subcapsular clouding. This modification of BSS Plus appears to be nontoxic.[99]

## TISSUE PLASMINOGEN ACTIVATOR (tPA)

Human recombinant tPA can dissolve experimental hyphemas and fibrin clots in the anterior chamber and vitreous of rabbits without apparent toxicity to the lens, cornea, or retina, and with no increase in IOP or inflammation.[100–103] Intracameral injection of tPA (25 μg) has been used to treat successfully three aphakic patients who developed severe intraocular fibrin formation within 24 hours after vitrectomy surgery.[104] Subconjunctival tPA has also been successful in lysing a clot within a filtering bleb after trabeculectomy.[105] Some concerns for toxicity remain. Fibrin degradation products are toxic to rabbit corneal endothelial cells and are chemotactic for leukocytes.[106] Further studies of effects on human endothelium and lens are needed. Systemic hemorrhage is not expected with the low doses of tPA employed in intraocular therapy, but intraocular hemorrhage has been reported.[107]

## THROMBIN

Commercial preparations of bovine thrombin designed for topical application have been added to irrigation solutions and used during vitrectomy for diabetic retinopathy and retinopathy of prematurity, trabeculectomy for neovascular glaucoma, and keratoplasty in a vascularized recipient bed.[108–110] Although thrombin (100 U/ml) is effective for reducing intraoperative and postoperative bleeding, it is associated with a 20% incidence of severe postoperative inflammation with sterile hypopyon formation and fibrin deposition.[108]

McDermott and co-workers[111] investigated the toxicity of two commercially available thrombin preparations: Thrombinar® (Armour Pharmaceutical, Blue Bell, PA) and Thrombostat® (Parke-Davis, Morris Plains, NJ). Gel electrophoresis exhibited multiple peaks suggestive of proteins other than thrombin that might be immunogenic. Particulate analysis demonstrated from 700 (Thrombinar) to 21,000 (Thrombostat) 5–20-μm particles per ml of 100 U/ml solution. In addition, 100 U/ml solutions of Thrombostat contain 78 mg/dl of glycine. Serum glycine levels in excess of only 30 mg/dl have been associated with temporary graying of vision and electroretinographic changes in patients undergoing bladder irrigation after prostate surgery.[112] Therefore, Thrombostat should not be used inside the eye.

Sheep and rabbit corneas exposed to 100 U/ml and 1,000 U/ml concentrations of thrombin showed no damage with vital-dye staining in two studies.[110,113] However, thrombin solutions containing 1,000 U/ml are hyperosmotic, and perfusion of human donor corneas with this concentration causes intracellular vacuolization and disruption of junctions between endothelial cells. The pH and osmolality of a 100 U/ml solution of Thrombinar in BSS Plus are physiologic. Perfusion of human donor corneas with this solution significantly inhibits corneal deswelling but does not cause ultrastructural damage to endothelial cells.[111]

Human thrombin (80 U/ml) has been infused continuously during vitrectomy in eight patients without a marked increase in inflammation or development of sterile hypopyon after surgery.[114] Although this solution was free of nonhuman proteins, it was not tested for presence of nonthrombin proteins, particulate contamination, or endothelial toxicity. There is also the need to ensure against transmission of hepatitis and human immunodeficiency virus when thrombin derived from human blood is used.

Concern for the purity, immunogenicity, and toxicity of currently available thrombin preparations has led Aaberg[115] to comment that intraocular thrombin must be used prudently as an adjunct during uncontrolled hemorrhage or as prophylaxis to prevent hemorrhage. Intermittent injection of limited quantities of thrombin at sites of uncontrolled bleeding, followed by thorough washout, may reduce but will not eliminate the potential for inflammatory reactions and endothelial toxicity. Therefore, conventional techniques for control of bleeding, such as tamponade, are preferred.

## TISSUE ADHESIVES

Fibrin, thrombin, collagen, muscle-activated protein, and cyanoacrylates all have been considered as tissue glues. At present, Histoacryl Blue (n-butyl-2-cyanoacrylate) is commonly used in the treatment of small wound dehiscences and corneal perforations. The product is not available in the United States. Krazy Glue® (methyl-2-cyanoacrylate), which is available, is considered too toxic for clinical applications.[116] Polymerization of cyanoacrylate adhesives is initiated by water or weak bases on the surface to which it is applied. The polymer then gradually degrades into formaldehyde and an alkylcyanoacetate. Lower-order cyanoacrylates degrade faster than the higher-order molecules, resulting in more rapid release of formaldehyde. This is presumed to be the reason for the increased toxicity associated with the lower molecular weight cyanoacrylates.[117,118] Impurities may also contribute to the toxic effects.[118] A localized polymorphonuclear inflammatory response followed by a foreign body granuloma occurs in the cornea after topical or intracorneal application,[119–121] and may result in corneal neovascularization.[122] Results of experimental anterior chamber injections of cyanoacrylates have been variable, including no anterior chamber reaction,[123] self-limited iritis with fibrovascular plaque formation on the the cornea and iris with endothelial cell damage,[124] and severe inflammation with corneal opacification, vascularization, and deformation and obliteration of the chamber angle.[125] The range of toxicities is probably dose related.

Accidental anterior chamber instillation of cyanoacrylate during repair of a corneal transplant wound dehiscence resulted in corneal graft failure. However, remaining ocular structures were intact after removal of the adhesive and repeat grafting.[126] Cataract formation due to polymerization of the adhesive directly over the lens in an eye with a flat anterior chamber can be avoided by using a small corneal or scleral tissue patch to close a large perforation with adhesive.[127] This will also prevent significant amounts of adhesive from entering the anterior chamber.

## SILICONE OIL

Silicone oils comprise a variety of silicone fluids with various radical side chains and chain lengths that may be used as vitreous replacements. Low molecular weight constituents and other chemical impurities are present in clinically used silicone oils. No single standard defines medical-grade silicone oil, so comparisons of clinical and experimental results are difficult and must be considered in light of the source of the silicone oil used. Early reports of ocular tolerance of silicone oils have been supplanted by reports of keratopathy, glaucoma, lens opacification, and retinopathy. Anterior chamber injection of silicone oil in rabbits and cats resulted in retrocorneal membrane formation, endothelial cell loss of 40%, and corneal thinning.[128] The mechanism of damage may be the presence of a barrier to nutrition from the aqueous humor. Band keratopathy, stromal opacification and vascularization, and bullous keratopathy have been reported clinically after the use of silicone oil.[129–133]

## INTRAOCULAR AIR AND GAS

Air can be used to maintain the anterior chamber or, in posterior segment procedures, to facilitate closure of retinal breaks. Other gases, such as sulfur hexafluoride and the perfluorocarbons, are also used in the posterior segment. Experimental studies have demonstrated endothelial cell toxicity and cell loss associated with contact with air, sulfur hexafluoride, and perfluorocarbon gases.[134–139] The mechanism of damage may be related to surface tension at the edge of the gas bubble or to a mechanical barrier to nutrients.[134]

## INFLAMMATION

Inflammation can affect endothelial function by reversibly interfering with the endothelial pump and barrier functions or by destroying endothelial cells. In most cases of uveitis there is temporary compromise of endothelial function, with increased corneal thickness but no decrease in cell density.[140] Polymorphonuclear leukocytes can release prostaglandins, hydrolytic enzymes, and superoxides, all of which can adversely affect the endothelium

(Fig. 8.11). Steroids can prevent the loss of endothelial pump and barrier function associated with intraocular inflammation.[141] Control of inflammation in the postoperative period is important because the endothelium may be more susceptible to the toxic effects of inflammatory mediators during the early wound-healing response.

## METABOLIC DYSFUNCTION

The effects of hypoxia and toxic metabolites produced by the epithelium and endothelium are commonly seen in contact lens wearers. Contact lenses that do not provide enough oxygen permeability to maintain normal aerobic metabolism cause a shift to anaerobic pathways, with build-up of stromal lactic acid and $CO_2$ and a decrease in pH. Hypoxia induced by contact lens wear also stimulates production of the cytochrome P450 arachidonate metabolite 12(R)HETE, a potent inhibitor of corneal $Na^+$,$K^+$-ATPase.[142] The resulting clinical changes include the endothelial bleb response, endothelial dysfunction, and increased corneal thickness (Fig. 8.12).[143–146] These acute changes are reversible when normal oxygen levels are restored. However, chronic hypoxia may cause the formation of epithelial microcysts, which take months to resolve, and endothelial polymegathism and pleomorphism, which appear to be permanent.[147–158] The precise pathophysiology of altered endothelial morphology is not well understood. Changes in the cell's cytoskeleton may account for pleomorphism and polymegathism. There is mounting evidence that cells exposed to chronic hypoxia are functionally impaired. Animal studies have demonstrated a decrease in endothelial pump-site density.[159] Human studies indicate that there may[157,160] or may not[158] be decreased endothelial barrier function after long-term contact lens

**8.11** | Polymorphonuclear leukocytes are a prominent component of the anterior chamber inflammatory reaction. They release prostaglandins, superoxides, and hydrolytic enzymes which can disrupt endothelial tight junctions or directly attack the cell membrane.

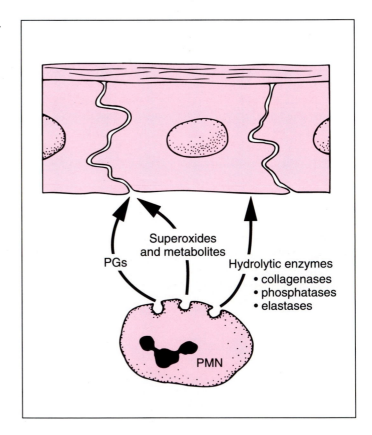

wear. Polse and colleagues[155] have shown that chronic hypoxic exposure in humans alters endothelial morphology and reduces the cornea's ability to reverse induced swelling.

Increased endothelial pleomorphism and polymegathism have also been described in diabetics.[10] Dogs and rats with chemically induced diabetes mellitus show similar morphologic abnormalities. These experimentally induced changes can be prevented by administration of aldose reductase inhibitors,[161-163] which suggests that activation of the sorbitol pathway with accumulation of sorbitol or other metabolites plays a role in the development of the morphologic abnormalities.

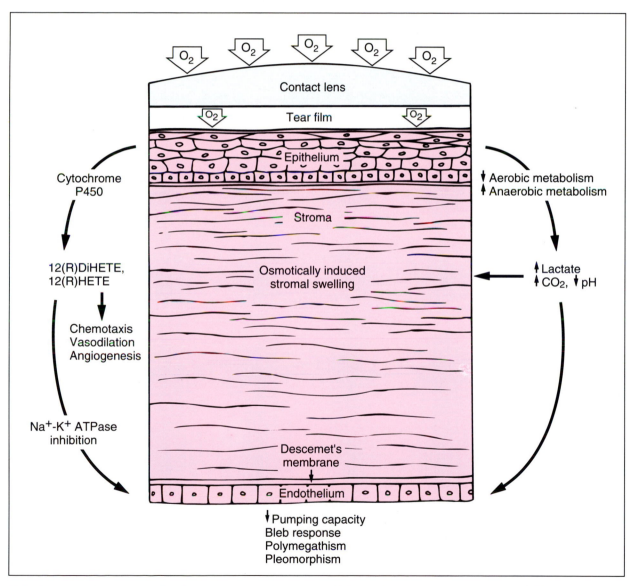

**8.12** | Decreased oxygen tension in the precorneal tear film due to presence of a contact lens causes a shift in epithelial metabolism to anaerobic pathways. The resulting increase in lactate can induce stromal swelling via osmotic effects. Epithelial production of the cytochrome P450 arachidonate metabolites 12(R)HETE and 12(R)DiHETE is also stimulated by contact lens-induced hypoxia. The 12(R)HETE and pH changes can affect endothelial morphology and function; 12(R)DiHETE has chemotactic, vasodilatory, and angiogenic effects.

# 9 | DEGENERATIVE CHANGES OF THE CORNEA

## John W. Chandler

The term "corneal degeneration" has been used in a variety of ways. Consequently, some disorders have been categorized in more than one way. This section describes corneal changes that either are associated with maturational and aging processes and are referred to as "primary" degenerations or occur after another primary process such as trauma or inflammation, or as a result of a systemic condition, such as endocrine abnormality, and are listed as "secondary" degenerations.

In most instances degenerations must be recognized and differentiated from conditions that require treatment. In other cases the underlying problem and the pathophysiology of the primary disorder, as well as the degeneration, must be appreciated to achieve successful management. Therefore, the ophthalmologist must be skilled in slit-lamp biomicroscopy and must possess a thorough knowledge of corneal pathophysiology. Primary and secondary degenerations can usually be recognized and categorized by their current slit-lamp appearance. Knowledge of the patient's general and ophthalmic medical histories is also necessary. A list of primary and secondary corneal degenerations is given in Figure 9.1.

## PRIMARY CORNEAL DEGENERATIONS

Primary corneal degenerations are usually bilateral but may occur unilaterally. They are quite common and, although seen occasionally in young adulthood, they are distinctly associated with older adulthood. When any of these conditions are noted in patients less than 30 years of age, the ophthalmologist should consider the possibility that the observed changes have a more important cause than an aging process.

Although not included here, changes in the appearance of the corneal epithelium are common and may or may not have familiar patterns of inheritance. The findings in some series of maps, dots, and fingerprint lines in up to 30% of the adult population suggest that in some instances these phenotypic changes are degenerations. In this setting they are typically asymptomatic. These changes will be discussed along with the corneal dystrophies (see Chapter 10). The remainder of the primary corneal degenerations present with distinctive slit-lamp biomicroscopic features.[1-27]

## Figure 9.1. Primary and Secondary Corneal Degenerations

**PRIMARY CORNEAL DEGENERATIONS (MATURATIONAL AND AGING CHANGES)**

Hudson–Stahli, Stocker, Fleischer, and Ferry corneal lines[2–6]
White limbal girdle of Vogt[7,8]
Corneal arcus[1,9–20]
Cornea farinata[21,22]
Mosaic shagreen[7,23–25]
Descemet's stria[26]
Hassal–Henle bodies[27]

**SECONDARY CORNEAL DEGENERATIONS (RESULT FROM INFLAMMATION, TRAUMA, OR SYSTEMIC DISEASES)**

Pterygium[28–46]
Spheroid degeneration[47–49]
Amyloid degeneration[50–52]
Salzmann's degeneration[53]
Band keratopathy[54]
Coats' white ring[55]
Pellucid marginal degeneration[56–59]
Senile marginal degeneration
Terrien's marginal degeneration[60–65]
Fuchs' superficial marginal keratitis[66]
Lipid degeneration[67–69]
Dellen
Exposure keratitis[70]
Traumatic recurrent erosion[71–73]
Keratitis sicca
Neuroparalytic keratitis[74–77]

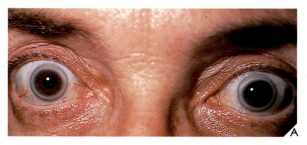
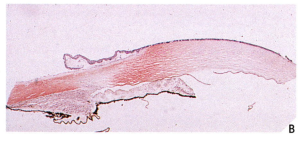

**9.2** | Corneal arcus. *A:* A peripheral corneal white ring separated from the limbus by a clear zone. *B:* Histologic section demonstrates lipid in the anterior and posterior portions of the corneal stroma seen as red triangles. The sclera also stains red due to its lipid content (oil red-O stain). (From Yanoff M, Fine BS: *Ocular Pathology. A Color Atlas*, ed 2. New York: Gower Medical Publishing, 1992, 8.11.)

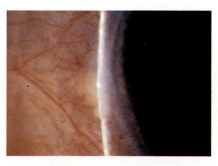
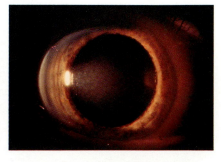

**9.3** | White limbal girdle of Vogt. A yellow-white line near the limbus in the interpalpebral zone which extends to the limbus (early band keratopathy has a clear zone) and is common in people after the age of 60 years.

**9.4** | Mosaic shagreen. Whitish opacities with shapes like crocodile leather can be seen in the anterior or posterior cornea. The cause is unknown.

## CORNEAL ARCUS

This condition represents the deposition of cholesterol esters, phospholipids, and neutral fats in the peripheral cornea, and therefore is not a true degeneration (Fig. 9.2). The accumulation starts in the upper cornea, then in the lower peripheral cornea, and finally becomes confluent in a ring. Deposition begins at the level of Descemet's then Bowman's membrane, and finally affects the intervening stroma. A clear interval exists between the deposition and the limbus. The prevalence of corneal arcus increases with advancing age and probably has no pathologic significance in individuals over age 40.[1]

## VOGT'S LIMBAL GIRDLE

This condition was originally described in two forms. Type I probably represents early band keratopathy. Type II (Fig. 9.3), vastly more common, consists of fine radial white lines, most frequently seen at the nasal limbus. This represents elastotic and hyaline changes and affects the majority of normal eyes over the age of 40, approaching 100% of eyes in the very elderly.[8]

## MOSAIC SHAGREEN

Also known as anterior and posterior crocodile shagreen of Vogt, this condition is characterized by the presence of polygonal hazy areas in the stroma, separated by clear lines (Fig. 9.4). The anterior variety is seen commonly in the anterior peripheral cornea bilaterally and is of no visual significance. Posterior crocodile shagreen has a similar appearance in the central deep stroma and again is of little or no visual significance. The pattern appears to be created by obliquely running collagen fibers bridging corneal lamellae.[25]

## CORNEA FARINATA

This condition represents a degenerative accumulation of pre-Descemet's fine particles that resembles farina ("cream of wheat"). These are of no practical significance (Fig. 9.5).

## IRON LINES

Many descriptions of iron deposits in the cornea have been published. The Hudson–Stahli line (Fig. 9.6) is a normal finding in the horizontal lower third of the cornea where lid closure takes place. A similar line, the Fleischer ring, is seen at the base of the cone in keratoconus. Stocker's line is central to a pterygium and Ferry's line at the leading edge of the filtering bleb. A similar deposit of iron is also seen central to radial keratotomy incisions. All of the lines appear to represent areas of tear pooling with deposition of iron from the tears in the basal epithelium.

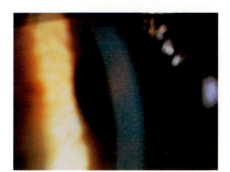

**9.5** Cornea farinata. Deep stromal small "flour-like" opacities are sometimes noted in older patients. The exact biochemical nature of these opacities is unknown.

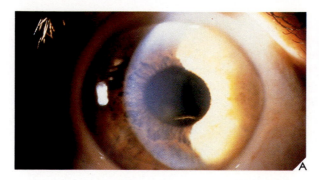

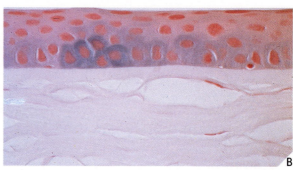

**9.6** I Hudson–Stahli Line. *A:* A horizontal brown line is located just below the center of the cornea within the epithelium. *B:* Histologic section demonstrates iron deposition within the epithelium (Perl's stain). (From Yanoff M, Fine BS: *Ocular Pathology. A Color Atlas*, ed 2. New York: Gower Medical Publishing, 1992, 8.20.)

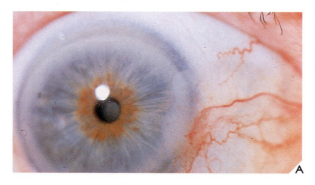

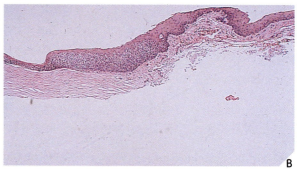

**9.7** I Pterygium. *A:* The nasal limbal conjunctiva and the contiguous cornea are involved by a vascularized lesion, a pterygium. *B:* The histologic section shows basophilic degeneration of the substantia propria of the conjunctiva (identical to that seen in a pingueculum) towards the right and invasion of the cornea with destruction of Bowman's membrane towards the left. It is the invasion of the cornea that distinguishes a pterygium from a pingueculum. (From Yanoff M, Fine BS: *Ocular Pathology. A Color Atlas*, ed 2. New York: Gower Medical Publishing, 1992, 98.)

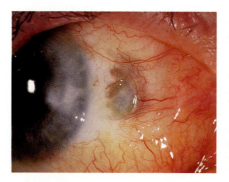

**9.8** I Scleral necrosis 12 years after pterygium excision and limbal radiation treatment.

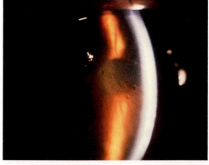

**9.9** I Spheroid degeneration (climatic droplet keratopathy). Yellow-brown interpalpebral zone deposits are extracellular and contain protein. The deposits often begin in the periphery and spread centrally.

The secondary corneal degenerations are almost all capable of producing symptoms as well as reducing best corrected visual acuity as the result of opacifications or of regular or irregular astigmatism.

## SECONDARY CORNEAL DEGENERATIONS

### PTERYGIUM

Actinic exposure of the ocular surface can lead to degeneration of limbal subepithelial structures that give rise to pingueculae in the conjunctiva[28] (Fig. 9.7), which in some cases progress to involve the cornea.[29,30] In combined involvement of conjunctiva and cornea, pterygia have a predilection for the interpalpebral zones, especially the nasal aspect. The fibrovascular membrane is triangular in shape and has a grayish central avascular edge. These pterygia are most common in warm, sunny climates and in persons who spend their time outdoors. For example, pterygia are common in agricultural workers in the southern part of the United States.[31] A recent study in Australia showed increased risk for pterygium in those with an outdoor working environment, who worked on a sandy surface, and who spent their early life at less than 30° latitude. Wearing of glasses or a hat also reduced the risk of pterygium development.[32]

Histologically, changes occur in the subepithelial connective tissue of the conjunctiva (i.e., elastoid degeneration); fibroblastic tissue migrates onto the cornea beneath the epithelial basement membrane and destroys Bowman's layer.[33] With time, the overlying epithelium undergoes degeneration and the fibroblastic tissue becomes vascularized.

Pterygia may remain small and cause only cosmetic blemishes or may spread across the cornea to encroach on the visual axis. Photographs and specific measurements of the horizontal and vertical lengths of pterygia are useful for follow-up. Keratometry can often demonstrate changes in the corneal curvature when there is progression.

Because the recurrence rate for pterygia after surgical removal is significant, up to 40% in some studies,[34,35] excision should be considered only for blatant cosmetic problems, documented progression, or encroachment on the visual axis. When surgery is undertaken it should be a precise microsurgical procedure rather than a quick peeling and amputation. The grayish central extent can be outlined with a blade or trephine to the level of Bowman's layer and removed in a lamellar fashion. The limbus is cleaned and the subconjunctival fibroblastic tissue carefully removed, including fibroblastic tissue that is adherent to the horizontal rectus muscles. In some cases the fibroblastic tissue restricts ocular motility. Some surgeons combine excision with other interventions, including local beta-irradiation,[36,37] topical thiotepa drops,[38,39] mitomycin-C,[40,41] conjunctival autologous grafts,[42] and lamellar corneal grafts.[43–46] Despite all of these approaches, recurrences are frequent and the selection of a technique is usually based on experience. Conjunctival or lamellar corneal grafts appear to give the lowest recurrence rates. Radiation and antimetabolites have been associated with scleral necrosis in some patients (Fig. 9.8).

### SPHEROID DEGENERATION

The appearance of spherical, subepithelial golden-brown material occurs in a variety of situations, most commonly in populations exposed to considerable ultraviolet light or in corneas that have sustained traumatic insults[47–49] (Fig. 9.9). Spheroid degeneration goes by a variety of names (e.g., Labrador keratopathy, climatic droplet keratopathies). The changes have a predilection for the interpalpebral limbal areas and spread towards the central cornea. At first the deposits are translucent but later become opaque. Ultraviolet exposure appears to play a major role in causation, and the process often is bilateral. Symptoms may include foreign body sensation, irritations, and eventually decreased visual acuity.

The nature and source of the golden-brown deposits are not completely elucidated. The material is protein containing, extracellular, and acidophilic. The deposits may represent breakdown of collagen and other extracellular matrix components in the superficial stroma or plasma proteins that have diffused into the stroma and have been degraded by UV exposure.[49]

In most cases no therapy is required. When removal is necessary, lamellar or penetrating keratoplasty is indicated.[49]

## AMYLOID DEGENERATION

Secondary amyloid corneal degeneration (Fig. 9.10) has been reported in association with a number of conditions. It is probably most common after trauma and is usually localized to areas of preexisting scar. Figure 9.11 lists other associations. Amyloid deposition may also be seen in lattice corneal dystrophy,[50,51] polymorphic stromal dystrophy,[52] and in association with primary systemic amyloidosis,[51] but is not observed in secondary systemic amyloidosis.

The clinical appearance of amyloid corneal deposition is not distinctive and may be seen as grayish haze, as clear, glass-like opacities in the cornea, or as nodular or flat subepithelial opacities that range in color from white to yellowish to pinkish. The latter form is common after corneal trauma or chronic inflammation. A distinct clinical appearance of localized corneal amyloid degeneration is the presence of punctate and linear transparent deposits at any depth in the stroma but often most pronounced deep in the stroma. The rest of the stroma is spared. The condition is usually bilateral and occurs in people of 40 to 60 years or older without evidence of hereditary transmission. These deposits cause minimal visual decrease.[52] The conjunctiva also may have amyloid depositions. The absolute recognition of amyloid is made by histological examination. It has a characteristic dichro-

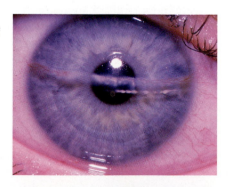

**9.10** I Amyloid degeneration. Linear amyloid deposit across cornea at site of previous trauma.

## Figure 9.11. Chronic Ocular Conditions Associated with Localized Secondary Amyloid Deposition

| | |
|---|---|
| Trachoma | Uveitis |
| Leprosy | Glaucoma |
| Sarcoidosis | Keratoconus |
| Interstitial keratitis | Retinopathy of prematurity |
| Phlyctenulosis | |

ism and birefringence in polarized light after staining with Congo red. It can also be identified with the fluorescent marker thioflavin-T and by electron microscopy.

If the deposits are associated with visual loss, keratoplasty is indicated.

## SALZMANN'S DEGENERATION

Whitish, raised subepithelial nodular opacities may occur in any area of the cornea, usually at or adjacent to previous corneal conditions (e.g., trachoma, phlyctenulosis) (Fig. 9.12).[53] They are seen in adults and may be bilateral. The surface of elevated epithelium is atrophic and the subepithelial tissue is hyalinized collagen, often replacing Bowman's layer and the superficial stromal lamellae. The lesions are sometimes vascularized.

Salzmann's degeneration may be asymptomatic or may cause irritation and foreign body sensation. The epithelial surface may break down, especially in the dry-eye syndrome. Visual symptoms can include glare, photophobia, and decreased acuity.

When the patient is asymptomatic no therapy is required. Lamellar or penetrating keratoplasty is indicated in patients who have lesions in the visual axis and significant loss of visual acuity. Some of these lesions are now being removed with excimer laser photoablation.

## BAND KERATOPATHY

The deposition of calcium salts and calcification of Bowman's layer known as band keratopathy (Fig. 9.13) can occur in a variety of conditions, most commonly associated with local inflammation, topical ophthalmic medications, and systemic disorders that cause hypercalcemia (Fig. 9.14). The process typically originates near the limbus in the nasal and temporal interpalpebral zones and moves from both sides towards the center of the cornea. Usually a clear zone exists at the limbus, and small holes occur in the deposits across the cornea. These holes may or may not coincide with the sites at which corneal nerves pass through Bowman's layer.

The histologic picture demonstrates a basophilic, stippled staining of the corneal epithelial basement membrane after hematoxylin and eosin staining in the milder cases. With progressive changes, calcium salts deposit

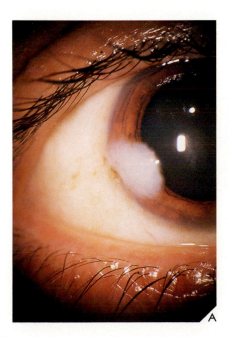

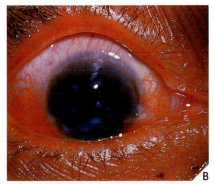

**9.12** I Salzmann's degeneration. *A:* Whitish raised subepithelial changes that include hyalinized collagen and atrophic epithelium. They are often adjacent to sites of previous corneal conditions. *B:* More typical multiple lesions in patient with a history of phlyctenulosis.

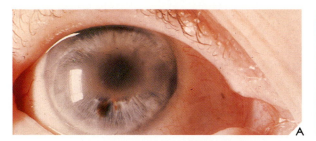

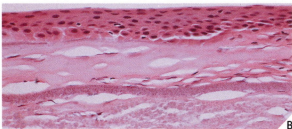

**9.13** | Band keratopathy. *A:* Clinical appearance of the band occupying the central, horizontal zone of the cornea and typically sparing the most peripheral clear cornea. *B:* A fibrous pannus is present between the epithelium and a calcified Bowman's membrane. Some deposit is also present in the anterior corneal stroma. (From Yanoff M, Fine BS: *Ocular Pathology. A Color Atlas*, ed 2. New York: Gower Medical Publishing, 1992, 8.12.)

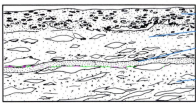

Corneal epithelium
Degenerative pannus
Calcified Bowman's membrane
Corneal stroma containing granular deposits

### Figure 9.14. Conditions Associated with Band Keratopathy

**LOCAL OCULAR CONDITIONS**
Nongranulomatous uveitis (especially in juvenile rheumatoid arthritis)
Interstitial keratitis
Longstanding glaucoma
Chronic corneal edema
Phthisis
Spheroid degeneration
Norrie's disease

**TOPICAL OPHTHALMIC MEDICATIONS**
Medications containing mercury
Solutions containing phosphate

**SYSTEMIC DISORDERS THAT CAUSE HYPERCALCEMIA**
Hyperparathyroidism
Idiopathic hypercalcemia
Excess vitamin D ingestion
Osteoporosis, acute
Renal failure
Sarcoidosis
Lymphoma, leukemia, multiple myeloma
Bone metastasis
Milk–alkali syndrome
Thiazide medications

**OTHER ASSOCIATED CONDITIONS**
Gout
Discoid lupus erythematosis
Tuberous sclerosis
Ichthyosis
Parry–Romberg syndrome (progressive facial hemiatrophy)
Rothmund–Thomson syndrome

**9.15** | Coats' white ring. A subepithelial irregular white ring outlines the site of a previous corneal foreign body.

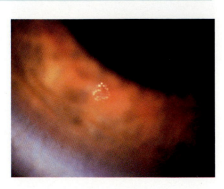

in Bowman's layer, which may be destroyed and fragmented.[54] Occasionally the anterior stroma is involved. In systemic disorders of calcium metabolism, intracellular calcium deposition occurs. The other causes are associated with extracellular deposits of calcium.

If the band keratopathy is causing painful erosions or decreased vision or both, removal is indicated. After topical anesthesia, the overlying corneal epithelium is removed. Disodium EDTA 1% or 2% can be applied locally to chelate the band for approximately 1 minute and then gentle scraping with a blade is carried out. These cycles are repeated until removal is complete. The EDTA can be toxic to the remaining corneal and conjunctival epithelium and in patients with poor wound healing (e.g., diabetes mellitus) care must be exercised. Alternatively, scraping can be performed without EDTA.

## COATS' WHITE RING

When a metallic corneal foreign body has been observed, slit-lamp examination may reveal a subepithelial or anterior stromal circular white ring with a granular appearance[55] (Fig. 9.15). Histopathology demonstrates the presence of iron. Treatment is not necessary.

## PELLUCID MARGINAL DEGENERATION

This condition is characterized by inferior peripheral corneal thinning and usually presents as decreased vision associated with against-the-rule astigmatism (Fig. 9.16). The precise cause is unknown, although some argue that this is an unusual form of keratoconus. However, some clinical differences exist (Fig. 9.17), and the approaches to treatment are somewhat different. Because the exact cause of pellucid marginal degeneration is unknown and because it does have some important features that distinguish it from keratoconus, it seems reasonable to designate it as a secondary degeneration.

The site of corneal thinning is usually 1 mm to 2 mm central to the limbus and in the inferior one third of the cornea. The zone of thinning is usually 1 mm to 2 mm in vertical diameter by 3–4 mm horizontally. The area otherwise appears normal and is avascular. Stromal thinning with localized destruction of Bowman's layer is evident on histologic examination.[56,57]

Because pellucid marginal degeneration is a reasonably uncommon condition, optimal treatments have not been conclusively determined. Usually, neither glasses nor contact lenses are satisfactory for correction of the marked refractive error. Several surgical approaches have been described, including the placement of large eccentric penetrating grafts, resection of the thinned region, and crescent-shaped peripheral lamellar keratoplasty.[58,59]

## SENILE MARGINAL DEGENERATION

Marginal thinning may be seen in the peripheral cornea with advancing age. Typically this occurs superiorly or inferiorly in the clear interval between an arcus and the limbus (the clear interval of Vogt). At times the normal clear

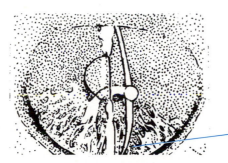

Thinning and ectasia

**9.16** I Pellucid marginal degeneration. Note the inferior thinning and ectasia.

interval may be misinterpreted as thinning, but true noninflammatory thinning does occur and can even rarely lead to perforation (Fig. 9.18). There is usually minimal or no vascularization or evidence of inflammation. The cause is unknown.

## TERRIEN'S MARGINAL DEGENERATION

This clinical condition (Fig. 9.19) was described in 1900,[60] and is usually categorized as a noninflammatory peripheral corneal thinning with a central edge of opacification, which appears to be lipid, in the corneal epithelium and superficial vascularization. However, it has been described in association with ocular inflammation.[61] It is often a stable condition that does not cause symptoms. In some eyes, the thinning spreads circumferentially, centrally, or both and causes significant astigmatism. Perforation is uncommon but can occur spontaneously or with minor trauma.

The condition is most commonly noted in adults of age 50 or older but can occur at any age. It appears to affect men more often than women. There

### Figure 9.17. Characteristics of Pellucid Marginal Degeneration and Keratoconus

|  | PELLUCID | KERATOCONUS |
| --- | --- | --- |
| Location | Inferior near limbus | Central or paracentral |
| Astigmatism | Against the rule | Irregular |
| Fleischer ring | No | Yes |
| Vogt striae | No | Yes |
| Hydrops | Rare | Uncommon |
| Scarring | Yes | Yes |
| Age at appearance | 20–40 years | 10–30 years |
| Correct with glasses | Sometimes | No |
| Correct with contact lens | Sometimes | Yes |
| Family history | No | +/– |

**9.18** I Senile marginal furrow with small perforation sealed by iris.

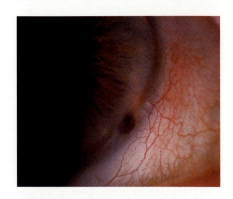

is often bilateral involvement that is more advanced in one eye. The pathophysiology is unknown. There are local absences of Bowman's layer, and fibrillar degeneration of stromal collagen occurs.[62] There is a paucity of inflammatory cells. However, phagocytosis of collagen by histiocytes has been reported with the use of electron microscopy.[63]

Treatment is required for eyes with vision-reducing astigmatism, or threatened or actual perforation. In most instances, a partial or full-thickness crescent-shaped corneal graft can be overlaid in the thinned area.[64,65] By careful free-hand sizing and appropriate suturing, the astigmatism can be reduced.

This disorder, of unknown cause, should perhaps be considered an inflammation rather than a degeneration. Its similarity to Terrien's, however, prompts its discussion here. In this disorder recurrent ocular inflammation, usually at the inferior limbus, is associated with superficial corneal inflammation peripheral to which there is pseudopterygium formation overlying corneal thinning (Fig. 9.20). Unlike Terrien's, there is an irregular central bor-

## FUCHS' SUPERFICIAL MARGINAL KERATITIS

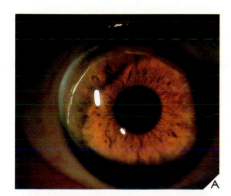
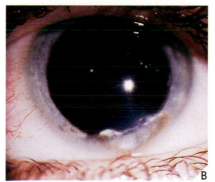
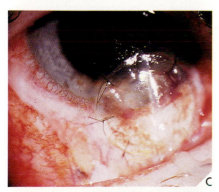

**9.19** | Terrien's marginal degeneration. *A:* Peripheral thinning with a lipid line along the central edge of thinning. This patient had 19 diopters of astigmatism with the flat axis at 110°. *B:* A more localized but progressive area of thinning that perforated. *C:* A lamellar keratoplasty has covered the site of perforation.

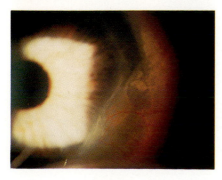

**9.20** | Fuchs' superficial marginal keratitis.

der without lipid deposition. In addition, there is usually no corneal ectasia or induced astigmatism.[66] Our preference is to treat with topical corticosteroids during active inflammation.

**LIPID DEGENERATION**

Lipid deposition can occur at any time in a cornea with stromal vascularization from any cause (Fig. 9.21). The events that lead to the extravasation of lipid from blood vessels into the cornea are unknown. It may occur suddenly without other concurrent events.[67] When lipid deposits in the visual axis, sudden visual decrease may be the presenting complaint. The lipid depositions are yellowish-white and may have feathery edges.[68] Sometimes cholesterol crystals can be seen.[69]

No specific treatment exists. Laser photocoagulation has been used to attempt to ablate corneal vessels but usually is not successful. Over time the lipid may gradually return to the vessels whence it came, leaving perivascular "clearing lines." Penetrating keratoplasty can be done for visual restoration if warranted by the condition of the rest of the eye.

**DELLEN**

Localized compacting of the cornea (or sclera) can occur as the result of water loss beneath an area of surface drying of the corneal epithelium (Fig. 9.22). A delle or dellen typically occur in the peripheral cornea adjacent to conjunctival swelling (e.g., after surgery) that has resulted in failure of the lid margin to wet the area and subsequent localized drying.

These areas return to normal thickness when appropriate eyelid–cornea surface contact is reestablished, and can be aided by frequent applications of artificial tears and lubricants. When the conjunctival elevation does not subside, excision of the abnormal conjunctiva may be necessary.

**EXPOSURE KERATITIS**

Drying of other areas of the corneal epithelium may be associated with incomplete blinking and lagophthalmos.[70] Breakdown of the corneal epithelium leads to decreased visual acuity and photophobia. The epithelial breakdown can predispose the cornea to microbial keratitis and even to perforation.

Treatment is directed primarily towards surgical correction of the eyelid positional abnormalities. Taping the eyelids, as well as temporary or permanent tarsorrhaphies may be beneficial. Artificial tears and ointments help to maintain a moist ocular surface and to restore the corneal epithelium to nor-

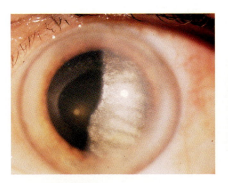

**9.21** | Lipid degeneration. Yellow-white deposition of lipid with feathery edges spreading away from old corneal blood vessels rapidly occurred several years after the vascularization.

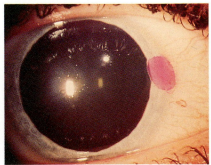

**9.22** | Delle. Rose bengal staining of devitalized corneal epithelial cells outlines an area of compacting of the cornea. The staining and thinning resolved once artificial tears kept the area lubricated.

mal. Therapeutic soft contact lenses can be successful in selected patients but are often the cause of additional complications. Correction of the underlying problems is less risky than therapeutic lenses.

Corneal abrasions, especially those caused by fingernails, paper, and vegetation (e.g., pine needles), are often associated with prolonged abnormalities of the epithelium–basement membrane adhesion complex (basement membrane, hemidesmosomes, and anchoring filaments) which may persist for 2 to 3 months and even for years in some cases[71] (Fig. 9.23). During this time, recurrent slippage or loss of the involved corneal epithelium may occur. Additional impediments to complete epithelial healing include damage to Bowman's layer or its disruption, damage to the superficial stroma, inflammation, and preexisting epithelium–basement membrane dystrophy. Nontraumatic causes of recurrent corneal epithelial erosions include epithelial or superficial stromal dystrophies, corneal edema, herpetic infections, diabetes mellitus, epidermolysis bullosa, and Cockayne syndrome.

The classic presentation includes pain that may awaken the patient in the early morning hours, foreign body sensation, photophobia, and tearing.[72] The symptoms may be preceded by a vague sensation several hours earlier. On slit-lamp examination, an epithelial defect or subtle wrinkles in the epithelium that move slightly can be seen. Within the epithelium, microcysts or bullae may occur. Occasionally subepithelial haze, anterior stromal inflammation, or both can be observed. Retroillumination may be more revealing than focal slit illumination.

Treatment is initially directed towards healing the abrasion with patching and cycloplegics. Once the surface is covered, attention must be directed to concomitant conditions. Dry-eye status and exposure problems are handled in standard ways. Stromal inflammation is treated with topical corticosteroids. Inter- and intraepithelial edema is treated with hypertonic saline solutions. Therapeutic soft contact lenses can be used for 3 to 4 months to allow healing. The lenses must fit very well and constant attention must be given to the fit. In patients with multiple recurrences due to lesions out of the visual axis, several anterior stromal punctures with the bent tip of a 25-gauge needle (the length of the bent tip is no more than 25% depth of the corneal thickness) may be useful.[73] This treatment appears to entrap the

## TRAUMATIC RECURRENT EROSION

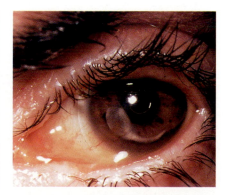

**9.23 |** Traumatic recurrent erosions. If the recurrent erosions are not prevented, the area of involvement becomes scarred and vascularized.

**9.24 |** Neuroparalytic keratitis. A persistent corneal epithelial defect with rolled edges is present in a patient after transection of the V cranial nerve. Low-grade iritis is also present.

basal epithelial cells in the anterior stroma and is carried out only in the area of recurrent erosion. Early results using the excimer laser to treat this condition are promising. Note: the treatment of recurrent erosion in epithelial basement membrane dystrophies is somewhat different and is discussed in the section on corneal dystrophies.

## KERATITIS SICCA

Corneal epithelial degenerations occur along with similar changes in the conjunctiva in all dry-eye states. These changes are discussed in Chapters 2 and 14.

## NEUROPARALYTIC KERATITIS

The essential importance of sensory corneal innervation via the V cranial nerve is clearly demonstrated by the devastating effects of its loss[74] (Fig. 9.24). The earliest clinical indications of neuroparalytic keratitis are corneal haze and conjunctival hyperemia. Experimentally, this coincides with increased corneal permeability and reduced metabolic and mitotic rates, along with reductions in the levels of acetylcholine and choline acetyltransferase in the epithelium.[75-77] Soon afterwards, persistent corneal epithelial defects develop, along with anterior segment inflammation. In some cases, stromal melting and perforations occur. Vascularization is another common finding.

The list of possible causes of neuroparalytic keratitis is long (Fig. 9.25), and care should be taken to make an accurate diagnosis because some causes are life-threatening, potentially treatable, or both.

Treatment should be initiated immediately and comprehensively. The ocular surface must be protected with artificial tears, ointments, and tarsorrhaphies. In carefully selected cases, therapeutic soft contact lenses may be useful. Once the epithelium is healed, it may be possible to partially open the tarsorrhaphy.

## Figure 9.25. Potential Causes of Neuroparalytic Keratitis

**V CRANIAL NERVE PALSY**
Tumors
Aneurysms
Trauma

**V CRANIAL NERVE SURGICAL ABLATION**

**CONGENITAL DISEASES**
Riley–Day syndrome (familial dysautonomia)
Goldenhar syndrome
Möbius syndrome
Parry–Romberg syndrome
Bassen–Kornzweig syndrome

**SYSTEMIC DISEASE**
Diabetes mellitus

**LOCAL OCULAR CONDITIONS**
Infections
    Herpes simplex virus
    Varicella-zoster virus
    Leprosy

**CHEMICAL BURNS**

**TOXIC EXPOSURES**

**CORNEAL DYSTROPHIES**
Lattice
Granular

**SURGICAL OR LASER DAMAGE TO SENSORY NERVES**

**TOPICAL MEDICATIONS**
Anesthetic abuse
Atropine
Sulfacetamide, 30%

# 10 | Congenital Anomalies and Inherited Dystrophies of the Cornea

John W. Chandler

Joel Sugar

This section will review a number of disorders of congenital and/or genetic origin involving the cornea.[1] The distribution between these groups is at times arbitrary, because some of the congenital anomalies are heritable and some of the dystrophies are present at birth and, therefore, congenital. The term dystrophy will be applied to disorders that are generally bilateral, progressive, inherited, and isolated to the cornea. They may also appear to involve only a single corneal layer and predominate in the central cornea. A large number of systemic inherited disorders may also cause corneal changes, which are referred to in Chapter 15.

## DEVELOPMENTAL ANOMALIES OF THE CORNEA

By the end of the fifth week of gestation, the lens vesicle has separated from the surface ectoderm. The optic cup margins advance and the mesenchymal neural crest migrates between the surface ectoderm and the optic cup, filling what is to become the anterior chamber. The first wave of mesenchyme forms the corneal endothelium and trabecular meshwork, the second forms stromal keratocytes, and the third forms the anterior iris stroma. Separation of this mesenchyme leads to the formation of the anterior chamber.[2] Genetic, teratogenic, and infectious insults can lead to alterations in this development and be conducive to various congenital corneal anomalies. The timing and nature of the insult determine the anomalies that occur.

### SIZE AND SHAPE ANOMALIES

Anomalies of size and shape of the cornea include *microcornea* and *megalocornea.* Microcornea appears as part of microphthalmos (see Chapter 13), but true microcornea refers to a small cornea, less than 10 mm in adults, in a globe of normal size (Fig. 10.1). There appears to be completed corneal development but arrested corneal growth. Angle-closure glaucoma may occur as the lens enlarges. A number of genetic syndromes have microcornea associated with them. A syndrome of autosomal dominant microcornea with cataract and associated mild steepening of the corneal curvature, Peters' anomaly, and sclerocornea has also been described.[3]

Megalocornea, or anterior megalophthalmos, is a disorder in which the anterior segment of the globe is bilaterally enlarged and the corneal diameter 13 mm or greater (Fig. 10.2). Astigmatism, iris atrophy, lens subluxation, and miosis due to poor dilator function have all been associated with this sex-linked recessive disorder. Corneal endothelial cell densities are normal despite the large corneal endothelial area, which suggests that this disorder involves total corneal hyperplasia rather than distention of the cornea after it has developed as in congenital glaucoma.[4]

*Keratoglobus* is the term used to describe a rare congenital disorder with bilateral limbus to limbus corneal thinning and protrusion (Fig. 10.3). A variant has been described with associated blue sclera, hyperextensible joints, and hearing, as well as dental problems.[5] Corneal perforation and hydrops may occur, although the disorder is generally stable throughout life. Keratoconus may progress to limbus to limbus thinning that resembles keratoglobus.

*Cornea plana* is probably the same as *sclerocornea*, which is described below.

## ANOMALIES OF CORNEAL CLARITY

A broad spectrum of developmental anomalies involving migration of the mesenchyme of neural crest origin leads to congenital alterations of corneal clarity. Those involving the first wave of mesenchyme lead to endothelial and angle anomalies, whereas alterations in the second wave lead to stromal disorders. Alterations in the third wave lead to iris changes. Not uncommonly, the genetic or intrauterine environmental factors leading to developmental defects act over a period of time and encompass more than one of the events, leading to anomalies involving more than one neural crest-derived tissue.

*Posterior embryotoxon*, a thickening of Schwalbe's ring often seen most readily temporally at the slit lamp, occurs commonly in the general population (Fig. 10.4). The term *toxon* comes from the Greek word for

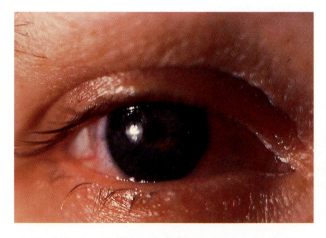

**10.1 | Microcornea.** Corneal diameter is 9 mm horizontally. The patient has angle closure glaucoma.

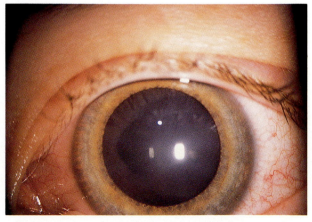

**10.2 | Megalocornea.** Horizontal corneal diameter is 14 mm in each eye.

bow and refers to the crescent of Schwalbe's line. The isolated presence of this finding is of no clinical significance. *Embryotoxon* or *anterior embryotoxon* refers to a congenital broad limbus (Fig. 10.5).

*Axenfeld's anomaly* refers to bilateral, prominent, anteriorly displaced Schwalbe's line with multiple adherent peripheral iris strands. Axenfeld's anomaly may or may not be associated with glaucoma (Fig. 10.6).

*Rieger syndrome* has the changes of Axenfeld's with the addition of iris atrophy, corectopia, and iris holes. A fine membrane may be seen extending from Schwalbe's to the peripheral iris or covering the chamber

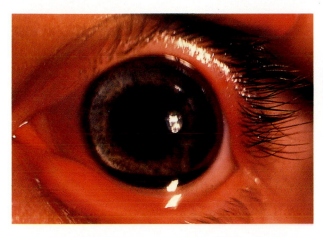

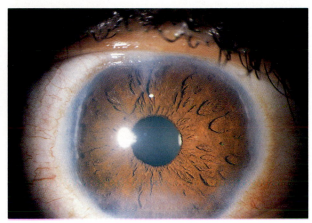

**10.3** | Keratoglobus. The cornea is thin and protruberant limbus to limbus.

**10.4** | Posterior embryotoxon.

**10.5** | Anterior embryotoxon.

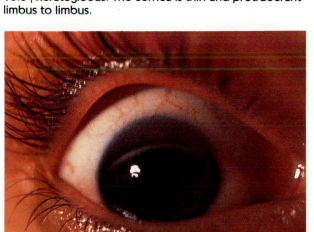

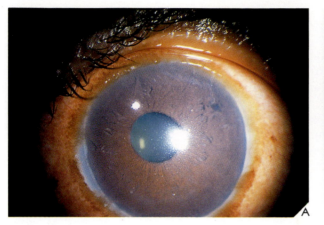

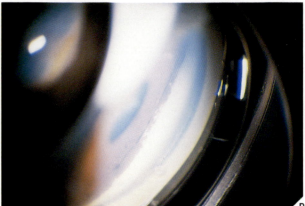

**10.6** | Axenfeld's anomaly. *A:* Anterior view with prominent Schwalbe's line. *B:* Gonioscopic view showing numerous iris processes to Schwalbe's line.

**10.7** | Axenfeld's anomaly. *A:* Especially prominent and centrally displaced Schwalbe's line. *B:* In this photograph Schwalbe's line is anteriorly displaced 360°. *C:* Histologic section of another case shows an iris process attached to the anteriorly displaced Schwalbe's ring. (*B,* courtesy of Dr. WC Frayer. *C,* courtesy of Dr. RY Foos. *B* and *C* from Yanoff M, Fine BS: *Ocular Pathology. A Color Atlas,* ed 2. New York: Gower Medical Publishing, 1992, 8.4.)

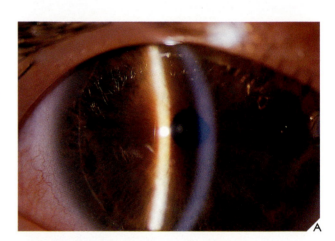

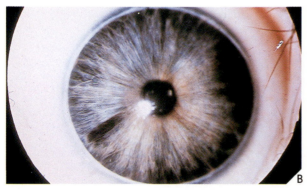

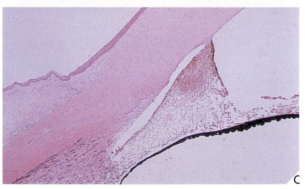

angle (Fig. 10.7). Associated systemic abnormalities include dental anomalies and flattening of the midface and nasal bridge (Figs. 10.8, 10.9). Shields and co-workers have postulated that the ocular component of Rieger's and Axenfeld's are variants of the same disorder and result from an arrested development in late gestation with retention of neural crest remnants and primordial endothelium on the iris and chamber angle.[6] The differential diagnosis includes the iridocorneal endothelial syndrome and a variant of posterior polymorphous corneal dystrophy which has associated iridocorneal adhesions, iris abnormalities, and glaucoma (Fig. 10.10).

*Peters' anomaly* involves a variable spectrum of findings. Peters' anomaly Type I refers to the presence of a corneal stromal opacity in the visual axis in which adherent iris strands arise from the collarette and extend to the periphery of the opacity (Fig. 10.11). A defect in Descemet's membrane and the corneal endothelium is present. In Type II Peters' anomaly the lens is also involved either with adherence to or lack of separation from the cornea or with cataract (Fig. 10.12). Type I is usually unilateral whereas Type II is more commonly bilateral.[7] Peters' anomaly has been described as part of the fetal alcohol syndrome and presumably is the result of other teratogens as well[8] (Fig. 10.13). It has been our experience that the corneal clouding often improves with time in Peters' Type I as the corneal edema surrounding the denser opacity resolves. Posterior keratoconus and the posterior ulcer of von Hippel are

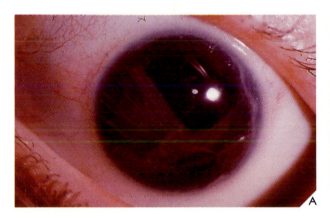
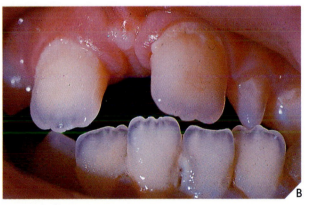

**10.8** | Rieger syndrome. *A:* Note extensive iris changes as well as prominent Schwalbe's line. *B:* Dental anomalies in the same patient shown in *A.* (Courtesy of Dr. H. Saul Sugar.)

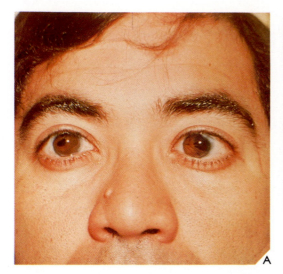

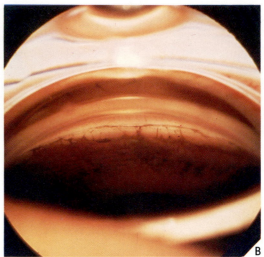

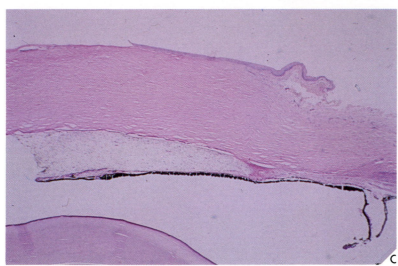

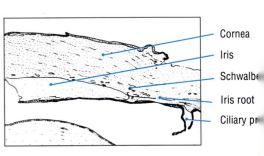

Cornea
Iris
Schwalbe
Iris root
Ciliary pr

**10.9** | Rieger syndrome. *A:* The patient has numerous iris abnormalities and bilateral glaucoma. Note the hypertelorism. *B:* The patient's daughter has similar abnormalities. Note the iris processes attached to an anteriorly displaced Schwalbe's line (posterior embryotoxon). *C:* Histologic section of an eye from another patient shows an anteriorly displaced Schwalbe's ring. A diffuse abnormality of the iris stroma is present. (*A* and *B,* courtesy of Dr. HG Scheie. From Yanoff M, Fine BS: *Ocular Pathology. A Color Atlas,* ed 2. New York: Gower Medical Publishing, 1992, 8.5.)

## Figure 10.10. Comparison of Axenfeld Anomaly-Rieger Syndrome, Iridocorneal Endothelial Syndrome, and Posterior Polymorphous Dystrophy

|  | AR | ICE | PPD |
|---|---|---|---|
| Laterality | Bilateral | Unilateral | Bilateral |
| Age | Birth | Adult | Birth |
| Inheritance | Dominant | Sporadic | Dominant |
| Systemic findings | Yes | No | No |
| Corneal edema | No | Yes | Sometimes |
| Corneal endothelium | Normal | Abnormal | Abnormal |

AR = Axenfeld anomaly-Rieger syndrome.
ICE = iridocorneal endothelial syndrome.
PPD = posterior polymorphous dystrophy.

Modified from Shields MB, Buckley E, Klintworth GK, Thresher R: Axenfeld-Rieger syndrome: a spectrum of developmental disorders. *Surv Ophthalmol 1985; 29:387–409.*

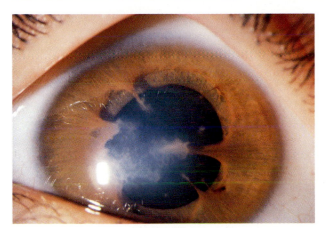

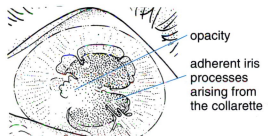

**10.11** | Peters' anomaly, Type I. Note central opacity and iris processes extending from the collarette to the cornea.

opacity

adherent iris processes arising from the collarette

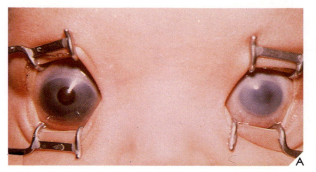

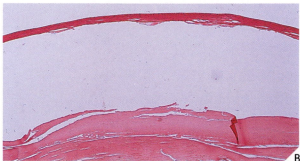

**10.12** | Peters' anomaly, Type II. *A:* The right eye shows an enlarged cornea, secondary to glaucoma. The left eye shows a small cornea as part of the anomalous affliction. *B:* Histologic section shows considerable corneal thinning centrally. The space between the cornea and the lens material is artifactitious and secondary to shrinkage of the lens cortex during processing of the eye. *C:* Increased magnification shows lens material attached to the posterior cornea. Centrally, no endothelium, Descemet's membrane, or Bowman's membrane are present. Lens capsule lines the posterior surface of the cornea. (*B* and *C,* PAS stain. From Yanoff M, Fine BS: *Ocular Pathology. A Color Atlas,* ed 2. New York: Gower Medical Publishing, 1992, 8.4.)

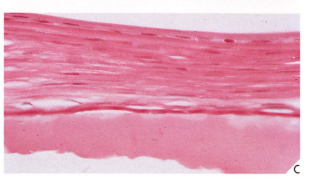

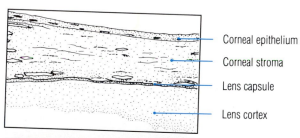

Corneal epithelium

Corneal stroma

Lens capsule

Lens cortex

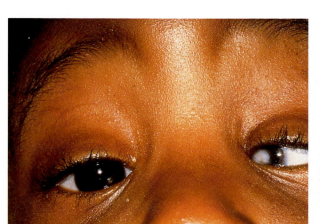

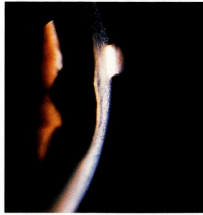

**10.14** | Posterior keratoconus. Note normal anterior corneal contour with focal increased concavity of posterior surface.

**10.13** | Unilateral Peters' anomaly in a child with fetal alcohol syndrome. (Courtesy of Dr. Marilyn Miller.)

terms that appear to apply best to the presence of the endothelial and Descemet's defects seen in Peters' anomaly without the iris adhesion (Fig. 10.14). Congenital anterior staphyloma with corneal thinning and protrusion and multiple anterior segment developmental anomalies occurs as an isolated entity or may be associated with contralateral Peters' anomaly (Fig. 10.15).

*Sclerocornea* refers to peripheral (Fig. 10.16) or diffuse (Fig. 10.17) sclera-like opacification of the cornea. Sclerocornea appears to result from a defect in the second wave of mesenchymal migration and is often associated with corneal flattening as the mesenchymal condensation that forms the limbus fails to develop normally and the corneal contour is more continuous with that of the sclera. The disorder is usually bilateral and sporadic, although familial cases have been reported as have associations with chromosomal

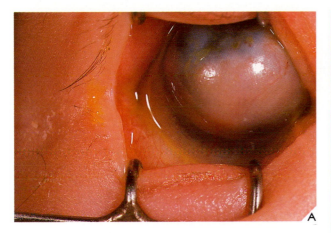

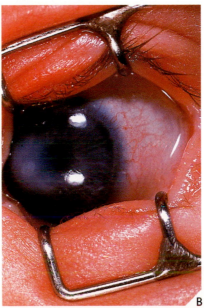

**10.15 |** *A:* Congenital anterior staphyloma. *B:* Contralateral eye of patient in *A* with Peters' anomaly Type I.

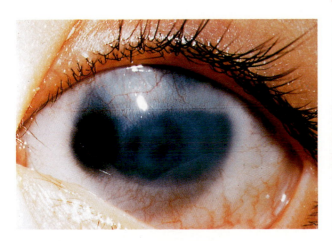

**10.16 |** Peripheral form of sclerocornea.

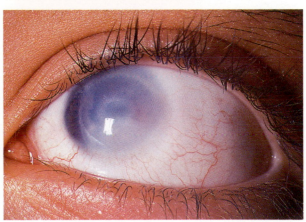

**10.17 |** Sclerocornea with associated microcornea and Peters' Type I anomaly.

anomalies. Peters' and Axenfeld's-like anterior segment anomalies as well as glaucoma often are present. Response to keratoplasty is usually poor.

## EPITHELIAL DYSTROPHIES

This section refers to dystrophies that clinically appear to involve predominantly the epithelium, as opposed to dystrophies which clinically show a stromal predominance or those involving primarily the endothelium. Obviously, the stromal dystrophies may lead to epithelial changes as do the endothelial dystrophies, and the epithelium may play a major pathogenetic role. This portion will discuss disorders that appear to be limited to the epithelial layer of the cornea.

### MAP-DOT-FINGERPRINT DYSTROPHY

This disorder includes a number of entities described in the literature, including the epithelial basement membrane dystrophy,[9] Cogan's microcystic dystrophy,[10] and some cases of dystrophic recurrent erosion syndrome. It is characterized by the presence of a number of patterns of epithelial change which may occur singly or in various combinations. Maps are grayish thickenings of subepithelial collagen and basement membrane collections which are seen in broad focal illumination and take varied patterns resembling the geographic boundaries on conventional maps (Fig. 10.18). They may elevate the epithelium sufficiently to cause thinning of the overlying tear film creating "negative" staining with fluorescein. Dots are cyst-like spaces in the corneal epithelium containing degenerated cellular debris. They may appear clear, gray (Fig. 10.19), or putty-colored (Fig. 10.20) and vary in size and shape. Histopathologically they are often seen posterior to abnormally positioned basement membrane. Fingerprint lines are seen as fine, often parallel, clear lines in the deep epithelium (see Fig. 10.19) on retroillumina-

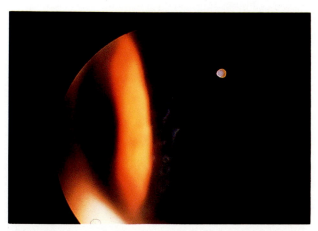

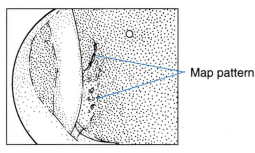

Map pattern

10.18 | Map-dot-fingerprint dystrophy, map pattern.

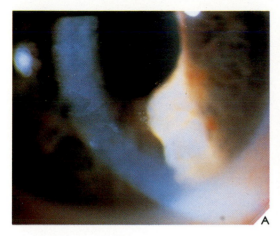

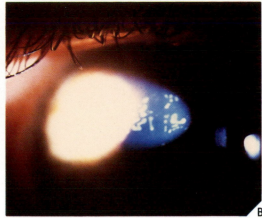

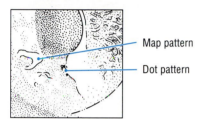

Map pattern
Dot pattern

**10.19** | Dot, fingerprint, and map patterns. *A:* The dot pattern is shown in the lower central cornea. A map pattern is seen above and to the left of the dot pattern. *B:* The dot pattern resembles "putty" within the epithelium. *C:* The fingerprint pattern, best seen with indirect lighting, is clearly shown. (*B,* courtesy of Dr. WC Frayer. From Yanoff M, Fine BS: *Ocular Pathology. A Color Atlas,* ed 2. New York: Gower Medical Publishing, 1992, 8.14.)

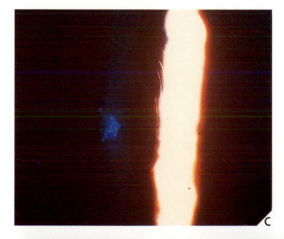

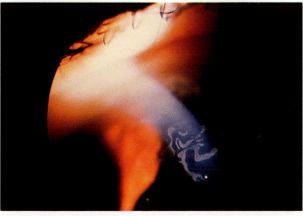

**10.20** | Map-dot-fingerprint dystrophy, putty-like opacities.

**10.21** | Dot, fingerprint, and map patterns. *A:* Histologic section shows that the dot pattern is caused by cysts that contain desquamating surface epithelial cells. *B:* The fingerprint pattern is caused by extensive aberrant production of basement membrane material within the epithelium (red lines).

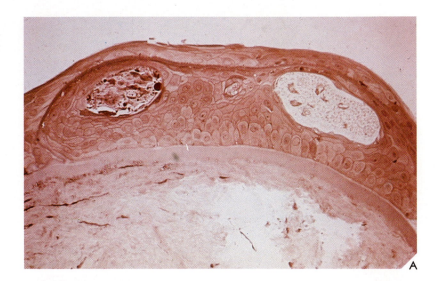

A

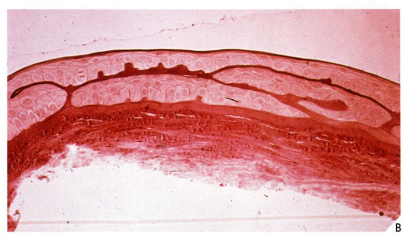

B

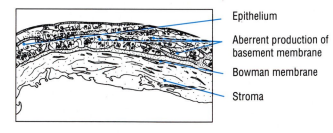

Epithelium

Aberrant production of basement membrane

Bowman membrane

Stroma

tion, especially with a dilated pupil. These represent projections of thickened epithelial basement membrane into the epithelium (Fig. 10.21).

Clinically, the most common presentation is an asymptomatic finding on routine slit-lamp examination. Recurrent painful erosions are the next most frequent presentation, with patients complaining of spontaneous episodes of tearing and foreign body sensation. These episodes most commonly occur in the early morning and awaken the patient from sleep, or they occur on the first opening of the eyes after awakening. The least common presentation is with decreased vision from the anterior irregular astigmatism caused by the irregular epithelial surface.

The pathogenesis of this disorder is incompletely understood but involves abnormal basal layer epithelial proliferation and excess production of epithelial basement membrane. The familial nature of this disorder has been demonstrated. Laibson and Krachmer[11] have reported two families with three generations involved and eight families with two generations involved. Nonetheless, the majority of patients have no family history and map-dot-fingerprint corneal changes have been noted to occur in 43% of a general population and in 76% of those over age 50, suggesting that this may be a degeneration.[12]

Treatment of recurrent corneal erosions in these patients calls for hypertonic saline ointment at bedtime. This is sufficient in most patients. Occasional use of soft lenses may be necessary to get a patient through a particularly troubling episode. Patients with continuing recurrences appear to benefit from corneal epithelial debridement, which includes scraping off the redundant epithelial basement membrane or from excimer laser phototherapeutic kerate-

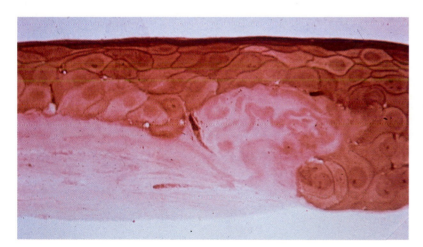

**10.21 |** *C:* The map pattern is caused by accumulated subepithelial basement membrane and collagenous tissue that resembles a subepithelial fibrous plaque. (*A* and *B,* PD stain. From Yanoff M, Fine BS: *Ocular Pathology. A Color Atlas,* ed 2. New York: Gower Medical Publishing, 1992, 8.14.)

ctomy. Superficial keratectomy has also been suggested.[13,14] Reduced vision from anterior irregular astigmatism due to the irregular epithelial thickness and the redundant epithelial basement membrane is effectively treated by removal of the epithelium and the underlying basement membrane.

## MEESMANN'S DYSTROPHY

Also called juvenile epithelial corneal dystrophy, this is an autosomal dominant disorder characterized by the presence of multiple cysts in the corneal epithelium. The cysts are regular in size and appear grayish in direct illumination and clear on retroillumination (Fig. 10.22). They often appear to have irregular material partially filling them. The lesions may be seen anywhere in the corneal epithelium but are often most prominent in the corneal periphery and in the interpalpebral region. The cysts can be seen early in life and appear to increase in number and density throughout life. Patients are usually asymptomatic until their teens or 20s, when they develop the symptoms of recurrent erosions caused by the abnormal epithelium.

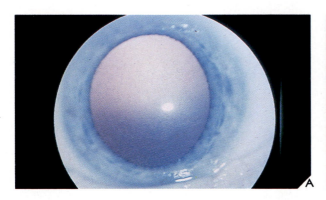

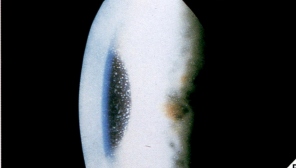

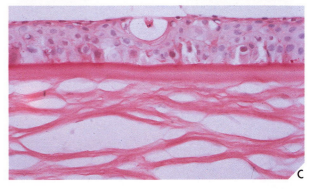

**10.22** | Meesmann's dystrophy. *A* and *B:* Tiny, fine punctate, clear vacuoles within the corneal epithelium. *C:* Histologic section shows an intraepithelial cyst that contains debris. (*C*, PAS. From Yanoff M, Fine BS: *Ocular Pathology. A Color Atlas,* ed 2. New York: Gower Medical Publishing, 1992, 8.13.)

Histopathologic evaluation of specimens from patients with Meesmann's dystrophy shows a fibrillogranular "peculiar substance" that stains for mucopolysaccharide in the epithelial cells. In addition, a vacuolated dense homogeneous material is present in the cysts.[15]

Treatment is the same as for other recurrent erosive disorders, although symptoms are usually less severe. Daily soft contact lens wear has been associated with decreased number of cysts.[16]

Other epithelial dystrophies have been described, although usually with very little subsequent information in the literature. Recently an epithelial dystrophy was described with progressive cystic intraepithelial lesions in a whorl-like pattern. Patients had no erosions of the cornea but some developed decreased vision. Marked vacuolation of the epithelium was noted on pathologic examination.[17]

These disorders have both epithelial and anterior stromal involvement, and Bowman's layer is particularly involved. Because of differences in the descriptions of these disorders in European and American literatures, there has been confusion in the eponymal terminology used. Figure 10.23 provides a framework for better defining these disorders.

## ANTERIOR MEMBRANE DYSTROPHIES

### FIGURE 10.23. Anterior Membrane Dystrophies

| Dystrophy | Symptoms | Clinical Appearance | Pathology |
| --- | --- | --- | --- |
| Reis-Bücklers | Painful erosions early in life | Subepithelial sheet and map-like opacities | Rod-shaped bodies on EM |
| Superficial granular | Less frequent erosions, more visual symptoms early in life | Discrete granular subepithelial and anterior stromal opacities | Rod-shaped bodies on EM |
| Honeycomb (Thiel and Benke) | Painful erosions early in life | Irregular honeycomb pattern protruding into epithelium | Curly filaments on EM |

EM = transmission electron microscopy.

## REIS-BÜCKLERS' DYSTROPHY

Reis[18] and later Bücklers[19] reviewed the same family and described a disorder characterized by recurrent painful corneal erosions starting in infancy. Subepithelial opacities in the Bowman's region are seen in a map-like pattern and they become more confluent in sheets over the years (Fig. 10.24). Painful erosions become less frequent but decreased vision occurs by the second or third decade of life. By this time corneal sensitivity is also decreased. Histopathologic examination shows destruction of Bowman's layer and accumulations of eosinophilic material which can also be found in the epithelium. Electron microscopy shows the presence of "rod-shaped bodies" between the epithelial cells and replacing Bowman's layer.[20] The microscopic findings are the same as those seen in superficial variants of granular dystrophy. Treatment consists of lamellar keratectomy with peeling off of the superficial accumulated material. Recurrence may be found relatively fast, but in patients who have undergone keratoplasty, can be readily scraped off.

## SUPERFICIAL GRANULAR DYSTROPHY

Superficial granular dystrophy presents less frequently with corneal erosions but commonly with superficial granular subepithelial and anterior stromal opacities (Fig. 10.25). Histopathologic and electron microscopic evaluation show the same changes noted above in Reis-Bücklers' dystrophy. Some investigators feel that the entities are variants of the same disorder.[21] Others have demonstrated superficial granular dystrophy in relatives of patients with classic stromal granular dystrophy.[22]

Grayson-Wilbrandt dystrophy and Stocker-Holt dystrophy appear to be variants of Reis-Bücklers' dystrophy.[23]

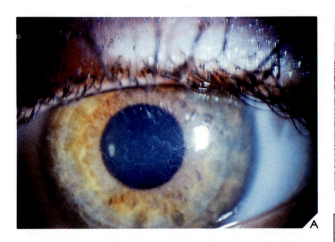

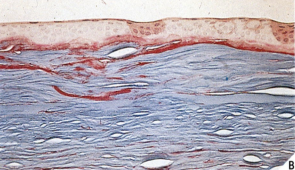

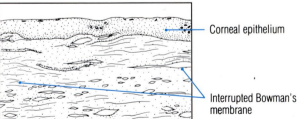

Corneal epithelium

Interrupted Bowman's membrane

**10.24** | *A:* Reis-Bücklers' dystrophy. *A:* The characteristic, corneal map-like pattern is apparent. *B:* Histologic section shows disruption of Bowman's membrane by fibrous tissue, along with a fibrous plaque between Bowman's membrane and the epithelium. (*B*, trichrome. From Yanoff M, Fine BS: *Ocular Pathology. A Color Atlas,* ed 2. New York: Gower Medical Publishing, 1992, 8.15.)

## HONEYCOMB DYSTROPHY

Also known as Thiel and Behnke's dystrophy, Waardenburg and Jonkers' dystrophy, honeycomb-type Reis-Bücklers' dystrophy, and "English literature Reis-Bücklers" dystrophy, honeycomb dystrophy refers to an entity with recurrent corneal erosions beginning early in life. Corneal opacities have a honeycomb pattern at the level of Bowman's layer (Fig. 10.26) with irregular protrusion into the epithelium in a "saw-tooth" pattern.[24] Histopathology shows irregular fibrous tissue replacing Bowman's layer. Electron microscopy shows replacement of Bowman's layer with electron-dense "curly filaments."[25] Treatment is the same as in Reis-Bücklers' dystrophy.

## PRIMARY (FAMILIAL) BAND KERATOPATHY

Primary band keratopathy is rare. Most band keratopathy is due to ocular degenerative and inflammatory disease or is secondary to systemic disorders. A few reports exist, however, of familial band keratopathy both in a childhood form occurring at puberty and in an adult form. Most reports have been in siblings, although parent to child transmission has also been reported, and the inheritance pattern is uncertain.[26] Treatment is the same as for band keratopathy of any other cause.

## DYSTROPHIES OF THE CORNEAL STROMA

Stromal opacities may be caused by a variety of stimuli such as inflammation, trauma, and as a result of systemic metabolic diseases. In addition, hereditary and congenital disorders may cause corneal stromal bilateral opacities that often have distinguishing clinical features as well as specific histopathologic findings. These conditions cause opacities that are not

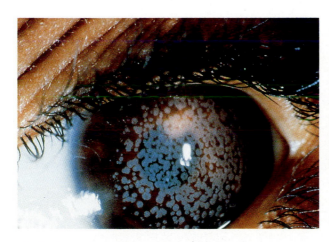

10.25 | Superficial granular dystrophy.

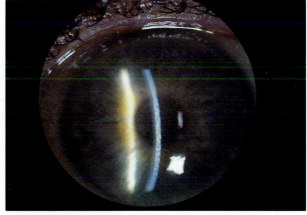

10.26 | Honeycomb dystrophy.

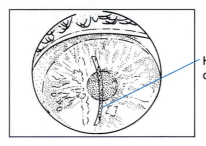

Honeycomb opacities

related to inflammation, may or may not reduce visual acuity, may cause glare and photophobia and other conditions such as recurrent erosions. Some of these conditions require treatment by penetrating keratoplasty when there is significant visual impairment and many have more than one name (Fig. 10.27). In most instances there is an abnormal accumulation of some substance in the stroma that leads to localized or diffuse stromal opacification. In most cases, the precise pathogenesis remains to be determined. The interplay between stromal keratocytes and the abundant extracellular matrix of the stroma is a unique site for the study of such interactions.

In embryologic development, the second wave of migration of neural crest cells results in the positioning of cells anterior to the endothelium (from the first wave of migration from neural crest cells) that become stromal keratocytes and produce the stromal extracellular matrix.[27,28] Abnormalities of neural crest cell migration and development can account for such abnormalities as posterior embryotoxon or sclerocornea. In contrast, biochemical abnormalities involving stromal keratocytes can lead to corneal opacifications due to accumulations of abnormal material in the keratocytes, extracellular matrix, or both. Because the corneal endothelium is also derived from neural crest cells, it is not surprising that both stromal keratocytes and corneal endothelial cells demonstrate the same biochemical abnormalities in patients with some stromal dystrophies.

## GRANULAR DYSTROPHY

Granular corneal dystrophy is transmitted as an autosomal dominant disorder and causes discrete, whitish, irregular opacities often with clear centers that are most abundant in the anterior portion of the central cornea.[29] The opacities are seen in very young children and typically remain stationary throughout life, or slowly additional opacities develop in deeper stroma or towards the corneal periphery, or both. With time, the centers of the opacities may become more whitish and take on the appearance of commonly recognized objects such as trees or snowflakes (Figs. 10.28, 10.29). When examining several affected people of various ages in a single family, it is relatively common to note the progression toward solid opacities with advancing age.

Most people with granular dystrophy have no visual changes until at least age 40 and a minority of patients with this dystrophy require penetrating keratoplasty. Some patients with superficial stromal opacities develop

### FIGURE 10.27. More Common Corneal Stromal Dystrophies, Their Other Names and Patterns of Inheritance

| DYSTROPHY | OTHER NAMES | INHERITANCE PATTERN |
|---|---|---|
| Granular | Groenouw I | Autosomal dominant |
| Lattice | Biber-Haab-Dimmer | Autosomal dominant |
| Macular | Groenouw II | Autosomal recessive |
| Central crystalline dystrophy of Schnyder | | Autosomal dominant |
| Fleck | Speckled, Francois | Autosomal dominant |

painful recurrent erosions. These problems may require superficial keratectomy or penetrating keratoplasty.

Most of the histopathologic specimens for the study of granular dystrophy have come from patients with disease severe enough to necessitate corneal transplantation. The discrete lesions have characteristic appearances in light microscopy using multiple stains. With hematoxylin and eosin staining, the discrete lesions of eosinophilic hyaline-like deposits are noted in the stroma and occasionally under the epithelium (see Fig. 10.28). The lesions are bright red with Masson's trichrome stain, sometimes weakly PAS-positive,

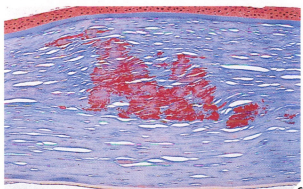

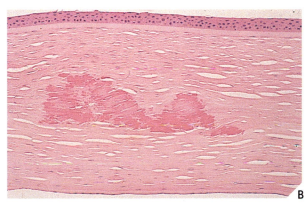

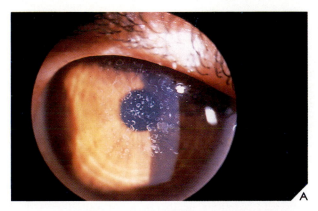

10.28 | Granular dystrophy. *A:* Clear cornea is present between the small, white, sharply outlined stromal granules. *B:* Histologic section shows that the granules stain deeply with H&E and, in *C,* stain red with the trichrome stain. The PAS stain and stains for acid mucopolysaccharides and amyloid are negative. The condition is inherited as an autosomal dominant trait. (From Yanoff M, Fine BS: *Ocular Pathology. A Color Atlas,* ed 2. New York: Gower Medical Publishing, 1992, 8.16.)

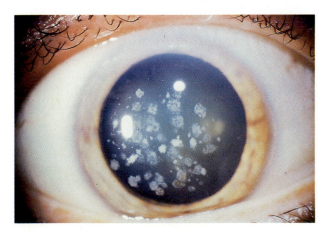

10.29 | Granular dystrophy. Patient with prominent opacities and normal visual acuity.

and the periphery of each lesion may stain with Congo red.[30,31] The deposits have been shown to contain tyrosine, tryptophan, sulfur-containing amino acids, and sometimes arginine on the basis histochemical studies.[32] The lesions are not birefringent when viewed with polarizing microscope optics. On electron microscopy there are rod and trapezoid shaped deposits that are electron-dense and measure 100–500 nm wide and are of variable lengths.[30,31] Other studies have revealed that the lesions contain microfibrillar proteins and phospholipids. In some instances, the deposits have been identified inside of corneal epithelial cells as well as keratocytes.[33,34] The deposits have been noted to develop within the donor cornea following transplantation to recipients with granular dystrophy. Some of the recurrences have been limited to the epithelium.

Despite these findings, the exact nature and biochemical pathway abnormality in granular dystrophy remain elusive. It seems possible that both corneal epithelial cells and stromal keratocytes may participate in the formation of the deposits.

Most people with granular corneal dystrophy have minimal symptoms and no decrease in visual acuity until age 40 years or older. After that time, some develop recurrent erosions with pain. These can be managed with patching or therapeutic bandage soft contact lenses. Occasionally, superficial keratectomy may be successful if there are just a few deposits beneath the epithelium. Significantly decreased visual acuity is an indication for penetrating keratoplasty. As mentioned above, recurrent granular deposits may appear in the donor cornea. Those that recur just beneath the epithelium can be managed by superficial keratectomy.

A variant of granular dystrophy with amyloid deposits in the stroma and lattice-like opacities as well as granular opacities on slit-lamp examination has been described in patients who originate from the Italian province of Avellino.[35]

## LATTICE DYSTROPHY

Lattice corneal dystrophy is inherited as an autosomal dominant trait with variable penetrability.[36,37] The clinical features are typically bilateral and symmetrical, although unilateral as well as asymmetrical cases can be found.[38] In affected persons, the earliest findings are often noted before 10 years of age. By age 30 years decreased visual acuity, recurrent epithelial erosions, or both, often dominate the clinical course and are accompanied by increased deposits in the stroma of the cornea and in subepithelial sites. This classic type of lattice dystrophy has been called Type I and other forms are referred to as Types II and III.

The corneal deposits in Type I lattice dystrophy begin as thin, irregular lines and dots in the central anterior stroma and at the level of Bowman's layer. As the dystrophy progresses the deposits enlarge and become branched. Deposits also become evident in the deep corneal stroma and towards the periphery. The deposits are highly refractile and the superficial ones cause anterior irregular astigmatism and recurrent corneal erosions. In the advanced stages the central cornea becomes hazy (Fig. 10.30).

On histopathologic examination, the deposits are fusiform in the stroma and stain with Congo red, periodic acid-Schiff, and Masson's trichome[39] (Fig. 10.31). Additionally, the deposits that stain orange-red with Congo red also exhibit dichroism and birefringence when examined with a microscope fitted with a polarizing lens[40] (see Fig. 10.31). The deposits also

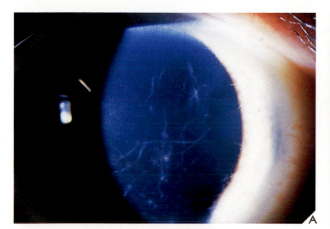

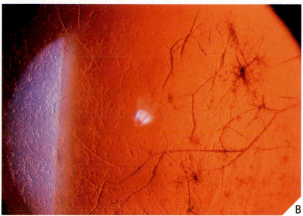

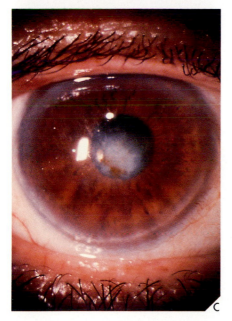

**10.30** | Lattice dystrophy. *A:* Direct illumination of characteristic, refractile lattice lines in the corneal stroma. *B:* The same area viewed in retroillumination. *C:* Central corneal opacity late in the clinical course of lattice dystrophy complicated by recurrent epithelial erosions.

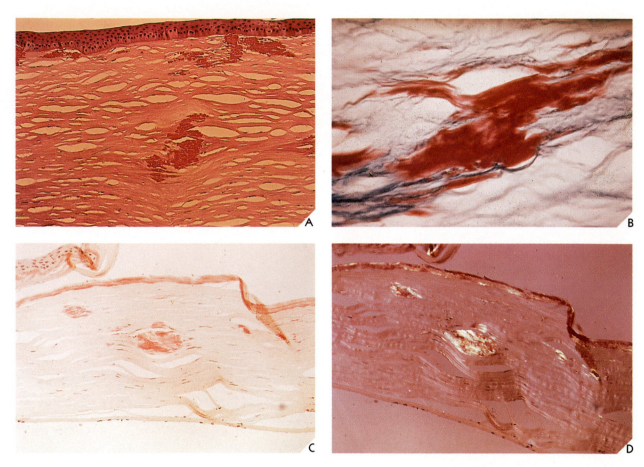

**10.31** | Histopathologic characteristics of lattice dystrophy. *A:* PAS stains the deposits a bright red throughout the stroma and beneath the epithelium. *B:* Masson's trichrome stains the lattice deposits red. *C:* Congo red stains the deposits an orange-red color. *D:* The same Congo red-stained deposits exhibit dichroism when viewed through a polarizing filter.

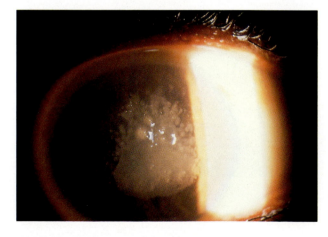

**10.32** | Gelatinous drop-like dystrophy.

fluoresce when stained with the fluorochrome thioflavin-T and examined with a fluorescence microscope. Collectively these findings indicate that the deposits are amyloid. Deposits with the same histochemical characteristics may also be found beneath the corneal epithelium in association with thinning or thickening of the epithelium, breaks or thickening of its basement membrane, breaks in Bowman's layer, and loss of hemidesmosomes in the basal layer of the epithelium.[41]

Transmission electron microscopy demonstrates that the deposits are electron-dense 8–10 nm aligned fibrils.[42] Amyloid is a protein that has been found in several forms in patients with either primary or secondary systemic amyloidosis. In persons with elevated immunoglobulins, the deposits appear to be similar to prealbumin. Both primary and secondary systemic amyloidoses have a protein designated as protein AP in their deposits and secondary forms also have another protein designated as protein AA. The corneal stromal deposits in Type I lattice dystrophy contain protein AP.

Type II lattice corneal dystrophy is seen in association with dominant hereditary amyloidosis of the Meretoja type, a form of familial amyloid polyneuropathy (Type IV or Finnish Type).[43] This disorder appears to be due to a mutation in the gene for gelsolin, an actin-binding protein found in normal plasma.[44] More recently, gelsolin reactivity has been found in the amyloid deposits of lattice dystrophy of all types as well as in some secondary forms of amyloidoses and drop–like corneal dystrophy.[45] The clinical findings and symptoms in Type II appear to be milder. The pathologic examinations of corneas with this form of lattice dystrophy reveal a layer of amyloid posterior to Bowman's layer and possibly the replacement of corneal nerves by amyloid. Many of the patients with Type II lattice dystrophy come from Scandinavian countries. Type III lattice dystrophy is characterized by autosomal recessive inheritance and no evidence of systemic amyloidosis.[46,47] Thick, ropy, corneal opacities are present and corneal erosions are absent. A variant of Type III with dominant inheritance and corneal erosions has been described.[48]

The management of patients with decreased visual acuity is penetrating keratoplasty. Recurrent erosions often can be managed in the early stages of lattice dystrophy with patching or therapeutic bandage soft contact lenses, but later they require corneal transplants. Recurrence of lattice deposits in donor tissue is a significant problem that begins approximately two years after the transplant surgery and may occur in up to one-half of these recipients.[49,50]

Another dystrophy involving corneal accumulation of amyloid is gelatinous drop-like dystrophy or primary familial corneal amyloidosis. This disorder is probably autosomal recessive in nature and is characterized by nubbly or mulberry mounds of grayish material accumulating beneath the corneal epithelium and in the anterior stroma (Fig. 10.32). Recurrence in corneal grafts is rapid and our treatment of choice has been repeated superficial keratectomy.

## MACULAR DYSTROPHY

Macular dystrophy is inherited as an autosomal recessive disorder in which both corneas are equally involved. Until recently, it was thought that patients with macular corneal dystrophy did not have involvement of other ocular tissues or other body sites.[51] However, it is now evident that patients with macular corneal dystrophy have abnormal synthesis of keratan sulfate proteoglycan, possibly involving sulfotransferases required for the sulfation of lactosaminoglycans.[52] It also appears that this is a systemic abnormality because some patients lack any detectable keratan sulfate in serum or cornea,[53,54] and in one case, in cartilage as well as serum and cornea.[55] In some patients, monoclonal antibodies against the protein core of normal keratan sulfate proteoglycan detect presumably abnormal keratan in both cornea and serum of patients who have other histochemical evidence of macular corneal dystrophy. This heterogeneity has led to the designation of macular corneal dystrophy Type 1 and Type 2, respectively.[55,56] Photophobia and discomfort begin in the first decade of life and by the teenage years visual acuity has significantly decreased. Heterozygous carriers of the gene for macular dystrophy appear normal. The clinical features of the involved cornea are diffuse haze of the entire stroma with focal whitish stromal opacities, an irregular corneal epithelium due to superficial deposits, and irregularities of Descemet's membrane[51] (Fig. 10.33).

Histopathologic examinations of involved corneas are characterized by the accumulations of glycosaminoglycans within stromal keratocytes and corneal endothelial cells beneath the epithelium and within the stroma. Classically, the accumulations of glycosaminoglycans can be demonstrated by staining with alcian blue, colloidal iron, and periodic acid-Schiff[30,58] (Fig. 10.34). The accumulated glycosaminoglycans are known to be an abnormal keratan sulfate.[59] Electron microscopic examination demonstrates the accumulation of glycosaminoglycans within intracytoplasmic vacuoles.[60] The architecture of the stromal collagen appears normal. Endothelial cells have degenerative changes similar to stromal keratocytes, and guttae are evident on the posterior layer of Descemet's membrane.[61]

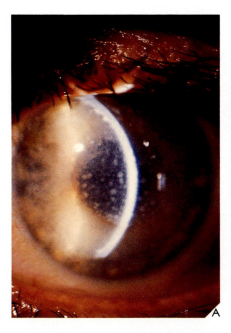
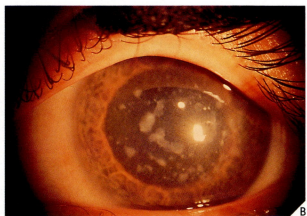

**10.33** | Macular dystrophy. *A:* Diffusely hazy cornea and small whitish dense opacities are seen at all depths over the entire cornea. *B:* Larger dense opacities but less diffuse haziness are noted in another patient with macular dystrophy.

Penetrating keratoplasty is the treatment for macular dystrophy when visual acuity becomes significantly impaired. Recurrence of the deposition of the abnormal keratan sulfate has been noted several years after transplantation.[62] This happens after recipient stromal keratocytes repopulate the donor tissue. The recurrence spreads from peripheral to central portions of the donor cornea.

Central crystalline dystrophy is an autosomal dominant disorder.[63] After having clear corneas at birth, the characteristic crystals appear at approximately one year of age or later. By 30 years of age, a significant corneal arcus and Vogt's limbal girdle are often present along with disc- or ring-shaped crystalline deposits.[64] Significantly elevated levels of serum cholesterol and triglycerides have been found in some patients as well as family members without corneal crystals.[65] Other findings in some affected individuals include genu valgum and xanthelasma.

The crystals are needle-shaped and appear as brightly colored iridescent deposits. Often there is a diffuse central stromal haze as well. These changes are most evident in the anterior portion of the corneal stroma but often involve its full thickness. The corneal arcus and Vogt's limbal girdle are not distinctive in appearance but are evident at a younger age than normal.

Histopathologic studies demonstrate that the crystalline deposits are cholesterol crystals and the more diffuse opacities consist of cholesterol esters, triglycerides, and noncrystalline cholesterol. Electron microscopy shows notched crystalline structures randomly distributed among normal collagen fibrils.[66,67] Occasionally the crystals are seen within stromal keratocytes.[68] The lipids dissolve with normal tissue fixation but staining of frozen sections with oil red O shows neutral fats as red.

CENTRAL CRYSTALLINE DYSTROPHY OF SCHNYDER

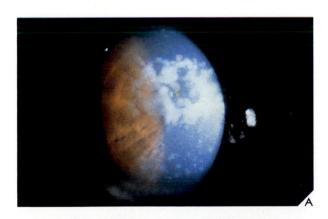 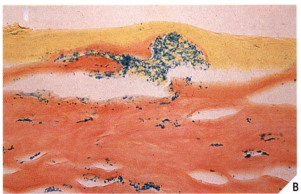

**10.34** | Macular dystrophy. *A:* The corneal stroma between the opacities is cloudy. *B:* Histologic section shows that keratocytes and vacuolated cells beneath the epithelium are filled with acid mucopolysaccharide. In this condition, the trichchrome stain and stains for amyloid are negative, but the PAS stain is positive. The condition is inherited as an autosomal recessive trait. (*B,* AMP. From Yanoff M, Fine BS: *Ocular Pathology. A Color Atlas,* ed 2. New York: Gower Medical Publishing, 1992, 8.16.)

Any patient found with crystalline corneal dystrophy and any unstudied family members should have blood drawn for cholesterol and triglyceride levels.[69] If hyperlipidemia is present, it is important to manage it medically. Visual acuity is usually satisfactory. In some patients age 50 or older, penetrating keratoplasty may be necessary to improve vision. Most reports describing this condition have been published in American and European literature. Two reports describe large pedigrees from central[64] and southeastern[70] Finland.

FLECK DYSTROPHY

Also known as speckled dystrophy, fleck dystrophy is uncommon. The condition is transmitted as an autosomal dominant,[71] and has been noted in association with a variety of other eye conditions which apparently are not genetically related. Vision is normal.

Fleck dystrophy is bilateral and exhibits discrete, small, whitish deposits at all depths in the stroma from limbus to limbus (Fig. 10.35). The intervening stroma is normal. Some of the deposits appear as rings with clear centers, but most are solid and vary in shape from round to granular.

On histologic examination, the abnormalities are restricted to the stroma of the cornea. The extracellular matrix appears normal but, within it, some keratocytes are distended and stain positively with oil red O for lipids and with colloidal iron and alcian blue for glycosaminoglycans. Other stromal keratocytes appear normal.[72] Electron microscopy shows distended stromal keratocytes with membrane-bound vacuoles filled with electron-dense lamellar deposits.[71]

Patients with fleck dystrophy have normal vision and the diagnosis is usually an incidental finding. No treatment is required. The precise pathogenesis of this condition is not known. Stromal keratocytes are of neural crest origin. This dystrophy exhibits autosomal dominant transmission. Together, these conditions suggest that fleck dystrophy is a minor structural alteration of a subpopulation of stromal keratocytes that does not prevent the production of normal corneal stroma extracellular matrix by cells derived from the second wave of migration of neural crest cells. Further, the neural crest cells from the first wave of migration are not affected and have led to a normal, healthy corneal endothelium.

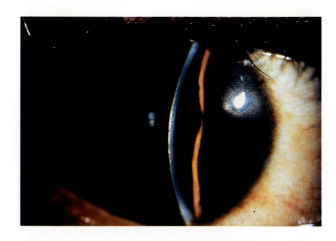

**10.35** | Fleck dystrophy. Collections of glycosaminoglycans seen as small white deposits at all depths throughout the corneal stroma.

Another syndrome with punctate opacities throughout the entire corneal stroma has been described[73] (Fig. 10.36). The condition is bilateral and occurs in a variant of spondyloepiphyseal dysplasia. Vision is normal. Collagen fibers in the dermis have intermittent unpacking and give the appearance of the frayed end of a rope. The cornea has not been studied in this condition. No treatment is required.

A rare, autosomal dominant disorder has been called posterior amorphous corneal dystrophy.[74] Patients present with thinning of the central corneas, flattened keratometric readings, and diffuse opacities slightly anterior to Descemet's membrane. They also have hyperopic refractions. Histopathologic examinations have demonstrated two types of pathologic changes. One patient had collagen alterations anterior to Descemet's membrane as well as in its anterior portion.[75] In another, these changes were accompanied by an abnormal posterior collagenous layer of Descemet's membrane and abnormalities of the epithelial basement membrane and Bowman's layer.[76]

There are some other unusual stromal dystrophies that result in opacities in the pre-Descemet's membrane area. Various patterns of gray to white deposits have been noted. They do not significantly reduce visual acuity. This group of dystrophies includes cloudy central corneal dystrophy,[77,78] congenital hereditary stromal dystrophy,[79] and pre-Descemet dystrophy of Grayson and Wilbrandt.[80] The exact causes and biochemical and structural alterations of this condition are not completely elucidated.

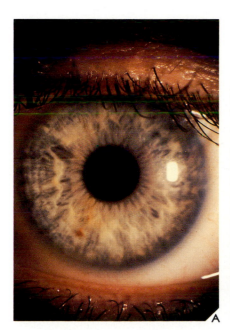
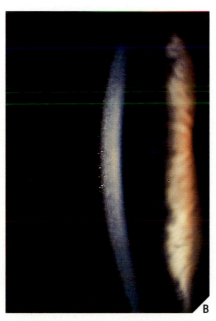

**10.36** | *A:* Punctate dystrophy associated with a variant of spondyloepiphyseal dysplasia and abnormal dermal collagen. *B:* The punctate lesions are small and white and are distributed throughout the entire stroma.

## ENDOTHELIAL DYSTROPHIES

The human corneal endothelium exists as a monolayer of hexagonal cells attached to Descemet's membrane. These cells function in two ways to maintain the relative deturgescence of the cornea. First, the endothelial cells and their intercellular junctions act as a barrier to the passage of significant volumes of aqueous humor into the stroma. Second, these cells have an active Na/K-ATPase pump that moves electrolytes and water back into the anterior chamber. Human corneal endothelial cells have very limited capacities to divide. Thus, normal aging, inflammation, and trauma are characteristically associated with decreased densities of normal endothelial cells. In some individuals this process occurs at an unexpected early age and without provocation, often with a family history of similar clinical findings and symptoms. These persons appear to have structural and/or biochemical abnormalities involving their endothelial cell population. Concomitant with decreased endothelial cell densities, there is production of excessive, abnormal, additional material adjacent to the normal Descemet's membrane. With slit-lamp biomicroscopy, discrete guttata or a more diffuse beaten metal appearance may be seen (Fig. 10.37). Histopathologic corneal examination shows the guttata as mushroom-shaped excrescences on Descemet's membrane and the latter as the generalized deposition of a posterior collagenous layer (Fig. 10.38). The end result of these histologic changes is corneal edema as the barrier and pump functions of the corneal endothelium progressively fail.

In addition to the endothelial dystrophies that are discussed below, various forms of insult to the endothelium can result in permanent corneal edema. Blunt trauma may directly injure or destroy endothelial cells, or rupture Descemet's membrane and subsequently result in corneal edema because of inadequate function of the endothelial cells that cover the area (Fig. 10.39). Descemet's membrane may be stripped away from the stroma

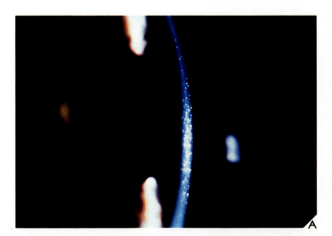

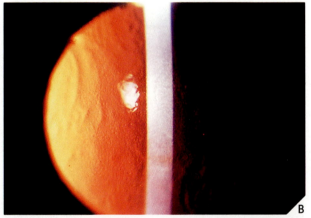

**10.37 |** Corneal guttata are present posterior to Descemet's membrane and seen with slit-lamp biomicroscopy as posterior protrusions with a narrow beam *(A)* or as a distinct irregular pattern in retroillumination *(B)*. Guttata may cause sufficient posterior irregular astigmatism to reduce visual acuity to 20/40.

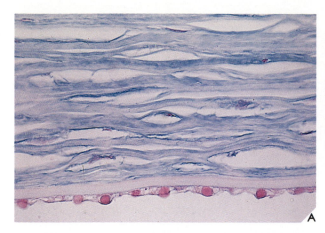

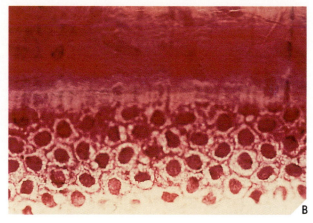

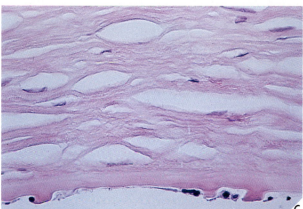

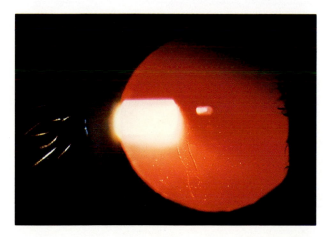

**10.38** | Histologic sections of the posterior stroma, Descemet's membrane, and endothelium. *A:* Normal cornea with normal-thickness Descemet's membrane and regular, healthy endothelium. *B:* Oblique section of normal cornea with normal density and shape of endothelial cells. *C:* Corneal guttata with reduced density of flattened endothelial cells.

**10.39** | Traumatic rupture of Descemet's membrane viewed in retroillumination. Vertically oriented scrolled edges of tear are evident.

during surgery and result in localized edema (Fig. 10.40). Bending the cornea, touching it with surgical instruments, or irrigation of the anterior chamber with a toxic chemical can all result in endothelial dysfunction and corneal edema (Fig. 10.41). Likewise, vitreous apposition against the endothelium may result in a similar sequence of events. Vitreous touch was much more common when intracapsular extractions were the standard approach to cataract surgery (Fig. 10.42). Corneas with any degree of endothelial dystrophy are very susceptible to further damage by any of these modalities. However, normal, healthy endothelial cell populations may also be permanently damaged by these types of insult.

There are four clinically distinct corneal endothelial dystrophies that appear to have their own unique pathophysiologic mechanisms. It is possible that these dystrophies are not as separate as our clinical categories.

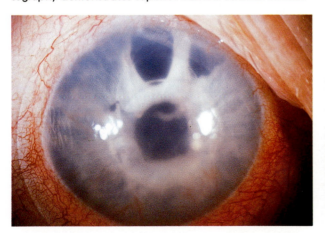

A

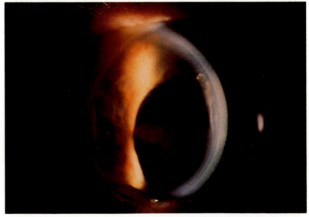

B

**10.40** | Descemet's membrane has been stripped at the time of cataract surgery. *A:* Lower power slit-lamp photography demonstrates superior corneal stromal edema.

*B:* Higher power examination shows detached Descemet's membrane.

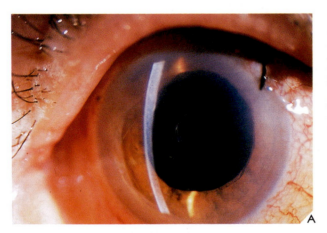

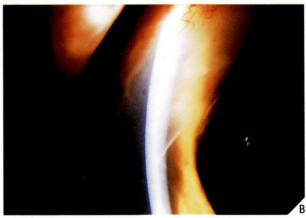

**10.41** | Corneal edema following cataract surgery that has caused damage to the endothelial cell layer. A therapeutic bandage soft contact lens is in place.

**10.42** | Slit-lamp photograph demonstrates corneal edema in association with vitreous touch.

Because corneal endothelium and trabecular meshwork are derived from the first wave of neural crest cells, it is possible to relate these conditions to one another and to some forms of glaucoma and congenital anomalies involving the cornea, trabecular meshwork, and iris (Fig. 10.43). The second and third waves of neural crest cell migrations give rise to corneal keratocyes and anterior iris, respectively[81-84] (Fig. 10.44). The common embryologic derivations of all of these structures from neural crest cells also explains the close resemblance of ICE syndrome and posterior polymorphous dystrophy in histologic specimens.[85] The demonstration of ocular neural crest cell anomalies (e.g., Peters' anomaly and Axenfeld's anomaly) in association with fetal alcohol syndrome suggests that disturbances late in fetal life can profoundly affect tissues derived from neural crest cells.[8]

## FIGURE 10.43. Neural Crest Cell Abnormality and Corresponding Clinical Disorder

| ABNORMALITY | DISORDER |
|---|---|
| Deficient formation | Brain-eye-face malformations |
| Abnormal migration | Congenital glaucoma<br>Posterior embryotoxon<br>Axenfeld's anomaly<br>Rieger syndrome<br>Peters' anomaly<br>Sclerocornea |
| Abnormal proliferation | Essential iris atrophy<br>Chandler syndrome<br>Iris-nevus syndrome |
| Abnormal terminal induction (final differentiation) | Nonprogressive corneal gutta<br>Congenital hereditary endothelial dystrophy (CHED)<br>Posterior polymorphous dystrophy<br>Fuchs' endothelial dystrophy |
| Acquired abnormalities | Metaplasia<br>Abiotrophy (hypertrophy)<br>Proliferation |

## NONPROGRESSIVE CORNEA GUTTATA

A number of individuals and family pedigrees have been reported who exhibit bilateral cornea guttata but do not progress to corneal edema.[86-89] It is not certain whether this represents a clinical dystrophic condition or is simply a description of the appearance of cornea guttata as part of the spectrum of the normal aging process. Cornea guttata have been described in presumably normal populations at frequencies of 5–70% and with higher prevalences at advanced ages. Leaving aside the issue of whether or not these changes represent a dystrophy, it is important to recognize that corneal guttata are common and that in a vast majority of patients they are nonprogressive and do not threaten vision.

## FUCHS' ENDOTHELIAL DYSTROPHY

Fuchs' classic description of advanced endothelial dystrophy (which was not recognized by Fuchs because the slit-lamp biomicroscope had not yet been invented) included marked epithelial edema and stromal edema with haziness.[90] It is generally believed that Fuchs' endothelial dystrophy is transmitted as an autosomal dominant.[91] Early symptoms of reduced vision, initially transient, due to corneal edema, usually begin between 40 and 50 years of age. The condition is typically more common and more severe in women. Fortunately, the progression of the endothelial dysfunction and subsequent

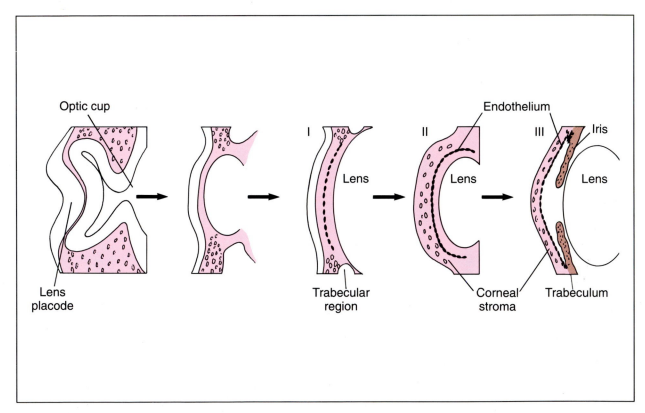

**10.44 |** Schematic depiction of the three waves of neural crest cells during development of the eye (after Bahn et al,[84] Hay,[82] and Meier[83]).

corneal edema is usually asymmetric and corneal transplantation can be performed in the eye in which the condition is more advanced while good vision remains in the other.

The first clinical findings are the guttata on Descemet's membrane along with pigment phagocytosis by the endothelium. At this stage, the patient is usually asymptomatic. However, a high density of guttata may be associated with glare and mild reduction in visual acuity to 20/30 or 20/40 due to posterior corneal irregular astigmatism. As the corneal endothelium loses more of its physiologic functions, mild degrees of stromal edema along with intermittent epithelial edema develop. Patients notice blurred vision upon awakening that clears throughout the day. As the barrier and pump functions of the corneal endothelium deteriorate further, constant epithelial and stromal edema is present. The edema eventually leads to epithelial bullae and a markedly thickened stroma with wrinkles in Descemet's membrane. Both markedly reduced visual acuity and pain are predominant symptoms. Finally, subepithelial fibrosis, often with vascularization, develops and the pain from rupture of bullae subsides (Fig. 10.45).

The histopathologic correlates of Fuchs' endothelial dystrophy parallel the clinical course. The endothelial cells become progressively thinner in histologic sections and are enlarged on specular microscopy. Guttata become larger and reach a greater density. They are positively stained with periodic

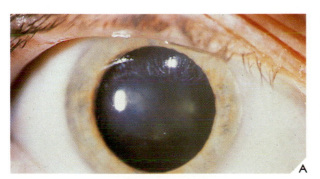
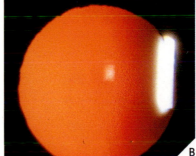
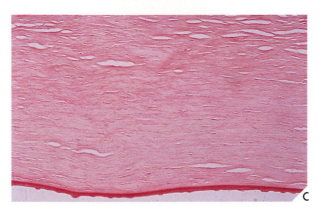
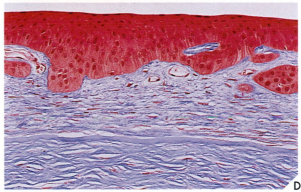

**10.45 | Fuchs' endothelial dystrophy.** *A:* The cornea shows central thickening and haze. *B:* The characteristic appearance of cornea guttata is shown in the fundus reflex. *C:* Typical wart-like bumps are present on Descemet's membrane. The primary endothelial defect leads to secondary epithelial and stromal edema and degeneration. The edema may spread between and under the epithelial cells, resulting in bleb formation (bullous keratopathy). *D:* Fibrous tissue may proliferate between the epithelium and Bowman's membrane, forming a degenerative pannus. (*C,* PAS. *D,* trichrome. From Yanoff M, Fine BS: *Ocular Pathology. A Color Atlas,* ed 2. New York: Gower Medical Publishing, 1992, 8.19.)

acid-Schiff (PAS) as is Descemet's membrane (see Fig. 10.45). Guttata are new collagenous tissues produced by the abnormal endothelium. Waring et al[92] have named this multilaminated collagenous tissue the "posterior collagenous layer" and have emphasized that it may appear as polymorphic excrescences or gray sheets as well as guttata. As these changes progress, the corneal stroma becomes thickened and fewer keratocytes are noted. Bowman's layer remains intact for the most part, but occasional focal breaks are present and filled with connective tissue. When subepithelial connective tissue is present, it consists of active fibroblasts, variable-sized small collagen fibrils, and a basement membrane-like collagen.[93,94] This tissue may reach a thickness that is seven times that of the normal epithelium (see Fig. 10.45). The spectrum of changes in the corneal epithelium also reflects the progressive increases in edema. Initial intracellular edema of the basal layer of cells is followed by intercellular edema and finally by bullae development. The thickness of the epithelial layer becomes irregular throughout the process, including the stage of subepithelial connective tissue deposition.

Ultimately, treatment for Fuchs' endothelial dystrophy is corneal transplantation. However, a number of other palliative measures can be effectively

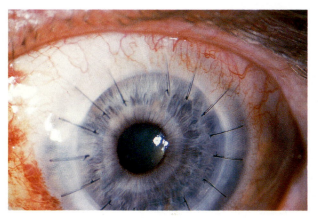

**10.46** | Postoperative photograph showing clear corneal transplant in patient with Fuchs' endothelial dystrophy.

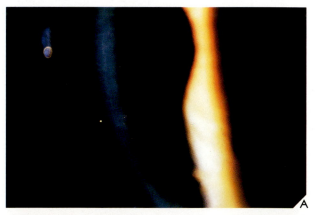

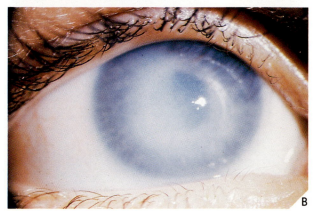

**10.47** | Posterior polymorphous dystrophy. Twin sisters demonstrate variable presentations with clear cornea and posterior vesicular-like lesions in one twin (A), and opaque, edematous cornea in her sister (B).

used to reduce symptoms and improve vision in the earlier stages. Hypertonic preparations (e.g., 5% NaCl) can reduce epithelial edema. Some patients benefit from the instillation of 5% NaCl ointment at bedtime, while others prefer using 5% NaCl solutions during the day. A useful regimen is 1 drop of 5% NaCl solution every 15 minutes for 1 hour after awakening and then every 2 hours for the remainder of the day. Some patients use both the ointment and solution preparations. A hair dryer turned to low heat and held at arm's length from the eye can also reduce corneal edema. The pain associated with the rupture of epithelial bullae can sometimes be controlled with topical cycloplegic agents (e.g., 5% homatropine), therapeutic contact lenses, or both. Because there is a break in epithelial layer integrity, there is significant risk for microbial keratitis associated with the use of therapeutic contact lenses for this condition. In patients for whom the relief of pain is the only therapeutic goal, cautery of Bowman's layer or a conjunctival flap offer simple and predictable relief. However, penetrating keratoplasty is required for visual rehabilitation (Fig. 10.46). In excess of 80% of grafts remain clear for at least two years.[95] In patients with any degree of lens opacification, penetrating keratoplasty, extracapsular cataract extraction, and insertion of a posterior chamber intraocular lens implant should be performed.

## POSTERIOR POLYMORPHOUS DYSTROPHY

This condition presents as a spectrum of posterior corneal changes that occasionally involve the iris and angle. Posterior polymorphous dystrophy was first described by Koeppe[96] in 1916, and Theodore[97] noted its autosomal dominant transmission in 1939. The condition demonstrates widely variable clinical presentations including severe cases of corneal clouding that have been noted at birth[98–100] (Fig. 10.47). Although most findings remain stable and do not reduce vision, some patients develop progressive corneal clouding and visual loss. Posterior polymorphous dystrophy is usually bilateral but somewhat asymmetrical. Most people with posterior polymorphous dystrophy are asymptomatic and the diagnosis is made as an incidental finding on slit-lamp biomicroscopy.

The spectrum of clinical findings of this dystrophy includes isolated or coalescent small vesicular-like lesions at the level of the endothelium. They are most easily seen along the edge of narrow beam or in oblique broad beam illumination. Other types of involvement appear as whitish opacities that may be flat or linear. In other instances, a clear zone is outlined by linear irregular white bands (Fig. 10.48).

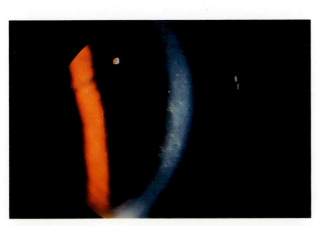

**10.48** | Posterior polymorphous dystrophy. The findings can be subtle; various types of slit-lamp illumination help highlight the changes.

In most cases, the face of the iris and the shape of the pupil appear normal. However, approximately 25% of patients with posterior polymorphous dystrophy have peripheral anterior synechiae that can be detected on gonioscopy. Raised intraocular pressure is found in approximately 15 percent of people with posterior polymorphous dystrophy.[101] Other findings that have been noted in association with some cases of posterior polymorphous dystrophy include prominent Schwalbe's ring, ectropion uveae, iridocorneal adhesions, and iris atrophy.

Histopathologic examinations reveal the presence of epithelial cell-like populations interspersed with seemingly normal endothelial cells. The epithelial-like cells are larger than normal endothelial cells, contain a high density of microvilli, and have a nonhexagonal, pleomorphic shape that is also evident by examination with specular microscopy. These nests of cells may be multilayered in contradistinction to normal endothelial cells. Additionally, the posterior layer of Descemet's membrane is abnormal in the areas where the epithelial-like cells are noted.[102] Specimens obtained from trabeculectomy operations show nests of these same cells on trabecular meshwork and iris.[103]

The precise source of the epithelial-like cells and the pathogenesis of posterior polymorphous dystrophy remain to be determined. It seems reasonable to hypothesize that the orderly migration of waves of neural crest cells[81–84] is disturbed in this condition, that the degree of the disturbance correlates with the severity of the wide spectrum of findings, and that the epithelial-like cells are, in fact, cells of neural crest origin.

Posterior polymorphous dystrophy usually does not require treatment. If significant corneal edema develops, it can be managed by the same approaches described for the treatment of Fuchs' endothelial dystrophy. Except in patients with extensive iridocorneal adhesions, glaucoma, or both, penetrating keratoplasty is usually successful. The glaucoma associated with posterior polymorphous dystrophy may also be difficult to control and may require surgery.

Posterior polymorphous dystrophy is clinically distinguished from iridocorneal endothelial syndrome (ICE syndrome) which includes Chandler syndrome, essential iris atrophy, and Cogan-Reese iris nevus syndrome. ICE syndrome is typically asymetrical and predominant in females with corneal edema, extensive iris atrophy, and ectropion uveae, and is invariably associated with glaucoma. The lesser involved eye most commonly has pleomorphism and decreased endothelial cell densities, iris transillumination defects, and abnormal aqueous outflow facility. Histopathologic specimens from ICE syndrome resemble those from posterior polymorphous dystrophy patients.[85]

Congenital hereditary endothelial dystrophy may occur as either an autosomal dominant or autosomal recessive disorder. The dominant form tends to have less severe corneal edema but may be associated with deafness.[104] In contrast, the recessive form is more common and displays more corneal edema, which is often present at birth, while in the dominant cases edema progresses slowly over the first few years of life.[105]

The corneal edema is bilateral. The stroma may be two to three times thicker than normal and opalescent or milk-glass in appearance over the entire cornea. The deep layers of the cornea and iris cannot be seen in detail. The corneal diameters are normal and the corneas do not vascularize (Fig. 10.49).

Endothelial cells are absent on histologic examination, or, if present, they are markedly atrophic over the entire posterior cornea. The anterior banded portion of Descemet's membrane appears normal, whereas the non-banded posterior portion that develops after the fifth gestational month is abnormal and thickened.[106,107]

Keratoplasty is the only treatment. It is difficult, but the bilateral nature of this condition mandates that corneal transplants be performed in both eyes as early as possible.

## CONGENITAL HEREDITARY ENDOTHELIAL DYSTROPHY

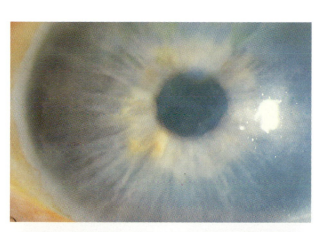

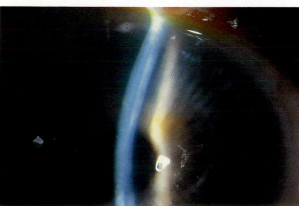

**10.49** | Congenital hereditary endothelial dystrophy. Corneal edema from shortly after birth with hazy cornea and poor visualization of iris *(A)* and thickened stroma and Descemet's membrane which is opacified *(B)*.

# 11 | KERATITIS AND ENDOPHTHALMITIS

## John W. Chandler

## OVERVIEW

Inflammatory corneal diseases, infectious and noninfectious, and endophthalmitis constitute vision-threatening conditions caused by a wide assortment of local or systemic diseases. Endophthalmitis, although usually caused by infectious agents, may be a noninfectious inflammatory process. In every instance, diligent efforts are essential to determine the specific causative agent or factor. In virtually all situations, appropriate therapy is contingent on laboratory data plus historical and physical examination data.

Physical findings are described in this chapter, but the emphasis is on other data that allow the ophthalmologist to make a specific diagnosis. The clinical findings of various conditions, including infections caused by various causative agents, often overlap or are indistinguishable.

To describe precisely the ocular features of these conditions, the examiner must be skilled at the use of the slit lamp biomicroscope and its accessories, and the direct and indirect ophthalmoscopes. Additionally, the indications for obtaining conjunctival or corneal cytology, biopsy or cultures, anterior chamber paracentesis, and vitreous biopsy must be understood and the procedures must be mastered. Knowledge of microbiology and pharmacology as they relate to ocular infections and inflammation is necessary for successful diagnosis and treatment. The clinician also should develop a system for carefully diagramming corneal disease processes, including specific measurements with the slit lamp biomicroscope and, if possible, to make photographs in order to follow corneal inflammations and infections.[1] In all cases of possible corneal infections or endophthalmitis, cytology and microbial cultures must be obtained before starting therapy to prevent problems related to partial treatment or masking of the specific diagnosis at later management points. Such an omission may lead to broad-based therapy rather than use of specific drugs, delayed appreciation of antibiotic resistance, or inappropriate antimicrobial therapy for a noninfectious inflammatory process. It is possible for people with a history of inflammatory corneal disease to develop microbial keratitis or for a person with recurrent herpetic keratitis to develop bacterial or fungal keratitis. For these reasons and the fact that these are all potential vision-threatening conditions, it is crucial that each episode of keratitis or possible endophthalmitis be thoroughly evaluated and appropriate laboratory studies performed.

This chapter will first cover microbial keratitis. The next portion will deal with noninfectious keratitis and, finally, endophthalmitis will be discussed. In infectious processes the host's inflammatory response often plays a significant role in the subsequent damage to ocular structures essential to visual function. In these infectious processes, eradication of the causative micro-organisms is only part of the therapy. Concurrent or subsequent management of inflammation and wound healing are vitally critical and equally or more challenging.

## Figure 11.1. Microbial Agents Causative of Infectious Keratitis

**BACTERIA**

**Gram-positive cocci**
*Peptostreptococcus sp.*
*Staphylococcus aureus*
*Staphylococcus epidermidis*
*Streptococcus faecalis*
*Streptococcus pneumoniae*
*Streptococcus pyogenes*
*Streptococcus viridans*

**Gram-negative bacilli**
*Aeromonas hydrophilia*
*Escherichia coli*
*Klebsiella pneumoniae*
*Morganella morganii*
*Proteus mirabilis*
*Pseudomonas aeruginosa*

*Pseudomonas acidovorans*
*Pseudomonas fluorescens*
*Pseudomonas pseudomallei*
*Pseudomonas stutzeri*
*Serratia marcescens*

**Gram-negative coccobacilli**
*Acinetobacter calcoaceticus*
*Branhamella catarrhalis*
*Moraxella lacunata*
*Moraxella nonliquefaciens*
*Neisseria gonorrhoeae*
*Pasteurella multocida*

**Gram-positive bacilli**
*Bacillus brevis*
*Bacillus cereus*

**Spirochetes**
*Borrelia burgdorferi*
*Treponema pallidum*

**Mycobacteria**
*Mycobacterium chelonei*
*Mycobacterium fortuitum*
*Mycobacterium tuberculosis*
*Mycobacterium leprae*

**Actinomycetes**
*Nocardia sp.*

**VIRUSES**
Adenovirus
Herpesvirus (herpes simplex, varicella-zoster, Epstein-Barr)
Poxvirus (variola, vaccinia, molluscum contagiosum)
Rubeola virus (measles)

**FUNGI**
*Acremonium sp. (Cephalosporium, Paecilomyces)*
*Aspergillus sp.*
*Candida sp.*
*Curvularia sp.*
*Drechslera sp.*
*Fusarium sp.*
*Neurospora sp.*
*Penicillium sp.*
*Phialophora sp.*
*Pseudallescheria boydii*

**PARASITES**
*Acanthamoeba castellani*
*Acanthamoeba polyphagia*
*Leishmania brasiliensis*
*Onchocerca volvulus*
*Trypanosoma sp.*

**CHLAMYDIA**
*Chlamydia trachomatis*

The causes and clinical pictures of ocular infections are numerous. Figure 11.1 lists the known microbial causes of infectious keratitis. There is some overlap with the myriad causes of infectious endophthalmitis (Fig. 11.2). In all cases, early and precise diagnosis and treatment depend on a high index of suspicion, thorough examination, and laboratory workup. Historical information, including pre-existing ocular conditions, occupation, type and situation of trauma, ocular surgery, contact lens wear, medication use, and general health or illness (e.g., deficiency or compromise of the immune system) are often useful. The ophthalmologist must resist the temptation to initiate therapy prior to a laboratory workup for all possible cases of microbial keratitis and endophthalmitis. Bacterial infections are the most likely to cause rapid destruction of the cornea or intraocular structures. However, bacteria can also cause mild, slowly progressive infections. Some rea-

## Figure 11.2. Microbial Agents Causative of Infectious Endophthalmitis

**BACTERIA**

**Aerobic gram-positive cocci**
Staphylococcus aureus
Staphylococcus epidermidis
Streptococcus pneumoniae
Streptococcus, other species

**Aerobic gram-positive bacilli**
Bacillus cereus
Bacillus subtilis
Bacillus, other species
Corynebacterium hofmannii
Corynebacterium xerosis
Corynebacterium, other species

**Aerobic gram-negative bacilli**
Acinetobacter sp.
Alcaligenes faecalis
Enterobacter sp.
Erwinia sp.
Flavobacterium meningosepticum
Klebsiella sp.
Moraxella sp.
Proteus sp.
Pseudomonas aeruginosa
Salmonella typhimurium
Serratia marcescens

**Anaerobic bacteria**
Clostridium sp.
Peptostreptococcus intermedius
Propionibacterium acnes

**Spirochetes**
Borrelia burgdorferi
Treponema pallidum

**Higher bacteria**
Actinomyces israelii
Mycobacterium avium
Mycobacterium intracellulare
Mycobacterium leprae
Mycobacterium tuberculosis
Nocardia sp.

**FUNGI**
Acremonium (Cephalosporium, Paecilomyces)
Aspergillus sp.
Blastomyces dermatitidis
Candida sp.
Cladosporium sp.
Fusarium sp.
Graphium sp.
Histoplasma capsulatum
Mucor sp.
Neurospora sitophila

Rhizopus sp.
Penicillium sp.
Pseudallescheria boydii
Sporothrix schenckii
Trichosporon sp.
Volutella sp.

**VIRUSES**
Herpesvirus (herpes simplex, cytomegalovirus, varicella-zoster)
Rubella virus
Rubeola virus

**PARASITES**
Onchocerca volvulus
Taenia solium (cysticercosis)
Toxocara canis
Toxocara cati
Toxoplasma gondii

sons for this variability are virulence of the infecting microbe, the health of the eye, and the patient's general health. Other classes of microbes usually are associated with infections that progress more slowly.

The laboratory workup is outlined in Figure 11.3. If organisms are identified on a careful and thorough microscopic examination of the Gram-stained slides, treatment can be targeted (Fig. 11.4). However, an experienced observer, clean and filtered stain solutions, and the avoidance of excessive destaining are vital to this workup. Extra slides can be used to look for microorganisms not identified by Gram stain or to repeat a Gram stain for confirmation of the original observation.

For a variety of reasons, including prior antibiotic therapy, excessively small inoculum, or laboratory mishandling, the culture may be negative. In these cases, the initial and subsequent selection of antibiotics is made to cover the gram-positive and gram-negative bacteria that are statistically most likely to be the cause (Fig. 11.5). The treatment of endopthalmitis is discussed later in this chapter.

In the following sections, infections are discussed by microbial classes (e.g., bacteria, viruses, fungi). Because the normal eye has many barriers to infections, the establishment of any infection usually requires antecedent

## Figure 11.3. Workup of Suspected Bacterial Ocular Infections

|  | KERATITIS | ENDOPHTHALMITIS |
| --- | --- | --- |
| **SMEAR** | | |
| Obtain 3–4 smears on slides for cytologic exam | Edge of infiltrate | Aqueous and vitreous aspirates* |
| Gram stain | Yes | Vitreous aspirate before infusion (1.0–1.5 ml)** |
| Giemsa stain (save two for special stains) | ± | Yes |
| **CULTURE** | **EDGE OF WOUND** | **ASPIRATE** |
| Blood agar | + | + |
| Chocolate agar | + | + |
| Sabouraud's media | + | + |
| Enriched broth | + | + |
| Antibiotic sensitivities (run on positive cultures) | + | + |
| **SPECIAL CULTURES** | | |
| E. coli-seeded agar | ± | ± |
| Viral transport media | ± | ± |
| **MATERIAL FOR SPECIAL STUDIES** | | |
| Polymerase chain reaction | ± | ± |
| Immunohistochemistry | ± | ± |

*Do immediately and begin antibiotic therapy, repeat vitreous aspirate at time of vitrectomy.     **Use initial aspirate for cytology plus culture.

events. For example, the normal corneal surface is covered with an intact epithelium that is covered by a mucin layer and flushed by tears that contain naturally occurring antimicrobial materials such as lysozyme and secretory antibodies as well as complement components. Very few micro-organisms can establish an infection unless the barriers have been violated by trauma, pre-existing disease states, contact lens wear, surgery, or other insults. Similarly, endophthalmitis is often associated with trauma or surgery and, less commonly, results from endogenous spread of infection from elsewhere in

## Figure 11.4. Gram Stain Cytology in Conjunctivitis and Corneal Ulcer

| | PROBABLE ORGANISM | |
|---|---|---|
| CHARACTERISTICS | CONJUNCTIVITIS | CORNEAL ULCER |
| **Gram-positive** | | |
| Cocci: singly, pairs, clusters | *Staphylococcus* sp. | *Staphylococcus* sp. |
| Cocci: chains | *Streptococcus* sp. | *Streptococcus* sp. |
| Diplococci | *Pneumococcus* | *Pneumococcus* |
| Rods | Diphtheroids | *Bacillus* sp. |
| | | Atypical mycobacteria |
| Filaments | Fungi | Fungi |
| | *Actinomyces* sp. | |
| **Gram-negative** | | |
| Diplococci | *N. gonorrhoeae* | *N. gonorrhoeae* |
| | *N. meningitidis* | *N. meningitidis* |
| | *Branhamella* sp. | *Branhamella* sp. |
| Diplobacilli | *Moraxella* sp. | *Moraxella* sp. |
| Rods | *Haemophilus* sp. | *Pseudomonas aeruginosa* |
| | | Other enterics |
| Filaments | Fungi | Fungi |

## Figure 11.5. Initial Therapy of Bacterial Keratitis Based on Cytological Findings*

| GRAM STAIN | TOPICAL ANTIBIOTIC |
|---|---|
| No organisms | Ciprofloxacin HCl 0.3% |
| | Cefazolin (50 mg/ml) and tobramycin (14 mg/ml) or gentamicin (14 mg/ml) |
| Gram-positive cocci | |
| Gram-negative cocci | Cefazolin (50 mg/ml) |
| Gram-positive bacilli | Penicillin G (100,000 U/ml) |
| | Tobramycin (14 mg/ml) or gentamicin (14 mg/ml) |
| Gram-negative bacilli | Tobramycin (14 mg/ml) or gentamicin (14 mg/ml) |
| Gram-positive filaments | Trimethoprim/sulfamethoxazole |
| Acid-fast bacilli | Amikacin (100 mg/ml) |

*Recommendations made at the time of writing. May change at later dates.

the body. Although inflammatory responses are often vigorous, once a microbe gains access to the vitreous, the growth of the organism usually cannot be controlled without the aggressive use of antimicrobial agents and therapeutic vitrectomy. Damage to the retina by the microbe and its enzymes and by the chemical products (e.g., enzymes and cytokines) of inflammatory cells starts early and, unless controlled promptly, will cause irreversible damage. The earlier in the infectious process the correct diagnosis is made and appropriate, specific therapy initiated, the greater the chance to prevent corneal scarring or damage, or retinal destruction.

## BACTERIAL KERATITIS

All corneal white blood cell infiltrates should be considered as possibly of microbial origin. The presence of purulent discharge, hypopyon, or loss of stromal substance are strong supporting clinical indicators. However, maximal effort should be made early in the process to establish laboratory evidence and then to initiate prompt, aggressive, targeted therapy. The ophthalmologist must avoid the pitfalls of waiting for definite clinical evidence of infectious causation, or of initiating therapy that may be adequate for conjunctivitis but inadequate for microbial keratitis and capable of rendering subsequent laboratory results inconclusive. Although virtually any microbe may cause keratitis, a few micro-organisms cause most cases. This must be kept in mind when the specific diagnosis cannot be made and the ophthalmologist is forced to select a "shotgun" approach (Fig. 11.5). Although data from different geographic areas differ with regard to the leading cause of bacterial keratitis, the short list presented here seems to include those that every area commonly encounters (Fig. 11.6).[1-4]

The cornea is a unique structure with regard to its lack of blood vessels and lymphatic channels as well as its clear optical properties. The mechanical action of the eyelid margins during blinking and the flushing action of the tearfilm help rinse away micro-organisms. In addition, the tearfilm contains lactoferrin, lysozyme, secretory immunoglobulins, ceruloplasmin, and complement components. The intact corneal epithelium plus glycocalyx and mucin constitute a strong barrier to the penetration of almost all bacteria. The only bacteria that appear to be able to penetrate an intact corneal epithelium and establish an infection are *Corynebacterium diphtheria*,

## Figure 11.6. Microbial Agents that Most Commonly Cause Infectious Keratitis

**BACTERIA**
**Gram-positive**
*Staphylococcus epidermidis,*
*S. aureus*
*Streptococcus pneumoniae,*
Group D streptococci
*Bacillus* sp.

**Gram-negative**
*Pseudomonas aeruginosa,*
other *Pseudomonas* species

*Haemophilus influenzae*
*Escherichia coli*
*Neisseria* sp.
*Proteus* sp.
*Klebsiella* sp.
*Serratia* sp.
*Moraxella* sp.

**VIRUSES**
Herpes simplex virus
Adenovirus

**PARASITES**
*Acanthamoeba* sp.

**FUNGI**
*Aspergillus* sp.
*Candida* sp.
*Fusarium*

*Haemophilus aegyptius, Neisseria gonorrhoeae,* and *Listeria.* The mechanisms by which these bacteria penetrate the intact corneal epithelium are unknown but may involve bacterial production of proteases.[5,6]

## PREDISPOSING CAUSES

Bacterial invasion through the corneal epithelium requires a number of conditions that may interfere with the normal defense mechanisms. For example, eyelid abnormalities such as lagophthalmos, entropion, ectropion, dry eye states, or trauma may cause disruption of the ocular surface and allow invasion of bacteria or other micro-organisms. Impairment of local or systemic nonspecific inflammatory processes or specific immune defense responses may also facilitate penetration of bacteria into the cornea. Likewise, denervation of the cornea, chemical injuries, or toxic insults including chronic topical medication disrupt the epithelial barrier to bacteria. Very young individuals, aged people, and those with long-standing diabetes mellitus are also more susceptible to bacterial corneal infections. The critical role of contact lens materials and wearing times in predisposing wearers to microbial keratitis has been demonstrated.[7,8] Once replicating bacteria have passed through the corneal epithelium, the strongest determinant of infection severity is the organism's virulence. However, the host's ability to initiate an inflammatory and subsequent immune response also plays a major role. The clinician's capacity to make an early and specific diagnosis and to initiate promptly appropriate therapy also is a key factor in the degree of tissue damage.

## LABORATORY DIAGNOSIS

Although it is sometimes inconvenient and time-consuming, laboratory workup is at the heart of decisions regarding specific treatment of infectious keratitis. Scrapings for cytology and appropriately obtained culture specimens that are promptly inoculated on suitable culture media are required before therapy is originally initiated. A sterile calcium alginate swab moistened with trypticase soy broth is superior to a platinum spatula for bacterial cultures from cases of keratitis.[9] Broad-spectrum treatment regimens work in a majority of, but not all, situations. Inappropriate therapy may prevent an accurate diagnosis later, in a situation that could lead to corneal perforation, endophthalmitis and, possibly, loss of vision. For these reasons, a thorough initial laboratory workup is in the patient's best interest. Careful microscopic examination of stained scrapings from the edge of a corneal ulcer yields valuable clinical information (see Fig. 11.4). For most purposes, the specimens should be placed on several slides. One or two slides with smeared material from the ulcer should be stored for possible use at a later date. The results of the examination of these scrapings will guide early therapy. The morphology and staining characteristics of the bacteria allow for the general categorization of bacteria and the selection of antibiotics (Fig. 11.5). In instances when no material for examination is available on the corneal surface, a 1- or 2-mm disposable skin trephine is used to remove overlying normal tissue and a portion of the deep infiltrate. This diagnostic step is carried out with the aid of a surgical microscope. The biopsy piece can be used for culture and direct cytology. It is then placed in fixative and prepared for light microscopy, electron microscopy, or both. Once the results from the cultures and sensitivities are known, the antibiotic therapy can be specifically refined.

## THERAPY OF BACTERIAL KERATITIS

The selection of antibiotics for broad spectrum coverage remains controversial. The new quinolone derivative antibiotics have been considered as a possible substitute for the combination of "fortified" aminoglycoside (either gentamicin or tobramycin) and cephalosporin (cefazolin) (Fig. 11.7). The use of frequent topical antibiotic solutions provides adequate levels of drug within the cornea. Subconjunctival injections are not required and intravenous antibiotics should not be used for treatment of bacterial keratitis. As noted above, the characteristics noted on the Gram stain of the corneal scraping can be utilized to specify the antibiotic selection. Some prefer simply to use either the combination of "fortified" aminoglycoside and cephalosporin or a fluoroquinolone preparation as initial therapy until the culture and sensitivity results become available.

While most infections can be adequately treated by the aforementioned drugs, there are very useful "second line" antibiotics that can be considered. Preparations for topical use of vancomycin, amikacin, or both made up from systemic preparations are particularly useful (see Fig. 11.7). Methicillin-resistant strains of staphylococci and penicillin-resistant streptococci, *Bacillus anthracis*, *Clostridium* species, and *Corynebacterium* species are best treated with topical vancomycin (50 mg/ml). Otherwise, cefazolin (50 mg/ml) is a good choice for gram-positive bacteria. Similarly, fortified topical aminoglycoside (gentamicin or tobramycin) is often appropriate for gram-negative bacteria, including *Pseudomonas* species, *Klebsiella*, *Proteus*, *Enterobacter*, and *E. coli*. However, some strains of these gram-negative bacteria, especially *Pseudomonas aeruginosa*, have become resistant to gentamicin and tobramycin. In these situations (as well as in the treatment of keratitis caused by mycobacteria) another aminoglycoside, amikacin (50 mg/ml), is more effective. All of these antibiotics must be made up from other formulations because they are not available as ophthalmic preparations. Gentamicin (3 mg/ml) and tobramycin (3 mg/ml) are available commercially but may not be potent enough to treat successfully many cases of established bacterial keratitis.

The newly available ophthalmic preparations of fluoroquinolones, ciprofloxacin (3 mg/ml), and norfloxacin (3 mg/ml), have broad-spectrum activity against a wide variety of gram-positive and gram-negative bacteria. The in vitro activities of ciprofloxacin are particularly suitable for *Staphylococcus aureus*, (including methicillin-resistant strains), *Staphylococcus epidermidis*, *Streptococcus pneumoniae*, other *Streptococcus* species, *Pseudomonas aeruginosa*, and *Serratia marcescens*, and this drug is approved for treatment of corneal

## Figure 11.7. Preparation of "Fortified" Topical Antibiotics to Treat Microbial Keratitis

| | |
|---|---|
| Cefazolin, 50 mg/ml | Add 10 ml of artificial tear to 500-mg vial of powdered cefazolin, mix, place in artificial tear dropper bottle |
| Gentamicin or tobramycin, 14 mg/ml | Add 2 ml of parenteral antibiotic (40 mg/ml) to 5-ml bottle of commercial ophthalmic antibiotic (3 mg/ml) |
| Vancomycin, 50 mg/ml | Withdraw 2 ml of artificial tear from a 10-ml bottle and inject into vial of powdered vancomycin (500 mg). Once in solution withdraw the entire volume and inject back into bottle containing 8 ml of artificial tears |
| Amikacin, 50 mg/ml | Withdraw and discard 2 ml from a 10-ml bottle of artificial tears, withdraw 2 ml from a vial of injectable amikacin (250 mg/ml) and add to the bottle of artificial tears |

ulcers caused by these organisms. Norfloxacin is currently approved for treatment of conjunctivitis for a similar group of bacteria (with the exception of *Pseudomonas aeruginosa*) but not for the treatment of keratitis. Thus, ciprofloxacin may be an acceptable alternative to the use of fortified antibiotics and offers the convenience of commercial availability and the instillation of a single antibiotic. However, it may cause ocular irritation and occasional white crystalline precipitates on the cornea that are reversible. Bacteria are capable of developing resistance to the fluoroquinolone antibiotics. In comparison studies ciprofloxacin appears to have good efficacy for treatment of bacterial keratitis caused by susceptible micro-organisms.

The frequency of antibiotic administration is varied over time. The initial instillation should be every 30–60 minutes around the clock for all antibiotics. If two different antibiotics are used, for example gentamicin and cefazolin, they should be given at least 5 minutes apart and preferably equally spaced. If each is being given every hour, one antibiotic can be instilled "on the hour" and the other "on the half-hour." There is also evidence that an initial loading dose can greatly increase corneal concentrations almost immediately by administration of 1 drop every minute for 5 minutes.[10] If two drugs are being used, load with the first and wait approximately 15 minutes to begin the loading dose of the second antibiotic.

As the intensive antibiotics are being used, the ophthalmologist must monitor for indicators showing that the infectious process is sterilized and for signs of toxicity. Detailed examination and recording of findings, including specific measurements made with the slit lamp, are crucial. The eyelids and conjunctiva must be given attention along with the cornea. The size of the defect and condition of surrounding corneal epithelium, the size, depth, and density of the infiltrate, and the amount of intraocular inflammation are important parameters. Along with sterilization of the infection, control of inflammation and promotion of wound healing are integral parts of the management of infectious keratitis.

Concurrent with antibiotic therapy, the use of cycloplegic medications helps to relieve pain and the use of mydriatics helps to move the iris to minimize the formation of synechiae. If there is raised intraocular pressure, topical beta blockers, oral carbonic anhydrase inhibitors, or both may be required. The use of topical corticosteroids remains unsettled. In *Pseudomonas* keratitis some data imply that corticosteroids can be used safely while other data suggest that they may potentiate the infection.[11-14] Additionally, epithelial wound healing may be impaired by the administration of topical corticosteroids. Despite these possible detrimental effects, corticosteroids do reduce inflammation and the possible scarring that may result from it.

Given these possible risks and benefits, topical corticosteroids should be used for specific purposes and the clinical course should be monitored. Patients already receiving topical corticosteroids at the time of initiation of antibiotic therapy should have them tapered to 1 or 2 applications per day but not stopped. When the corticosteroids have not been in prior use, 24–48 hours of antibiotic therapy and indications of antibiotic effectiveness will allow the ophthalmologist to consider use of topical corticosteroids. If the severity of inflammation within the cornea and anterior chamber warrants treatment, a potent corticosteroid 2 to 4 times daily may be used. In addition to its anti-inflammatory action, its effects on the infection and corneal epithelial wound healing must be evaluated and dosage appropriately adjusted.

The tapering of topical antibiotic(s) frequency is based on the clinical response. When there is a clear therapeutic effect, tapering can usually begin by 72 hours. The concentration in the tissues is high. A maintenance regimen that allows continued high concentration is 1 drop every 5 minutes for 15 minutes every 3 to 4 hours and then gradual decreases in frequency over the next 5–7 days. If the ulcer appears sterilized and fortified antibiotics are being used, it may be appropriate to switch to commercial ophthalmic preparations for the last stages of tapering. An important clinical dictum in bacterial keratitis is that the lack of progression of disease is a strong indication of success.

Although there are many exceptions to the typical clinical pictures used to describe the various causes of bacterial keratitis, the appearance and location of the keratitis, some concomitant findings, and knowledge of the circumstances leading to the development of the infection are often useful in the management of these vision-threatening problems. The following descriptions of the more common causes of bacterial keratitis emphasize the typical findings.

## SPECIFIC BACTERIAL ENTITIES

Streptococcal keratitis is most often caused by *Streptococcus pneumoniae*. Deep, central corneal stromal keratitis with an irregular, undermined edge is characteristic (Fig. 11.8). Rapid progression and hypopyon are common and often are associated with radiating folds in Descemet's membrane and a fibrin deposit on the endothelium immediately beneath the area of corneal infiltrate. Perforation may occur.[15]

Staphylococcal ulcers often occur in compromised corneas or as superinfections. *S. aureus* and *S. epidermidis* are most commonly isolated. The ulcer is round or oval, white or yellow-white, and is usually localized with distinct borders, although on occasion it is more diffuse because of the compromised state of the cornea. *S. aureus* causes deeper ulcers and greater anterior chamber reaction with hypopyon and endothelial plaque than *S. epidermidis*.

*Bacillus* species, especially *Bacillus cereus*, usually are associated with soil-contaminated trauma and their progress is rapid.[16] Severe pain begins at a time when the infiltrate may appear quite small, usually within 24 hours of

**11.8** | *A: Strep-tococcus pneumoniae* keratitis with whitish central infiltrate and hypopyon. *B:* Gram stain of corneal scraping is loaded with gram-positive paired cocci typical of *S. pneumoniae*.

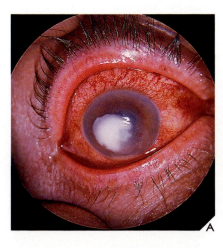

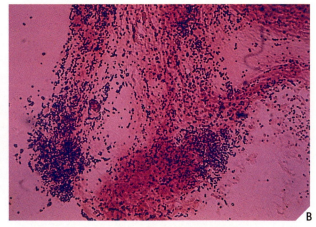

the injury. Marked lid edema, conjunctival chemosis, and circumferential corneal edema which rapidly progresses to a severe ring ulcer are seen.

*Neisseria gonorrhoeae* and *N. meningitidis* most commonly cause conjunctivitis and then progress to cause keratitis because of their capacity to penetrate intact corneal epithelium. Profuse purulent discharge is characteristic of *Neisseria* infections; intense conjunctival injection and chemosis are also common. The keratitis is characterized by an intense infiltrate and perforation often occurs. Early recognition and prompt treatment are essential. These infections may occur in newborns as ophthalmia neonatorum and in adults, often in association with other sexually transmitted diseases.

*Pseudomonas* corneal ulcers are quite common and of rapid progression. Trauma associated with contact lens wear is a frequent antecedent. However, *Pseudomonas* is found in water, many products such as mascara, contaminated eye drops, skin, saliva, and the gastrointestinal tract. Invasion of the corneal stroma requires some type of damage to the epithelium that allows adherence of *Pseudomonas*.[17] These bacteria secrete a variety of enzymes that include proteases and lipases as well as exotoxins. The virulence of a *Pseudomonas* isolate is determined by the volume of the chemicals it secretes plus the presence or absence of a glycocalyx that resists phagocytosis and destruction by antibody and complement.[18] Enzymes produced by inflammatory cells within the cornea also contribute to the tissue damage that occurs in *Pseudomonas* keratitis.[19]

*Pseudomonas* keratitis may be central or peripheral in location; progression is rapid and perforation often occurs in a few days (Fig. 11.9). Initially, there is a superficial ulceration with adherent mucopurulent material of a yellowish or greenish coloration. The ulcer and surrounding stroma become edematous and hazy. Dissemination of the dense infiltrate, including circumferential spread to develop a ring ulcer, endothelial plaques, perforation, and hypopyon are common. Marked conjunctival hyperemia and chemosis are typically part of the clinical picture. Even in the presence of appropriate antibiotics, progression of a well-established *Pseudomonas* keratitis is a distinct possibility.

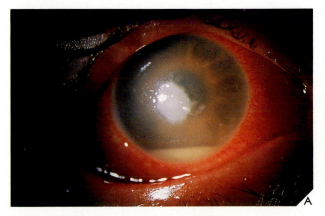
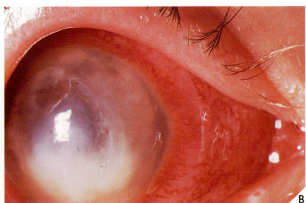

**11.9** | *A:* Central superficial keratitis with hypopyon 24 hours after the onset of pain and redness in a contact lens wearer. *Pseudomonas aeruginosa* was grown from the infiltrate. *B:* Central infiltrate, descemetocele, and hypopyon 72 hours after the onset of symptoms. Perforation occurred a few hours later and *Pseudomonas* sp. was isolated from the infiltrate.

*Moraxella* species typically cause a more chronic, indolent keratitis with a peripheral or paracentral infiltrate (Fig. 11.10). Chronically debilitated patients are more susceptible as are compromised corneas (including corneal transplants). In most instances the infiltrates are superficial and with over-hanging edges. At this stage the eye appears to have inflammation that is out of proportion to the infiltrate, which progresses over days or weeks and may eventually perforate.

Several other gram-negative bacteria including *Proteus, Klebsiella, Serratia,* and *Escherichia coli* may cause bacterial keratitis and need to be suspected during the laboratory workup.

In addition to causative considerations, some clinical appearances of the keratitis are unique and may help narrow down the most likely pathogen. A ring-shaped keratitis spreads circumferentially around the peripheral cornea. The most likely bacterial causes are *Bacillus* species, followed by *Pseudomonas* species, *Proteus, Streptococcus,* and *Listeria.* Another characteristic appearance is the so-called crystalline keratitis,[20] characterized by an infiltrate with a whitish crystalline appearance in the deeper stroma and seemingly normal stroma and epithelium overlying it (Fig. 11.11). The eye has minimal inflammation and progression is very slow. Specific diagnosis may require a corneal biopsy or a diagnostic penetrating keratoplasty. When bacteria have been identified, *Streptococcus* species and *Haemophilus* species have been most common.

In each instance of a patient with a corneal infiltrate due to infection, a bacterial cause is highly likely. However, viruses, parasites, and fungi may cause clinical pictures that are indistinguishable from bacterial keratitis and, therefore, all causes must be considered. The extra slides for cytologic examination should be saved for possible use if a specific etiology remains undetermined. The ophthalmologist must become familiar with special cultures and where they may be performed for situations in which the specific cause remains in doubt. Likewise, it is useful to obtain materials such as contact lenses and their solutions and cases early in the clinical evaluation and laboratory workup. They may play a crucial role in the search for a cause.

Another challenging problem in the management of infectious keratitis is the recognition and treatment of multiple pathogens. For example, herpetic keratitis that has secondarily become infected with bacteria. These are uncommon and the usual dictum is to look for a single cause. However, compromised corneas, immunocompromised hosts, or both, are sometimes infected with multiple organisms. A good knowledge of the natural history

**11.10** | A small, indolent peripheral infiltrate grew *Moraxella lacunata* in a patient with severe obstructive pulmonary disease and long-term oral prednisone treatment.

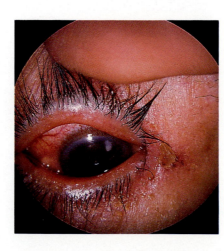

**11.11** | Crystalline keratitis with stromal opacities and a hypopyon. (Courtesy of Dr. David Meisler.)

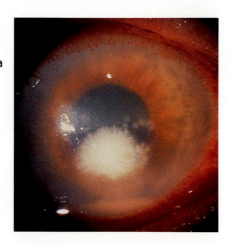

and typical response to therapy of the infectious causative agent give the clinician reference points for evaluating the process. Deviations from the expected response should alert the ophthalmologist to the possibility that this particular case of keratitis could best be explained by multiple organisms, or misdiagnosis of a single organism, drug resistance, or noncompliance on the part of the patient.

Surgery may be required in patients with bacterial keratitis, especially when perforation occurs. Before performing penetrating keratoplasty, aggressive antibiotic therapy should be used to sterilize the cornea. Lamellar keratoplasties and conjunctival flaps must be avoided during active infection but may be useful in postinfectious keratitis. Penetrating keratoplasties performed during active infection and inflammation are prone to failure whereas those done after the eye has become minimally inflamed are far more successful.

## FUNGAL KERATITIS

Fungal corneal infections are often not promptly diagnosed. As mentioned before, all organisms should be considered during the workup of all patients with presumptive microbial keratitis. Although mixed infections can occur, the finding of large numbers of bacteria on cytologic examination, culture, or both, are strong indicators against a fungal cause. However, the lack of bacteria should increase the suspicion about the possibility of fungal keratitis. A careful search of Gram- or Giemsa-stained slides may reveal fungal elements and their characteristics may help to classify the fungus (Fig. 11.12). However, classification is best done using the cultured material.

Virtually all fungi are capable of causing infectious keratitis, especially in patients with trauma in a setting where there is exposure to plants or soil. Additionally, immunocompromised individuals or eyes are more likely to develop fungal keratitis. Topical corticosteroids may potentiate the infections and hinder antifungal therapy. Environmental factors such as a hot, humid climate are associated with a greater possibility that fungal keratitis will develop following corneal trauma. However, no geographic area or particular type of climate is free of fungal keratitis. For example, approximately one third of microbial keratitis is associated with fungi in South Florida[21] and approximately 1 percent of suspected microbial keratitis cases are due to fungi in New York City.[2]

Fungi are eukaryotic and reproduce by the production of spores. They have cell walls with a high content of sterols, which accounts for their sus-

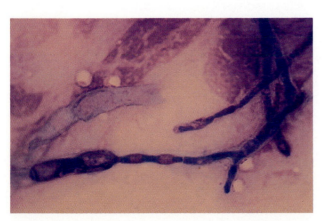

**11.12** | Giemsa stain of corneal infiltrate reveals branched septate hyphae that culture confirmed was Fusarium species.

ceptibility to polyene antibiotics. Fungi are classified as yeasts or filamentous fungi, or, in the case of those that cause systemic mycotic infections (blastomycosis, coccidioidomycosis, histoplasmosis), as diphasic (both yeast and filamentous phases). The yeasts are unicellular, round or oval, and reproduce by budding. Almost all the yeasts that cause keratitis are *Candida* species. The filamentous fungi are multicellular and consist of long branching hyphae that may have septae or be nonseptate.

### Figure 11.13. Fungi Most Commonly Isolated from Keratitis by Taxonomic Features

**YEASTS (UNICELLULAR)**
*Candida* sp.
**FILAMENTOUS (MULTICELLULAR, HYPHAE)**
Monociliaceae (nonpigmented)
*Acremonium (Cephalosporium, Paecilomyces)*
*Aspergillus* sp.
*Fusarium* sp.
*Penicillium*
Dematiaceae (pigmented)
*Alternaria*
*Curvularia*

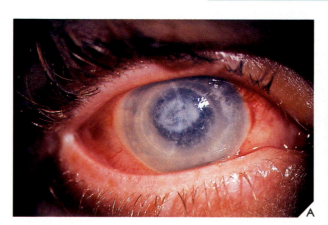

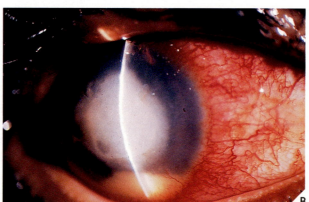

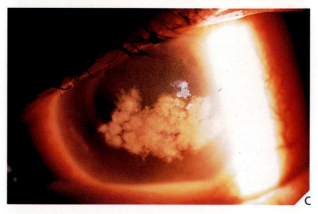

**11.14** | Typical clinical appearances of fungal keratitis. *A:* Slit-lamp photograph of central whitish infiltrate with radiating, hyphate-like edges and a surrounding immune ring. *B:* Similar findings plus an endothelial plaque and hypopyon. *C:* Keratitis caused by *Candida* sp. with characteristics more common for infections caused by yeasts with localized raised infiltrates that are coalescent, as well as a hypopyon.

Most of the fungi that cause keratitis are septate. The hyphae have cross-sectional walls that divide the hyphae into cells. Figure 11.1 lists fungi that have been found to cause keratitis. The most common causes of fungal keratitis are listed in Figure 11.13. Additionally, a wide variety of fungi have been cultured from eyes with endophthalmitis.

## CLINICAL FEATURES

The clinical features of established fungal keratitis caused by filamentous fungi were described by Kaufman and Wood.[22] The most distinctive features are: stromal infiltrates with feathery hyphate-like edges, and dry, dirty-white to gray infiltrates that appear to be slightly elevated above the corneal surface. The other typical features are immune rings, satellite lesions, and endothelial plaques (Fig. 11.14). Hypopyon is also quite common. Keratitis caused by yeasts appears somewhat different, with more localized infiltrates and small epithelial defects superficial to collar button-shaped stromal infiltrates.

## LABORATORY DIAGNOSIS

Fungal keratitis may appear as early as 48 hours following trauma. There may be granular infiltrates within the epithelium and minimal or no stromal keratitis or inflammation in the anterior chamber. Cytologic examination of corneal scrapings easily differentiates the fungal cause (see Fig. 11.12). Once the infection is more established, the edge of the stromal infiltrate is a better site for visualizing fungi and successfully culturing them. In some cases it may be necessary to perform a corneal biopsy to obtain stromal tissue from the edge of the infiltrate. The biopsy may be done with a 1.5 or 2.0 mm disposable skin biopsy trephine or with a microsurgical blade following lid and peribulbar or retrobulbar anesthesia. The biopsy will usually need to be one half to two thirds the thickness of the normal cornea. Whether a scraping or biopsy is performed, the most likely location to find fungal elements is at the edge of the infiltrate (Fig. 11.15). The biopsy can be pressed directly on clean, sterile glass microscope slides for impression cytology. Then the specimen is divided and one half is cultured on appropriate media and the other one half is fixed in formalin, sectioned, and stained with Gomori methenamine silver[23] or PAS to identify the walls of fungi (Fig. 11.16). Similar stains are used on the slides with impression cytology. Calcofluor with Evans blue counterstain[24] or 10 percent KOH wet mount preparations may also be used to identify fungal elements. Approximately two thirds of culture-proven

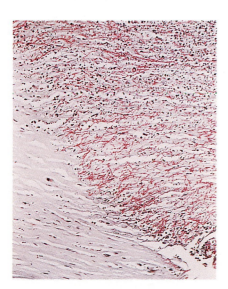

**11.15** | Corneal biopsy demonstrates fungi and inflammatory cells throughout (PAS stain).

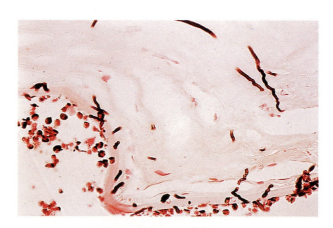

**11.16** | Corneal biopsy stained with Gomori methenamine silver reveals fungi in the stroma and protruding through Descemet's membrane.

cases have identifiable fungi on cytology.[2] In an experienced laboratory, the fungal cultures are often read as positive in 48–72 hours. Because only one quarter of fungal isolates grow in a single culture medium, it is important to use multiple media. A good combination includes blood agar at 25°C and another blood agar at 37°C, brain-heart infusion liquid at 25°C, and Sabaroud's agar with added gentamicin (50 mg/ml) but no added cyclohexamide at 25°C. An experienced mycologist is often necessary to identify accurately the specific fungal causative agent. This is important for the selection of optimal antifungal therapy. It is also prudent to save any positive culture for possible antifungal sensitivity testing.

## THERAPY OF FUNGAL KERATITIS

The lack of commercially available antifungal drugs for ophthalmic use mirrors the situation for bacterial keratitis therapy, and the lack of cases makes it difficult to conduct studies that can document therapeutic efficacy. In general, natamycin (5% microfine suspension) is the first-line antifungal for keratitis caused by filamentous fungi, and imidazoles (miconazole, 1%, or ketoconazole, 1–5%) or amphotericin B, 0.2–0.5% are second-line antifungals. In contrast, the first-line drug for keratitis caused by yeasts is amphotericin B, 0.2–0.5%, alone or in combination with flucytosine, 1%, whereas the imidazole preparations constitute second-line drugs. Flucytosine should not be used alone because of development of resistance.

These antifungal drugs, with the exception of natamycin, must be made up by a pharmacist. They often cause considerable ocular irritation and may lose potency during storage. Dosage schedules are not completely defined. A loading regimen as that described for topical antibiotics followed by applications every 30–60 minutes for 48 hours is an acceptable approach. Following this, the administration can be decreased to every 2 hours and gradually tapered as a therapeutic response is achieved. None of these drugs penetrates the cornea very effectively, especially if the epithelium is intact. In such instances, debridement of epithelium overlying the infiltrate is required to enhance penetration. Topical corticosteroids must be avoided.

The role of surgery in the management of fungal keratitis is usually secondary to medical therapy. When possible, the keratitis should be treated medically and, upon completion, be followed by a penetrating keratoplasty for visual purposes. Therapeutic penetrating keratoplasty may be required in progressive infection with or without perforation. The surgeon must keep in mind that the fungus may extend peripherally beyond the infiltrate into clear cornea. Therefore, a wide margin must be included when the diameter of the trephine is selected for removal of host tissue. Therapeutic transplants have a far lower probability of success as compared with those performed after infection is eradicated. While superficial keratectomy with debridement of necrotic tissue is often beneficial, lamellar keratoplasties and conjunctival flaps are contraindicated in active fungal keratitis.

## VIRAL KERATITIS

Virtually all viruses capable of infecting epithelial surfaces, especially mucous membranes, can cause conjunctivitis as well as keratitis (Fig. 11.17). With few exceptions, these are transient epithelial keratitides with no lasting sequelae. However, corneal infections caused by herpes simplex virus (HSV), varicella-zoster (VZV), Epstein–Barr virus (EBV), and adenovirus are capable of causing permanent corneal damage and loss of vision. Because of this potential, these four viruses are discussed in detail.

Herpes simplex virus (HSV) keratitis is the leading infectious cause of blindness in the United States. This virus infects almost all people by adulthood but very few have ocular involvement. HSV establishes latency in neurons including the trigeminal ganglion as a result of primary infection that rarely involves the cornea. At a later time, reactivation of latent virus and movement of virus via neurons to epithelial sites such as the lip or cornea lead to clinically evident lesions.[25] A wide variety of stimuli appear to trigger these events, including cold, ultraviolet, and emotional stress. Recurrent HSV keratitis may cause stromal opacities, corneal vascularization and perforation.

HSV is a DNA virus in the herpesvirus family as are VZV and EBV. HSV is divided into two major types, 1 and 2. Type 1 is most commonly seen in upper body infections and type 2 is associated with a vast majority of HSV genital infections. Within each type, individual isolates display highly unique variability with some isolates causing more severe clinical infections. Likewise, host responses to HSV infections vary and may partially explain differences in the inflammatory responses as well as frequency of reactivation of latent virus. Immunocompromised hosts may have unusual clinical presentations, prolonged infections, or develop disseminated disease and viremia. Newborns and infants, patients with AIDS, transplant recipients, or others on immunosuppressive drugs are especially susceptible to these more severe herpetic infections.[26] Healthy children and adults have more typical infections. The ocular involvements that may occur in patients with primary herpetic infections include vesicles on the eyelids, ulcerative blepharitis, and

## HERPES SIMPLEX VIRUS

### Figure 11.17. Types of Keratitis Caused by Viruses

| Virus | Type of Keratitis |
| --- | --- |
| Adenovirus | SPK, SEI |
| Herpes simplex virus | Dendrite, geographic, SK, DK |
| Varicella-zoster virus | Dendritic, SK, DK |
| Epstein-Barr virus | Dendrites, SEI |
| Vaccinia virus | SPK, IK, DK |
| Molluscum contagiosum | SPK |
| Rubella virus | SPK |
| Measles (rubeola) | SPK |
| Mumps | SPK, DK |
| Newcastle disease virus | SPK, SEI |
| Papilloma virus | SPK |

SPK = superficial punctate keratitis, SEI = subepithelial infiltrates, SK = stromal keratitis, DK = Disciform keratitis, IK = interstitial keratitis.

epithelial keratitis, and these involvements may be bilateral.[25](Fig. 11.18). Most cases of HSV keratitis occur in patients with a past primary infection, with or without ocular involvement. The clinical presentations are listed in Figure 11.17 and depicted in Figures 11.18 and 11.19. In most people, primary infection is asymptomatic or a nonspecific upper respiratory infection.

Dendritic epithelial keratitis is the most typical presentation (see Fig. 11.19). Active HSV replication occurs within epithelial cells along the edges of the dendrite. The explanation for the dendritic pattern of infections has not been elucidated. In most of these infections the dendrite disappears in approximately 10 days and leaves no scar. The use of an effective topical antiviral drug (e.g., idoxuridine, adenine arabinoside, trifluridine) leads to healing in approximately 5–7 days. Gentle debridement of the involved epithelium along the edges of the dendrite with a saline-moistened, cotton-tipped applicator decreases the healing time to approximately the same extent. Isolates of HSV type 1 have highly variable characteristics and perhaps some are more virulent than others, more prone to cause stromal scarring, or both. In addition, the development of stromal keratitis with a significant component of inflammation may be explained by the degree of immunologic responsiveness of the host.[27] In some instances recurrent HSV epithelial keratitis after some years will lead to stromal keratitis and scarring. The cause for this switch from epithelial to stromal disease is not yet understood. In other instances, especially immunocompromised or corticosteroid-treated hosts, corneas will have progressive active HSV replication, with the dendrite enlarging to a geographic epithelial keratitis. Among the available topical antiviral drugs, trifluridine seems to be the best for treatment of geographic forms of HSV epithelial keratitis.

**11.18** | Primary herpes simplex virus infection with vesicles involving the skin and margins of the eyelids along with conjunctivitis and fine epithelial keratitis.

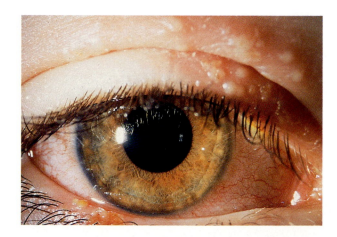

Recurrences of HSV keratitis are more common over time. In a study spanning 32 years, the recurrence rates increased from 10 percent at 1 year to 23 percent at 2 years to 63 percent at 20 years.[28] Multiple recurrences over time are likely to lead to significant loss of vision associated with scarring of the cornea.[29]

Stromal keratitis may occur at any point in these recurrent infections, but it is more likely after multiple episodes. Stromal disease may occur concurrent with epithelial disease or in its absence. In combination with epithelial disease due to active, replicating HSV, therapy needs to be selected that does not facilitate proliferation of live virus such as with topical corticos-

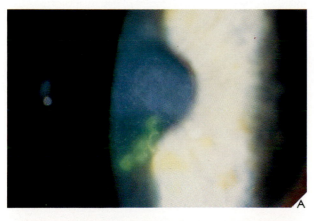

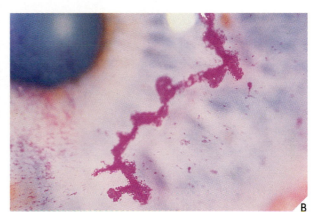

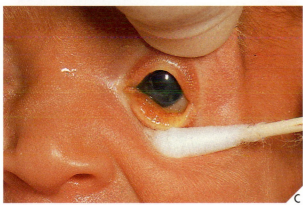

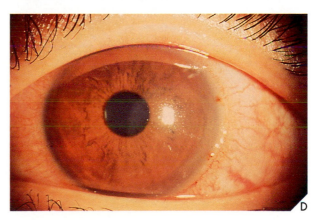

**11.19** | Herpes simplex virus epithelial keratits. *A:* Typical dendrite stained with fluorescein. *B:* Another dendrite stained with rose bengal. *C:* Dendrite in a 3-week-old baby caused by herpes simplex virus, type 2. *D:* Fluorescein-stained dendrite near limbus at 3 o'clock with a surrounding immune ring.

teroid alone. Similarly, the type of stromal keratitis that is manifest will further dictate the type of therapy (Fig. 11.20). In all cases of stromal keratitis, a constellation of pathophysiologic responses are possible, including inflammatory cell infiltration, stromal edema, vascularization, tissue necrosis, and anterior segment inflammation. In some instances the inflammation is localized to one site such as Descemet's membrane ("descemetitis") or corneal

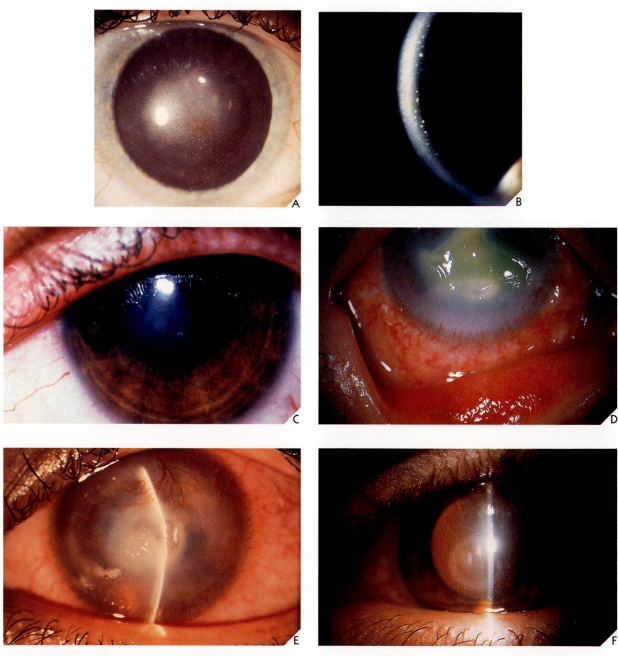

**11.20** | Herpes simplex virus stromal keratitis. *A and B:* Central corneal edema and haze associated with underlying keratic precipitates. Although immune-mediated disciform keratitis usually responds to topical corticosteroid applications, it also may resolve without any treatment. *C:* Stromal opacification without stromal loss. *D:* Stromal keratitis and necrosis. *E:* Descemetocele associated with necrotic herpes simplex virus keratitis. *F:* Stromal keratitis with associated uveitis.

endothelium (disciform edema). In all forms of stromal keratitis with the exception of necrotizing herpetic keratitis, inflammation appears to be directed towards previously infected cells that now express unique cell surface antigens that are encoded from HSV DNA. These cells are recognized as "foreign" in a manner similar to donor cells in a corneal allograft. In these situations, corticosteroid therapy appears to interrupt the inflammatory pathways and as a result edema, angiogenesis, and corneal scar formation are less likely to occur. While concomitant topical antiviral drugs are often administered, their exact role in the prevention of these sequelae remains speculative. Based on unmasked studies, the oral antiviral drug, acyclovir, has been judged to be beneficial in the management of patients with HSV stromal keratitis.[30] At present, it seems appropriate from a clinical standpoint to use topical steroids of such potency and with such frequency as to minimize or eliminate active inflammation in cases of nonnecrotizing HSV stromal keratitis. The decision on a concomitant topical antiviral drug should be guided by past experiences for a particular patient regarding the frequency of epithelial recurrences and patient reliability and compliance. The long-term use of a particular antiviral drug may cause the development of HSV resistance, toxicity of the ocular surface, or drug contact hypersensitivity. The corticosteroid will need to be tapered gradually and may require long-term instillation to prevent recurrence of stromal infiltrate and scarring. Such long-term use may cause cataract formation or steroid-induced glaucoma as well as predispose that cornea to fungal keratitis. All of these problems require diligent, regular, follow-up examinations and the agreement of the patient to seek immediate care if any new symptoms appear between scheduled appointments.

Necrotizing herpetic stromal keratitis is best explained by the concomitant occurrence of active stromal infiltration and replicating virus within the stromal keratocytes. The marked stromal inflammation and necrosis may mimic bacterial keratitis and delay specific diagnosis. However, the failure to find bacteria on microscopic examination of corneal scrapings, negative bacterial cultures, and previous history of herpetic keratitis are strong indicators of a correct diagnosis. Viral cultures are often positive within 48 hours. The laboratory workup should also include cytology, culture, or both for *Acanthamoeba* and fungi. Corneal perforation is not uncommon in herpetic necrotizing stromal keratitis. Treatment should initially focus on controlling the active viral infection with a topical antiviral drug. The possible benefits of oral acyclovir have not been determined. After approximately 5 days of topical antiviral drug, topical corticosteroids can be added 3–4 times daily or a short tapering dose of oral prednisone can be given beginning with 1 mg/kg body weight in single daily dose and tapering the dose by one half every third day for a course of 12–15 days. The therapeutic goals are to destroy the HSV, decrease inflammation, and regain an intact corneal epithelium. If the cornea perforates, the alternative treatments include sealing the perforation with cyanoacrylate glue and placing a therapeutic soft contact lens or collagen shield, conjunctival flap, or resorting to penetrating keratoplasty. If there is a good possibility that the active HSV infection is resolved, penetrating keratoplasty removes the necrotic tissue and helps bring the process under control. However, penetrating keratoplasty for all forms of herpetic stromal keratitis is significantly more successful when performed 6 months or longer after active keratitis.[31] A majority of these grafts remain clear long term. However, recurrent HSV keratitis may occur in up to 15 percent of these eyes within 2 years of surgery.[32] In many instances the recurrent epithelial keratitis occurs in the region of the graft-host interface and will only be visible with careful slit lamp biomicroscopic examination and staining with fluorescein or rose bengal (Fig. 11.21).

The commercially available topical antiviral drugs are quite similar in their actions and toxicities (Fig. 11.22). Different isolates are variable in their sensitivities. It is prudent to continue to use the same antiviral used in previous episodes unless there is a lack of response after 6–7 days or evidence of drug contact hypersensitivity. The latter problem may be due to the preservative in the preparation and must be given consideration when selecting an alternative antiviral. There are no data to substantiate therapeutic superiority of solutions versus ointments. Idoxuridine, adenine arabinoside, and trifluridine are nonselective in their actions that interfere with DNA synthesis. Therefore, uninfected conjunctival and corneal epithelial cells eventually are injured by these drugs and signs of toxicity such as diffuse superficial punctate keratitis develop. Likewise, after the virus has been destroyed, these drugs may prevent healing of the epithelium involved in the infection and

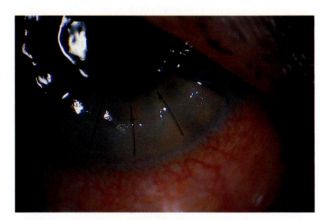

**11.21** | Recurrent herpes simplex virus epithelial keratitis following penetrating keratoplasty. The lesion is in the graft-host interface from 3:30-6:30 o'clock. These cases are often subtle and require careful examination. Frequently they are associated with subsequent slow stromal wound healing in the involved area.

## Figure 11.22. Commercially Available Topical Antiviral Drugs

| Generic Name | Trade Name | Composition | Preservative | Susceptible Viruses | Frequency |
|---|---|---|---|---|---|
| Idoxuridine | Herplex | 0.1% solution | Benzalkonium | HSV types 1 and 2 | During day every hour, during night every 2 hours |
| Trifluridine | Viroptic | 1.0% solution | Thimerosol | HSV types 1 and 2; in vitro some strains of adenovirus | 9 times daily for 14 days |
| Adenine arabinoside | Vira-A | 3.0% ointment | None | HSV types 1 and 2; varicella-zoster; vaccinia | 5 times daily (if no improvement by 7 days or failure of re-epithelization by 21 days, change therapy) |

what may be perceived as persistent infection is really drug toxicity. Stopping the antiviral in such cases becomes the correct action rather than continuing its use or switching to a different antiviral. Debridement is a very useful and successful treatment for epithelial dendrites and can be used with or without addition of topical antiviral therapy. It is especially valuable for the management of noncompliant patients.

Postinfectious keratitis or metaherpetic keratitis presents a diagnostic and therapeutic challenge. The clinical appearance usually includes a nonhealing defect with rolled edges of corneal epithelium, grayish nonadherent epithelium, and inflammation at the level of the basement membrane. Treatment includes gentle debridement of the loose epithelium (which can be submitted for viral culture), artificial tears without preservatives if there is an associated dry eye, and if necessary, mild, infrequent instillation of a topical corticosteroid. When eyelid pathology is also present, the use of a therapeutic soft contact lens or collagen shield may assist in the successful healing of the corneal epithelium. As mentioned previously, the topical antivirals inhibit wound healing and should be used very sparingly, if at all, in the management of postinfectious keratitis.

## VARICELLA-ZOSTER VIRUS

Varicella-zoster virus (VZV) is also a DNA virus in the herpesvirus family that causes systemic infections from chickenpox (usually in children) to herpes zoster (usually in adults older than 60 years). When the infection involves the V cranial nerve, ocular infection is often temporally related to diminished host cell-mediated immunity that allows reactivation of VZV latent since childhood chickenpox. Ocular involvement occurs in 8–17 percent of all zoster cases.[33] Among the several sequelae of zoster at any anatomic site, postherpetic neuralgia is often the most bothersome. It occurs in approximately 10 percent of patients and lasts for 8 weeks in approximately one half of them and a year or more in 20 percent.[34] Patients older than 60 years are at greater risk to develop this complication. Immunocompromised individuals including patients with lymphomas, immunodeficiencies, AIDS, and on immunosuppressive therapies are at increased risk and have more severe infections.

The onset of VZV infection is often insidious and the first symptoms include malaise, headache, and low-grade fever. Approximately one third of patients present with vesicles while others complain of paresthesias and burning sensations at the sites that subsequently develop vesicles. The clinical picture is usually so typical that the appearance of the lesions and their dermatome distribution allow diagnosis. Positive cultures can be obtained from fluid taken from fresh vesicles.

The ocular involvement in VZV infections of the V cranial nerve often involves several anatomic sites. In addition to epithelial involvement, VZV often causes damage to neurons and blood vessels. Some structures of the eye that may be involved include conjunctiva, cornea, sclera, trabecular meshwork with secondary glaucoma, uveal tract, optic nerve, extraocular and levator muscles. Keratitis may occur alone or in combination with scleritis or involvement of any of the aforementioned tissues.

Approximately 50 percent of people with VZV infection involving the ophthalmic (1) division of the V cranial nerve have ocular involvement, often in association with typical skin lesions.[35] Vesicular skin lesions involving the upper eyelid, conjunctivitis, and episcleritis are common. Corneal involvement is also common, especially epithelial keratitis manifested by dendritiform lesions that consist of raised, edematous cells, grayish in color.[36] These dendritiform lesions typically do not stain with fluorescein but do stain with rose bengal (Fig. 11.23). They contain live virus, appear early in the course of zoster infections, disappear spontaneously without antiviral therapy, and may reappear weeks or months later.

Stromal keratitis occurs in herpes zoster ophthalmicus in the same forms as in association with HSV keratitis (Fig. 11.24). The stromal inflammation is often intense and associated with vascularization, and occasionally

**11.23** | *A and B:* Grayish, raised dendritiform varicella-zoster virus epithelial keratitis lesions that do not stain with fluorescein.

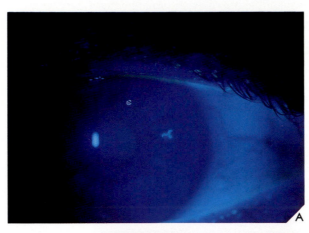

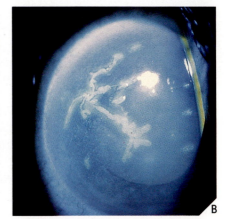

**11.24** | Varicella-zoster virus stromal keratitis. *A:* Non-necrotizing stromal keratitis. *B and C:* Necrotizing stromal keratitis. *D:* Paracentral immune ring surround area of quiescent stromal keratitis.

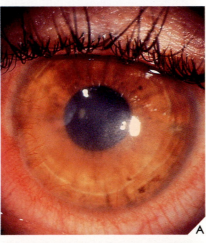

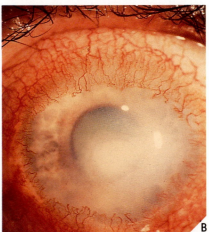

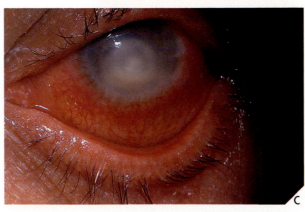

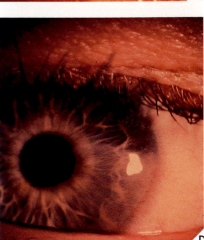

is followed by necrosis and perforation. Local or systemic corticosteroids are required to manage stromal keratitis. Peripheral keratitis in association with scleritis may mimic the appearance of Mooren's ulcer and is difficult to treat. Disciform keratitis may also occur in the weeks following epithelial disease.

The damage to neurons involved in herpes zoster ophthalmicus may lead to neuroparalytic keratitis with recurrent erosions, persistent epithelial defects, vascularization, secondary bacterial keratitis, and perforation. Therapy may include repair of eyelid abnormalities, artificial tears, therapeutic soft contact lenses, conjunctival flap, and therapeutic penetrating keratoplasty.

The management of corneal involvement requires constant attention to and treatment of glaucoma and intraocular inflammation. Topical beta-adrenergic blockers and cycloplegics along with corticosteroids are often used. In some instances, topical or systemic nonsteroidal anti-inflammatory drugs are also useful. Prolonged use of topical corticosteroids with slow tapering is usually necessary or the keratitis recurs. Episcleritis and scleritis are managed in a similar fashion.

The best treatment of acute herpes zoster ophthalmicus is systemic acyclovir initiated early in the course of the disease, ideally within 72 hours of the onset of skin lesions.[37] This treatment and other management decisions are made on the basis of the health and age of the patient. Figure 11.25 outlines the treatment of VZV infections. Other aspects of therapy are not as well defined. The optimal treatment of skin lesions is controversial. There is no conclusive demonstration that topical antivirals, acyclovir, or topical corticosteroids are beneficial for skin lesions. However, moisturizing preparations seem to help the condition. The use of prophylactic topical or systemic antibiotics is not required for immunocompetent VZV patients. Some investigators advocate the use of oral cimetidine for relief of pain and pruritis in the acute stage of the disease for all patients.[38] However, a recent masked study of nonophthalmic VZV infections failed to validate these findings.[39]

## Figure 11.25. Treatment of Varicella-Zoster Virus Infection with Ophthalmic Involvement Based on Immune Status and Age

| IMMUNE STATUS | AGE | SYSTEMIC CORTICOSTEROIDS | ANTIVIRALS | OTHER (OPTIONAL FOR ALL PATIENTS) |
|---|---|---|---|---|
| Immunodeficient | Any | None* | Intravenous acyclovir (15 mg/kg/day or 1,500 mg/m²/day) | |
| Immunocompetent | Under age 60 | None* | Oral acyclovir† (800 mg/5 times daily/10 days) | Cimetidine (300 mg/4 times daily/14 days) |
| | Over age 60 | Prednisone (60 mg/7 days; 40 mg/7 days; 20 mg/7 days; 10 mg/7 days) | Same as <60 | Perphenazine/amitriptyline (Triavil®) (2/25 mg/2 times daily) |

*Topical acceptable.   †Adult dosage; adjust for weight in children.

Likewise, antidepressants such as Triavil® (perphenazine-amitriptyline) may help patients with debilitating postherpetic neuralgia. Zostrix® cream (0.02% capsaicin) is available for painful skin lesions but not for application on the eye. It relieves pain by depleting sensory neurons of substance P. Oral corticosteroids are often given to immunocompetent people older than 60 years of age who are at higher risk to develop postherpetic neuralgia.

In the past, "Hutchinson's rule" has been used as a clinical dictum to determine whether or not there is a risk for intraocular VZV. The involvement of the tip of the nose, which has sensory innervation via the infratrochlear branch of the nasolacrimal nerve of the V cranial nerve which also has branches to the uveal tract, was supposed to signal intraocular involvement. There are numerous exceptions and careful, repeated examinations of all structures are essential to detect and aggressively treat all sites of involvement.

Eyes with previous ocular VZV infections are frequently considered for surgery, especially cataract extraction and corneal transplants. Because of the vasculitis that may cause anterior segment ischemia or changes in choroidal vasculature, these eyes may have excessive surgical complications including expulsive hemorrhages, choroidal effusions, and hypotony.

## EPSTEIN–BARR VIRUS

Epstein–Barr virus also belongs to the herpesvirus family and can cause keratitis. Most often it causes infectious mononucleosis. It is also seen in association with Sjögren syndrome, endemic Burkitt's lymphoma, nasopharyngeal carcinoma, and thymic carcinoma.[40] Ocular involvement of the cornea includes dry eye syndrome,[41] oculoglandular syndrome,[42] follicular conjunctivitis, epithelial (dendrites),[43] and stromal keratitis. Stromal involvement ranges from subepithelial infiltrates similar to those caused by adenoviruses

### Figure 11.26. Features of Pharyngoconjunctival Fever (PCF) and Epidemic Keratoconjunctivitis (EKC) Due to Adenoviral Infections

| FEATURE | PCF | EKC |
| --- | --- | --- |
| Adenovirus serotype | 3,7 | Primarily 8,19. Also 2,3,4,5,7,9,10,11,1 4,16,21,29,37 |
| Patient age | Children | All ages |
| Systemic features | Pharyngitis, fever, hepatospleno- megaly | Typically none |
| Preauricular adenopathy | + | + |
| Follicular conjunctivitis | + | + |
| Subconjunctival hemorrhages | + | + |
| Membranes/pseu- domembranes | – | ± |
| Epithelial keratitis (diffuse, later focal) | + | + |
| Subepithelial opaci- ties (usually at 2 weeks) | ± | ± |

to anterior stromal round infiltrates with a granular appearance to full-thickness, whitish, non-necrotic infiltrates.[44,45]

These involvements may resolve without treatment. Antivirals, including acyclovir, are not very active against Epstein-Barr virus. The stromal keratitis can be treated with topical corticosteroids if needed.

## ADENOVIRUS

Adenovirus is a well-recognized cause of viral keratitis that can occur in epidemics and cause significant corneal changes. The condition is highly contagious and easily spreads directly or indirectly person-to-person. Large outbreaks have occurred in the working place, such as the originally described outbreak in a shipyard.[46,47] However, many outbreaks have also been traced to spread within eye clinics.[48,49] Contaminated medication bottle tips, examination instruments (e.g., tonometer tips) and examiners' hands are the usual modes of transmission in the eye care setting. Adenovirus transmission can be prevented by good hygiene and hand washing, wearing gloves, discarding medication bottles that touch lids, globe, or tears, and cleaning instruments with alcohol and drying them.

Adenoviral infections with ocular involvements are most often caused by serotypes 3,7,8,10,19, and 37. The incubation period varies from 2 days to 2 weeks and some people remain infectious for 2–3 weeks after the onset of symptoms. There are two clinical forms of these infections: pharyngoconjunctival fever (PCF) and epidemic keratoconjunctivitis (EKC) (Fig. 11.26). The history, especially the relationship to others with red eyes, and the clinical pictures at various stages of the disease (Fig. 11.27) are virtually conclu-

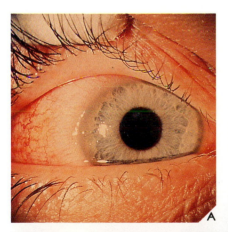
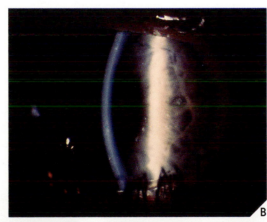
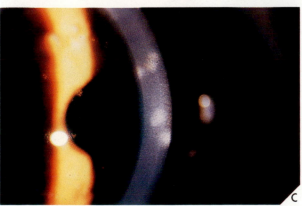
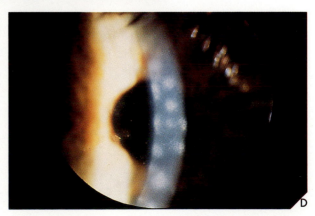

**11.27** | Adenoviral keratoconjunctivitis. *A and B:* Relatively mild involvements of conjunctiva and cornea caused by type 19 adenovirus. *C and D:* Subepithelial corneal infiltrates due to type 8 adenovirus.

sive causative evidence. During the first 1–3 weeks after ocular symptoms develop, adenovirus can usually be cultured from conjunctival swabs. However, this virus grows slowly and the clinical disease may resolve before the culture turns positive.

Adenoviral keratitis typically begins 3–5 days after the onset of tearing, foreign body sensation, tender and enlarged preauricular lymph node, and conjunctivitis with subepithelial hemorrhages. The initial corneal involvement is a diffuse, fine epithelial keratitis that may show fine white dots. This process resolves in approximately 2 weeks. In instances when keratitis persists, more focal epithelial lesions may develop with small central staining spots a week after the onset of diffuse keratitis. A week later subepithelial infiltrates that last for months develop in some.[50]

Currently, no specific antiviral therapy for adenoviral infections exists. Some believe that topical trifluridine is useful, but conclusive evidence is lacking.[51] Some patients develop secondary bacterial conjunctivitis and require topical antibiotics. Most find various degrees of relief during the epithelial keratitis from cool compresses and topical vasoconstrictors. The use of topical corticosteroids at this stage is debatable. If subepithelial opacities develop and reduce vision, topical corticosteroids may be useful. However, their use prolongs the time of resolution of inflammation once corticosteroids are stopped and they may be required for many months. Thus, the decision to use topical corticosteroids means monitoring for their complications, including steroid-induced glaucoma.

## POSSIBLE VIRAL KERATITIS

Thygeson's superficial punctate keratitis has the distinct clinical characteristics of a bilateral recurrent focal epithelial keratitis (Fig. 11.28). The lesion sites change almost daily. Its cause is unknown, although it has long been suspected to have a viral cause. The corneal findings consist of 1 to 20 or more coarse, granular, slightly raised, whitish opacities. These usually stain with fluorescein and tend to be located in the central cornea. While some patients are asymptomatic, others note mild decrease in vision, photophobia, foreign body sensation, and tearing. In some there is mild conjunctival injection.

Episodes often last 4–6 weeks, resolve, and reappear in another 4–6 weeks. This cycle lasts for 2–4 years and leaves without sequelae in all except a few in whom it lasts longer.

**11.28** | Thygeson's superficial punctate keratits with focal, irregular opacities whose locations shift almost daily.

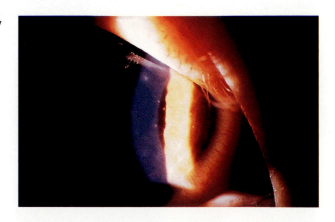

No therapeutic cure has been found. Soft or hard contact lenses as well as mild topical corticosteroids 2 to 3 times daily often relieve symptoms. The use of trifluridine 9 times daily for prolonged periods of weeks to months has been reported to prevent recurrences.[51] Regardless of the approach to therapy, the ultimate prognosis calls for resolution without sequelae.

# CHLAMYDIAL KERATITIS

The organisms belonging to the order known as the Chlamydiales include *Chlamydia trachomatis* and *C. psittaci*. They are non-motile, gram-negative, obligate intracellular bacteria. Ocular chlamydial infections and associated blindness represent an important problem worldwide. Chlamydial conjunctivitis and other ocular involvements have been described in Chapter 2. Most of the manifestations of trachoma have been described in the same chapter.

Chlamydial keratitis is estimated to be the cause of reduced vision or blindness in approximately 200 million people throughout the world, especially in less developed areas. Corneal involvements begin in stage I of the disease process (MacCallan's classification) (Fig. 11.29).

The corneal changes are quite distinct. In the early stages of trachoma, the punctate epithelial keratitis is predominantly located in the superior half of the cornea. The superior superficial pannus and the fibrovascular membrane extend from the superior limbus and destroy Bowman's layer (Fig. 11.30). An infiltrate at this level precedes the migration of the fibrovascular

## Figure 11.29. MacCallan Classification of Trachoma

| CLASSIFICATION | CHARACTERISTICS |
| --- | --- |
| Stage I: Incipient trachoma | Immature follicles of superior tarsal conjunctiva; papillary hypertrophy; diffuse punctate keratitis; superior corneal pannus; fibrovascular tissue destroying Bowman's layer |
| Stage II: Established trachoma | Increased pannus and subepithelial infiltrates |
| IIa | Mature follicles; limbal follicles |
| IIb | Intense papillary hypertrophy |
| Stage III: Cicatrizing trachoma | Conjunctival scarring (Arlt's lines); cicatrization of limbal follicles (Herbert's pits); lid scarring, symblepharon formation, trichiasis |
| Stage IV: Healed trachoma | Resolution of conjunctival and corneal inflammation; no follicles or papillae; corneal scarring, dry eyes; entropion, trichiasis, symblepharon; conjunctival scarring; corneal erosions |

membrane. Secondary bacterial keratitis is a common complication in areas of the world where trachoma is common. The more common causative bacteria are *S. aureus* and *Moraxella, Streptococcus,* and *Haemophilus*. These infections are often the final cause of blindness and are facilitated by the dry eyes, trichiasis, and entropion, as well as the corneal damage and scarring.

Acute chlamydial infections in newborns and adults in regions where trachoma is not present are most likely to cause conjunctivitis with minimal epithelial keratitis. Rarely, subepithelial infiltrates or superior corneal micropannus are noted.

The optimal management of chlamydial infections includes early specific recognition and laboratory diagnosis combined with systemic tetracycline, unless contraindicated, for 3–4 weeks. The selection of a specific drug is determined by cost, availability, and ease of dosing. Children and pregnant or nursing women must not receive systemic tetracycline. Alternatives for them include systemic erythromycin or triple sulfa. Surgical corrections of entropion and trichiasis are essential to prevent further corneal complications.

## PARASITIC KERATITIS

Worldwide parasitic infections have long been recognized as a major problem. In contrast, parasitic keratitis has been a curiosity in the United States until the 1980s when increasing numbers of cases of *Acanthamoeba* keratitis began to be recognized.

### ONCHOCERCIASIS

River blindness is a well-recognized clinical entity in people infected by *Onchocerca volvulus* in Central and West Africa, Central America, and the northern portion of South America. Larvae are transmitted to humans by black flies. The larvae develop into adults in subcutaneous nodules and migrate from them to involve any portion of the eye. The transparent microfilaria can be seen in the anterior chamber, but are hard to locate in the corneal stroma. As long as they are alive, microfilaria are well tolerated. At death, they incite inflammation. Conjunctival involvements are characterized by eyelid edema, chemosis, injection, limbal inflammation, and phlyctenules. Localized corneal stromal infiltrates consist of lymphocytes and eosinophils surrounding dead microfilaria (Fig. 11.31). Most are in the anterior stroma and tend to be transient, although some people develop marked corneal scars and loss of vision probably caused by very large amounts of microfilaria in the corneas.

**11.30** | Conjunctival subepithelial scarring in association with corneal pannus in patient with inactive trachoma.

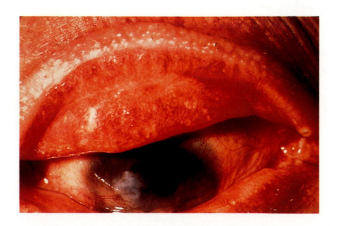

More than 60 million people are estimated to have onchocerciasis and more than 1 million are blind. In addition to conjunctival and corneal involvement, these people may have anterior uveitis, chorioretinitis, optic neuritis or atrophy. Treatment with ivermectin, 150 mg/kg repeated on a annual basis, appears to be the best approach. Systemic and/or topical diethylcarbamazine is also widely used to destroy microfilaria, but it may incite further ocular inflammation.

Leishmaniasis may also have ocular involvements and lead to blindness. *Leishmania* normally infects rodents and dogs and is transmitted to humans by infected sand flies found in Africa, Central and South America, India, and the Middle East. There are three clinical forms of systemic disease: cutaneous at the site of a bite; mucocutaneous with destructive lesions of the

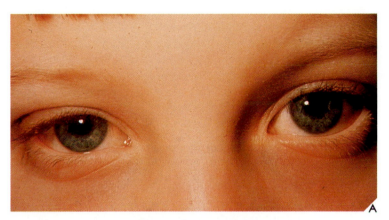

**11.31** | Onchocerciasis. *A:* This young girl had just returned from Africa. She had conjunctival injection and small corneal opacities at all levels. During examination at the slit lamp, a tiny thread-like worm was noted in the aqueous. *B:* Histologic section of a conjunctival biopsy shows a chronic nongranulomatous inflammation and a tiny segment of the worm in the deep substantia propia; this is shown under higher magnification in *C:*. (From Yanoff M, Fine BS: *Ocular Pathology. A Color Atlas,* ed 2. New York: Gower Medical Publishing, 1992, 8.7.)

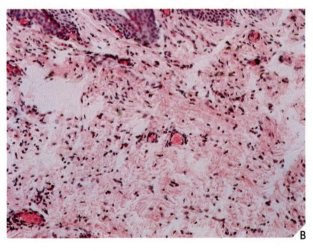

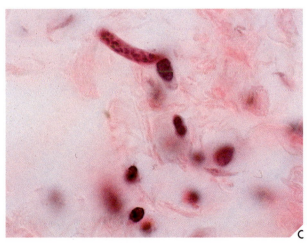

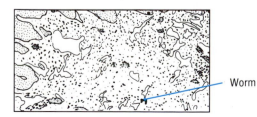

Worm

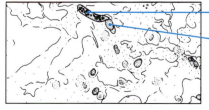

Worm with tiny nuclei

Human fibrocyte nucleus

mucous membranes and cartilage of the nasal septum, pharynx, and larynx; and visceral with spleen, liver, and bone marrow involvement.

Ocular involvements comprise the eyelids, conjunctiva, and cornea. Nodular granulomas of the eyelids and conjunctiva are reported. The cornea may develop phylctenules or interstitial keratitis, which may progress over 3–4 weeks until a perforation develops. Either sodium stibogluconate or meglumine antimoniate are given intravenously or intramuscularly to kill *Leishmania*.

## ACANTHAMOEBA

Acanthamoebic keratitis was first described in 1974 and since then only a few hundred cases have occurred.[52] *Acanthamoeba* species are found in water of any sort, from polar ice to fresh or salt water to boiled water. It can exist as a motile trophozoite or encyst by forming a double wall that contains cellulose and is resistant to many challenges including drugs. It seems likely that a break in the corneal epithelium assists in the initiation of infection. Trauma and exposure to contaminated water or contact lens solutions are often related to the establishment of infection.

The early symptoms and signs are foreign body sensation and irritation associated with redness, tearing, and photophobia. Preauricular adenopathy may be present. While most cases are unilateral, bilateral cases have been reported. The early corneal findings are variable. Some patients have normal epithelium and others develop pseudodendrites or punctate staining along

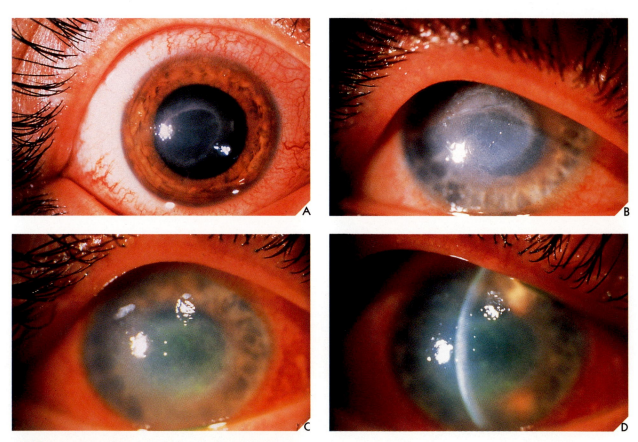

**11.32** | Acanthamoebic keratitis. *A–D:* Progression from epithelial disease with a "ring ulcer" to larger and deeper stromal involvement.

with variable stromal infiltrates and pain (Fig. 11.32). Whenever a patient is seen with this complex of findings, Acanthamoebic keratitis should be considered and a laboratory workup carried out. At this stage treatment has a far greater chance of being successful than when the later obvious signs are present. As the infection progresses, severe pain is common. The epithelium may show larger areas of involvement and recurrent erosions may develop. At this point there are often infiltrates surrounding corneal nerves (radial keratoneuritis) along with whitish stromal infiltrates of any size and at any location. With time the stromal infiltrate often becomes ring shaped and tiny satellite lesions form. Scleritis and secondary glaucoma may also develop.

Treatment is difficult because the trophozoites tend to encyst and become resistant to therapy. Therefore, early and aggressive approaches to diagnosis with scrapings of involved epithelium, corneal biopsies, and sometimes diagnostic penetrating keratoplasty for deep central lesions are mandatory. Cultures are done on nutrient agar overlain with *E. coli*. *Acanthamoeba* makes characteristic tracks in the culture. Microscopic examinations of clinical specimens are done following a variety of stains (Giemsa, trichrome, Gram), or counterstaining with calcofluor white and examination with a fluorescence microscope (Figure 11.33). Likewise, transmission electron microscopy can be used on biopsy or transplant sections (Fig. 11.34).

Treatment, surgical or medical, often fails. Virtually every imaginable topical medication has been tried.[53] Most clinicians use a multidrug, topical

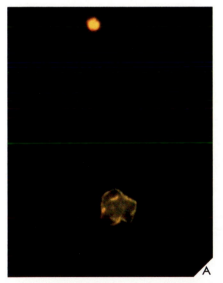
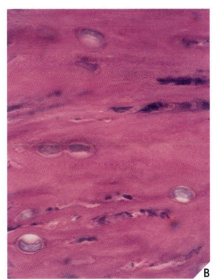

**11.33** | *A:* Calcofluor white with Evans blue counterstain reveals trophozoite when viewed in a fluorescence microscope. *B:* Round *Acanthamoeba* cysts within stroma of the cornea.

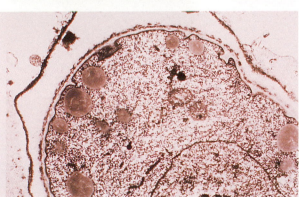

**11.34** | *Acanthamoeba* cyst in cornea with double wall can be found in biopsy or keratoplasty specimens using transmission electron microscopy.

shotgun approach using such medications as propamidine isethionate, polymyxin B-neomycin-gramicidin and an imidazole (ketoconazole, miconazole, clotrimazole). The role of topical corticosteroids remains controversial. They make the eye more comfortable, but cure may become more difficult. Likewise, the role and timing of penetrating keratoplasty remain to be determined. If perforation occurs, there are no alternatives. Recurrences in both the graft and the surrounding recipient cornea are quite common. Yet at other times corneal transplant seems curative. The best current approach remains early recognition and diagnosis followed by treatment with 0.02% polyhexamethylene biguanide in combination with other drugs (Fig. 11.35).

## INTERSTITIAL AND NONINFECTIOUS KERATITIS

There are many systemic conditions with associated corneal findings that have an inflammatory component in the absence of proven active infection at the site. It is possible that some of these responses are directed towards nonviable micro-organisms in the cornea. In other instances the cornea may accumulate immunologically active substances (e.g., cytokines) or cells that foster an inflammatory response in the cornea. Alternatively, inflammatogenic substances may gain access to the cornea via the ocular surface or adjacent structures and precipitate a corneal inflammatory response.

The clinical findings are quite similar in the cornea, including stromal infiltrates and scarring that often is associated with vascularization. Probably there are multiple pathways that lead to these findings. The corneal stroma is normally devoid of any types of immune or inflammatory cells. In contrast, the peripheral corneal epithelium of adults contains dendritic Langerhans cells that are capable of participating in immunologically mediated responses.[54] However, the uninflamed stroma may contain immunoglobulins, especially IgG and IgA, and complement components. Once the inflammatory response is initiated, a wide variety of inflammatory cells may migrate into the corneal stroma, accumulate at the limbus, and be present in the aqueous humor as well as settle out on the corneal endothelium. In these situations an array of soluble products (cytokines) may be released from cells, including interleukin-1 (IL-1) and interleukin-2 (IL-2). The cytokines have multiple functions. For example, IL-1 interacts with vascular endothelial cells

### Figure 11.35. Medical Treatment of Acanthamoeba Keratitis with Topical Medication

| | |
|---|---|
| Propamidine isethionate | |
| First 72 hours | Hourly around clock |
| At 4 to 7 days | Hourly waking hours and every 2 hours when asleep |
| At 1 to 3 months | Taper slowly to 4 times daily |
| Dibromopropamidine ointment | Substitute at night when administration of solution at night drops to every 4 hours |
| Polymyxin-B-neomycin-gramicidin solution | Same as propamidine isethionate |
| Polyhexamethylene biguandine, 0.02%* | Same as propamidine isethionate. Continue maintenance dose 6–12 months |

*Am J Ophthalmology 115:466-470,1993.*

to promote leukocyte adherence and extravasation, enhances the responsiveness of T-lymphocytes to antigens, and regulates fibroblast proliferation. Similarly, IL-2 has regulatory activity on virtually all types of cells participating in immune responses and stimulates the production and secretion of other cytokines. It is produced by antigen- or mitogen-stimulated T-lymphocytes. It has been shown that intrastromal injections of IL-2 can induce corneal vascularization in mice.[55] These and probably other immunologically mediated pathways are the likely mechanisms for corneal involvement in a vast array of conditions. At the present time, it is important to recognize the presence of noninfectious keratitis and its associated conditions. While current treatment of the cornea, if any, is likely to be nonspecific, specific therapeutic approaches are currently being devised on the basis of the biology of cytokines and include such strategies as blocking their cellular receptors or inactivating cytokines with specific antibodies. The current therapy for the corneal component of most of these conditions is topical corticosteroid administration for active inflammation and angiogenesis. Established blood vessels and scars are not amenable to treatment with corticosteroids or any other medical therapy. In instances when visual loss is associated with these processes, penetrating keratoplasty may be useful. It is important to have inflammation controlled and concomitant abnormalities of eyelids, conjunctiva, and tear production recognized, controlled, or continuously managed before and after performing a transplant.

## INTERSTITIAL KERATITIS

The classic example of these immunologically mediated processes is interstitial keratitis associated with congenital or acquired syphilis. The term "interstitial" implies midstromal inflammation, present or past. However, this pattern of clinical findings is not exclusively related to syphilis and may be seen in association with many other conditions (Fig. 11.36). The patterns of corneal cellular infiltration may be different in the various associations but still present a similar final clinical picture. Most patients present with an intact corneal epithelium regardless of the stage of keratitis and also lack other signs of active corneal infection.

**Cogan's syndrome** is a clinical constellation of bilateral stromal keratitis with blood vessel formation in association with vestibuloauditory symptoms which may lead to sensorineural deafness and profound balance and other vestibular abnormalities.[56] Pain may be felt in the eyes during the active process when corneal infiltrates are forming. Cogan syndrome is not caused by syphilis. Other involvements include arteritis and widespread

### Figure 11.36. Conditions Associated with Corneal Stromal Inflammation, Scarring, and Vascularization ("Interstitial Keratitis")

| | |
|---|---|
| Cogan syndrome | Ocular rosacea |
| Gold toxicity | Onchocerciasis |
| Herpes simplex virus keratitis | Rheumatoid diseases |
| Infectious mononucleosis | Rubeola |
| Lymphogranuloma venereum | Syphilis (congenital or acquired) |
| Leprosy | Tuberculosis |
| Lyme disease | Varicella-zoster virus keratitis |
| Mumps | Variola |

necrotizing lesions that lead to such problems as endocarditis and gastrointestinal hemorrhages.

**Systemic gold therapy** for connective tissue diseases such as systemic lupus erythematosus may lead to the accumulation of goldish-red substance in Descemet's membrane and the development of stromal keratitis with vascularization. This may necessitate switching the patient to other systemic treatments.

**Herpes simplex virus** keratitis and keratitis associated with infectious mononucleosis due to Epstein–Barr virus infection may have characteristics typical of those seen in syphilitic keratitis and be caused by similar immunologic responses without the involvement of live replicating virus in the stroma.

**Lymphogranuloma venereum**, a chronic sexually transmitted disease caused by certain serotypes (L1,L2,L3 of subgroup A) of *Chlamydia trachomatis*, is common in tropical regions of the world and uncommon in the United States. Genital infections lead to lymphadenitis followed by chronic fistulas and elephantiasis of genitalia in males and anorectal fistulas and strictures in females. Ocular involvements include Parinaud oculoglandular syndrome, elephantiasis of the eyelids and, less commonly, stromal keratitis, corneal vascularization, episcleritis, scleritis, uveitis, and optic neuritis.

**Leprosy, or Hansen's disease**, is a chronic granulomatous disease caused by *Mycobacterium leprae*. Disease in humans has clinical and histologic features that have been classified by Ridley.[57,58] The spectrum of systemic disease ranges from a few sharply marginated plaques in which the granulomas contain lymphocyes and Langerhans giant cells, so-called tuberculoid leprosy, to a condition in which many poorly defined nodules that contain few lymphocytes and no Langerhans giant cells predominate, so-called lepromatous leprosy. Ocular involvements are far more common towards the lepromatous leprosy end of the spectrum. Interstitial keratitis, often bilateral, occurs in a few patients along with corneal hypesthesia, superficial punctate keratitis, VII cranial nerve palsy, iritis, white opacities on the iris surface, subconjunctival lepromatous nodules, scleritis, entropion, and ectropion. Unlike the other causes of interstitial keratitis, live *M. leprae* is found in the sites of involvement including the cornea and corneal nerves. Other signs of leprosy include loss of eyelashes and eyebrows.

While topical corticosteroid therapy helps control the inflammation associated with keratitis, iritis, or scleritis, systemic treatment with clofazimine, rifampin, or dapsone alone or in combination is needed to control infection and eliminate the micro-organisms.

**Lyme disease** is caused by infection with the spirochete *Borrelia burgdorferi*. The bacterium is transmitted to humans by tick bites during outdoor activities. The systemic manifestations of Lyme disease are protean and the specific cause is often not detected in the initial stages. The disease process has been divided into three stages: Stage I (initial infection), Stage II (disseminated infection), Stage III (late immunologic sequelae) (Fig. 11.37). Stromal keratitis occurs late in Lyme disease and has been reported in a number of published papers.[59] On this basis, it seems likely that there is a specific relationship between the two. Lyme disease can be the cause of widespread systemic and ocular symptoms and findings. If the patient is having temporally related involvements, it is wise to inform the patient's other physicians that Lyme disease is a possible explanation for the ocular abnormalities. Laboratory diagnosis, especially serological tests, are rapidly being refined and local infectious disease experts and diagnostic laboratories can give advice on the current best test and interpretation of results. Some tests are cross-reactive with serologic tests for syphilis.

Treatment with topical corticosteroids is employed for ocular inflammation associated with Lyme disease. Treatment with antibiotics in all stages as well as with oral corticosteroids in cases of arthritis, cardiac and some neurologic involvements is best carried out by the internist or general physician.

**Mumps**, like most of the previous entities, may cause epithelial or stromal keratitis, episcleritis, scleritis, or uveitis.

**Rosacea** may involve the cornea and cause stromal keratitis with vascularization. The lesions are near the limbus, often are located inferiorly, and have superficial vascularization, stromal inflammation, and eventually scarring. More common and invariably present in patients with keratitis are marked blepharitis and meibomian gland dysfunction and often significant dry eye syndrome. Careful dermatologic examination usually detects typical vasodilation and telangiectasia of the nose and cheeks along with sebaceous gland hypertrophy.

Treatment of the general condition with systemic tetracycline, the local involvements with lid hygiene, warm compresses, and artificial tears, and the stromal keratitis with topical corticosteroid helps control the ocular manifestations. Isotretinoin has also been used to treat rosacea. However, this drug also causes a dose-dependent type of blepharoconjunctivitis. Another local therapy for the skin lesions on the face, but not for application on the eye, is metronidazole, 0.75% topical gel, twice daily to involved areas.

**Onchocerciasis** has been discussed on page 11.30. Stromal keratitis may occur as scattered nummular keratitis or as a diffuse process. In addition to appropriate systemic medications, topical corticosteroids are used to control inflammation in the cornea.

**Rubeola (measles)** may cause epithelial keratitis rather commonly and stromal keratitis infrequently.

**Syphilis** is caused by the spirochete *Treponema pallidum*. It has long been stated that approximately 90 percent of interstitial keratitis is associated with syphilis, most especially congenital syphilis. Although the preciseness of the incidence figure is not certain, interstitial keratitis, at any stage, should lead to consideration of this diagnosis and appropriate laboratory studies are indicated.

### Figure 11.37. Stages of Lyme Disease and Ocular Findings

| STAGE | OCULAR CONDITIONS |
|---|---|
| I. | |
| Skin: erythema migrans | Conjunctivitis |
| Lymphadenopathy | |
| II. | |
| Skin: erythema chronicum | Uveitis; anterior, posterior, or |
| Joints: arthralgia | both; optic neuritis or atrophy |
| Cardiac: myocarditis, heart | |
| block, other arrhythmias | |
| III. | |
| Skin: acrodermatitis chronica | Stromal keratitis, episcleritis |
| atrophicans | |
| Joints: arthritis | |

The complete evolution of untreated syphilitic keratitis may take months to 1–2 years. The earlier it is recognized and treated, the shorter the course and the smaller the damage. In its early stages there is a nonspecific infiltration with inflammatory cells and some edema. After a few weeks photophobia and discomfort are predominant symptoms, the intensity of the stromal inflammation increases, and new superficial and deep blood vessel formation begins from the periphery and then progresses. The inflammation adjacent to Descemet's membrane leads to wrinkle formation in it, which may be hard to appreciate due to an overall "ground glass" appearance. Finally, as the inflammation subsides, the vascular channels carry less blood and variable amounts of the haziness resolve to leave some degree of scarring and ghost vessels (Fig. 11.38). This residual group of findings, often with associated cornea guttata, are the most commonly recognized presentations. This stage does not require local therapy. However, many patients with old syphilitic interstitial keratitis still have viable *T. pallidum* many years after the acute infection, including many who have not had complete treatment. Serologic testing, including a rapid plasma Reagin test (RPR) for active or recent infection, fluorescent treponemal antibody absorption test (FTA-ABS), and lumbar puncture for studies for neurosyphilis may be indicated in some patients. Antibiotic type and dosage are based on the extent of systemic involvements and center on penicillin.

In patients with old interstitial keratitis, additional visual loss later in life usually occurs in association with cataract formation. In many instances cataract extraction without a penetrating keratoplasty gives a satisfactory visual result. In other situations a combined procedure may be more appropriate.

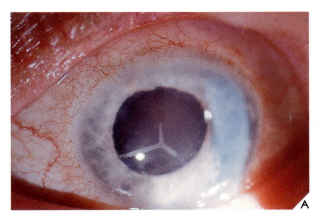
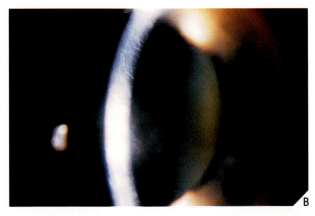

**11.38** | Syphilitic interstitial keratitis. *A and B:* Corneal stomal scarring and ghost vessels.

**Tuberculosis** is rarely associated with a type of stromal keratitis that may mimic that caused by syphilis.

**Varicella-zoster virus keratitis** was described on pages 11.23–11.26.

**Variola (smallpox)** stromal keratitis is seen only as old disease or scarring since the successful elimination of smallpox throughout the world.

Other noninfectious corneal infiltrates are seen in several conditions. A Wessely ring represents the collection of diffused antigen, specific antibodies against that antigen, complement components, and polymorphonuclear leukocytes (Fig. 11.39). It may be seen under a wide array of situations, including a response to herpes simplex virus antigen, fungal infections, or foreign bodies. A related phenomenon with a similar immunopathogenesis is seen in presumed staphylococcal marginal keratitis. In all of these, topical corticosteroids help eliminate the inflammation but their use must be judicious in the face of active herpetic and fungal infections.

**Vernal keratoconjunctivitis** is another noninfectious inflammatory disorder that may involve the peripheral cornea. The limbal form of vernal keratoconjunctivitis is extensively discussed in Chapter 2. The limbal lesions may occur in any position on the circumference of the limbus. Raised, semiopaque, rounded areas that sometimes merge with adjacent lesions may cover the peripheral cornea, which develops small opacities and superficial pannus (Fig. 11.40). In some cases whitish or yellowish dots develop on top of the limbal vernal lesions. Known as Trantas' dots, these small opacities contain aggregates of cellular debris and eosinophils and are more common along the superior limbus. The raised limbal papillae often have an overlying pseudomembrane and consist of large accumulations of eosinophils along

## NONINFECTIOUS KERATITIS

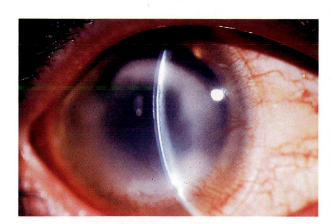

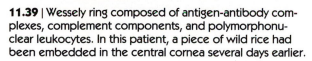

**11.39** | Wessely ring composed of antigen-antibody complexes, complement components, and polymorphonuclear leukocytes. In this patient, a piece of wild rice had been embedded in the central cornea several days earlier.

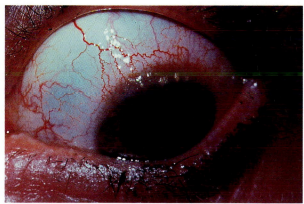

**11.40** | Limbal form of vernal keratoconjunctivitis with Trantas' dots.

with mast cells, basophils, and hyperplastic epithelial cells. Lymphocytes may be adjacent to blood vessels within the papillae.

There seems to be an association between a history of vernal kerato-conjunctivitis and keratoconus.[60] Another corneal involvement seen in a few patients is a chronic epithelial defect with opaque edges and slight loss of stromal substance. This so-called shield ulcer is most likely caused by mechanical contact and rubbing of superior palpebral papillae. Therapy has been discussed in the chapter on conjunctival diseases.

**Phlyctenular keratoconjunctivitis** is an immunologically mediated response to a number of stimuli (Fig. 11.41). These antigens probably cause a type IV or cell-mediated hypersensitivity of which a classic positive PPD skin response is the prototype. Phlyctenules may involve the conjunctiva, cornea, or both. As compared with conjunctival phlyctenules, those in the cornea develop more slowly and are associated with more symptoms. Some corneal phlyctenules result from movement of a conjunctival lesion and others occur alone. The natural history of the complete process to resolution takes approximately 1 to 2 weeks. As the inflammatory cells invade the cornea, irritation, tearing, photophobia, and blepharospasm are significant and dominant symptoms. The corneal phlyctenule usually has a small white superficial infiltrate with more diffuse infiltrate beneath it. A leash of superficial vessels extending directly from the nearest portion of the limbus surrounds the infiltrate and slowly the inflammation resolves. However, new lesions may occur at a later time and are often adjacent to the original one. Models of this disease process have been produced by immunizing rabbits with *Staphylococcus aureus* followed by corneal injections of ribitol teichoic acid (a cell wall antigen of *S. aureus*) and by injection of a cytokine from stimulated T lymphocytes, interleukin-2, into the corneas of mice.[61] These studies plus the clinical observations provide strong support for the hypothesis that phlyctenules represent type IV hypersensitivity responses. The histopathology of these lesions is also supportive. There is a lymphocytic infiltration at the level of Bowman's layer and the superficial stroma which elevates the overlying epithelium. Neovascularization occurs within this area and is followed by eventual clearing of inflammatory cells, scar formation, and localized destruction of Bowman's layer.

Therapy is two-pronged. The infection needs to be treated if it is active. Topical corticosteroids are utilized to minimize scar formation and angiogenesis. Penetrating keratoplasty can successfully restore visual loss due to

---

**Figure 11.41. Conditions and Putative Antigens that Can Cause Phlyctenular Keratoconjunctivitis via Type IV Hypersensitivity Response**

Staphylococcal antigen(s)
Tuberculosis (bacterial protein antigens)
Fungal antigens (*C. immitis, Candida albicans*)
Certain chemicals (e.g., cocaine)
Gonococcal antigens
Lymphogranuloma venereum
Adenovirus
Leishmaniasis

phlyctenular scars.

**Fuchs' superficial marginal keratitis** is an infrequent condition that was originally described in middle-aged or older patients and recently described in adults in their twenties.[62] The process begins as superficial inflammatory infiltrates in the peripheral cornea of one or both eyes. Involvement may be localized or comprise 360° of the peripheral cornea. Later, overlying epithelial defects and mild loss of stromal substance develop. This cycle of events tends to recur and eventually leads to subepithelial scar tissue formation and formation of blood vessels from the conjunctiva to cover the corneal lesions, giving the appearance of a pseudopterygium (Fig. 11.42). Typically, the process subsides and the central cornea remains clear. The cause, immunopathogenesis, and optimal therapy have not been completely elucidated.

Many systemic, immunologically mediated diseases have associated corneal inflammation as part of their involvement spectra. In most instances the systemic condition is already evident. In some of these diseases the types of immune mechanisms that best explain the immunopathogenesis are worked out for one or more target organs. The ocular involvements are presumably on the same basis but definite proof may be lacking.

**Rheumatoid arthritis** is relatively common with a prevalence of approximately 1–2 percent. Women are more often affected than men (3:2). Onset of disease occurs between 16 and 50 years of age. The specific cause is not known and a number of immunologic responses have been characterized. People with the HLA-DR4, specifically Dw4 and Dw14, markers have a much greater risk for disease. While arthritis is characterized by acute and later chronic lymphocyte (mainly T-cells) and plasma cell inflammation of joint synovial membranes along with erosion of adjacent cartilage and bone, many other tissues may be involved such as the eye, pleura, and cardiovascular system.

The ocular involvements include dry eye syndrome, episcleritis, scleritis including scleromalacia perforans, sclerokeratitis, and peripheral corneal furrow or melting (Fig. 11.43). In a few instances the peripheral corneal melting results in perforation. Acute stromal keratitis can also occur in the central cornea and progress to perforation. Ocular involvements occur in more than half of rheumatoid arthritis patients. The systemic therapy that controls the

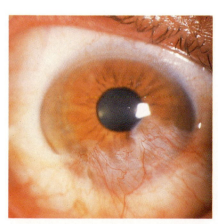

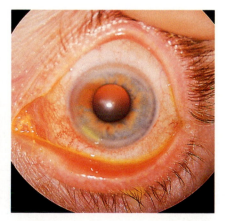

**11.43** | Peripheral corneal furrow with modest fluorescein staining is present in a patient with severe rheumatoid arthritis.

**11.42** | Fuchs' superficial marginal keratitis with superficial corneal infiltrates and the appearance of a pseudopterygium.

joint involvement often controls the ocular inflammatory components. Systemic corticosteroids and cytotoxic drugs are the most common treatments. Plaquenil® (hydroxychloroquine sulfate) and gold therapy are also used. Topical corticosteroids are avoided, because they often worsen the process as do periocular injections. Aggressive management of the dry eye syndrome that occurs in up to 25 percent of rheumatoid arthritis patients is necessary to avoid other complications.

**Systemic lupus erythematosus** typically affects many organs and tissues, including the musculoskeletal system (arthritis and myalgias), lungs (pleurisy and pleural effusions), heart (myocarditis), skin ("butterfly" rash on face), central nervous system (migraine headaches, depression, hemiplegia, seizures), kidney (glomerulonephritis), and blood (hemolytic anemia). There are notable racial and gender susceptibilities. The ratio of female to male is 9:1. Approximately 1 in 250 African-American women, 1 in 1,000 Chinese, and 1 in 4,000 Caucasian women have systemic lupus erythematosus. The exact cause is unknown. Approximately 10 percent of cases are drug-induced but usually lack antibodies to double-stranded DNA, and ordinarily the central nervous system and kidneys are spared. Virtually all the other patients have antibodies against double-stranded DNA and often other nuclear antigens. Circulating immune complexes consisting of DNA or other nuclear antigens and their corresponding antibodies deposit in involved tissues and cause damage. However, there are also notable cellular defects involving T- and B-cells as well. T-cells have an abnormal production of interleukin-2 and inappropriate response to this cytokine. B-cells are hyperresponsive due to a cellular defect and in addition they lack appropriate T-cell regulation.

The ocular manifestations in systemic lupus erythematosus include retinal hemorrhages, cotton-wool spots, retinal and disc edema, dry-eye syndrome, episcleritis, scleritis, uveitis, and stromal keratitis.

**Systemic sclerosis (scleroderma)** is a connective tissue disease of middle age that is more common in women. There is a widespread increase in fibrous tissue in skin, soft tissues, muscles, joints, and organs due to increased number of fibroblasts and collagen-containing connective tissue. Although the exact cause of this disease remains unknown, it is associated with antibody activity against nuclear and nucleolar antigens. Ocular involvements include keratoconjunctivitis sicca, symblepharon formation, corneal infiltrates, and vascularization.

**Wegener's granulomatosis** is a diffuse arteritis characterized by giant cells and fibrinoid necrosis. Sinuses, lungs, trachea, and kidneys are the most commonly involved sites. Patients with Wegener's granulomatosis usually have antibodies to cytoplasmic antigens present in polymorphonuclear leukocytes called antineutrophil cytoplasmic antigen (ANCA). Without aggressive systemic treatment with corticosteroids and cytotoxic (e.g., cyclophosphamide) agents, this is usually a fatal disease. Approximately one half of patients with Wegener's granulomatosis have ocular disorders including peripheral ulcerative keratitis, scleritis, conjunctivitis, uveitis, orbital vasculitis, and retinal artery occlusion.

**Polyarteritis nodosa** is a widespread vasculitis involving small and medium-sized arteries that frequently damages the kidneys and visceral organs. It has a poor prognosis unless treated with systemic cytotoxic agents and corticosteroids. Ocular involvements occur in up to 20 percent and include conjunctivitis, peripheral ulcerative keratitis, episcleritis, scleritis, uveitis, choroidal vasculitis, and retinal vasculitis.

**Relapsing polychondritis** is characterized by recurrent inflammation of cartilage of the nose, ears, trachea, larynx, and joints along with vasculitis. Eyes of patients with relapsing polychondritis may develop conjunctivitis, keratitis, episcleritis, scleritis, or uveitis.

**Behçet syndrome** is a vasculitis that causes recurrent oral ulcers, genital ulcers, arthritis, central nervous system abnormalities, and skin lesions. Uveitis has been described as the classic ocular involvement. However, conjunctival inflammation and ulceration as well as corneal infiltration, scarring, ulceration and vascularization have also been described. The immunologic characteristics of Behçet syndrome include the coating of epithelial cells with immunoglobulins and an underlying T cell infiltrate, circulating IgG immune complexes, high levels of circulating complement component C9, and acute-phase reactants (e.g., C-reactive protein). Systemic therapy includes corticosteroids and cytotoxic agents or cyclosporine.

**Inflammatory bowel diseases** include Crohn's disease and ulcerative colitis. Both conditions have been associated with various ocular inflammatory conditions. Among them are peripheral keratitis with infiltrates, ulcerations, or both, sclerokeratitis, scleritis, episcleritis, and uveitis. The therapies for the systemic conditions are the mainstay for control of the ocular inflammations.

In all these systemic conditions, the ocular manifestations are best controlled by appropriate systemic therapy and careful local therapy. Special attention must be paid to adequate therapy of dry eye syndrome, if present. It is best to have an intact epithelium prior to initiation of topical corticosteroid therapy. The roles, if any, of topical nonsteroidal anti-inflammatory drugs or topical cyclosporine are not yet clear. Other approaches, such as conjunctival resections for peripheral ulcerative keratitis, may be useful but definitive indications and predictable therapeutic responses are lacking. Because some systemic inflammatory diseases are life-threatening, their presence should be considered in all patients with these general ocular inflammatory lesions.

## INFECTIOUS ENDOPHTHALMITIS

The possible devastating effects on the neural retina and other intraocular tissues make endophthalmitis one of the most challenging and urgent problems for the ophthalmologist. The rapid onset of inexplicable intraocular inflammation or inflammation that is more intense than usual following surgery or trauma deserves to be considered as infectious endophthalmitis until proven otherwise. Trauma or excessive handling of intraocular tissues may cause excessive uveal tract inflammation. Likewise, sterile intraocular foreign bodies, microbial products such as endotoxin, and chemicals may all cause severe sterile inflammation that is not distinguishable from infectious endophthalmitis. In all cases, infectious causes must be suspected and laboratory workups performed. Although various micro-organisms destroy ocular tissues at different rates, the rapidity of workup and therapy are crucial outcome variables.

The vast majority of infectious endophthalmitis cases are associated with intraocular surgery and include cataract surgery, penetrating keratoplasty, and glaucoma filtering procedures. Some cases occur a long time after surgery, especially those caused by *Staphylococcus epidermidis* (which may occur 2 or more weeks postoperatively). Others may be associated with suture removal or spontaneous rupture of glaucoma surgery filtering blebs. Approximately 25 percent of infectious endophthalmitis cases are associated with trauma. In most instances, it appears that cases of bacterial exogenous endophthalmitis are caused by intraocular penetration of the identical organism from the patient's own eyelids or ocular surface.[63] A small portion of cases of endophthalmitis are caused by endogenous spread of a microorganism to the eye from another infected site (Fig. 11.44).

Regardless of the route of infection of the eye, marked anterior and posterior intraocular inflammation, rapid loss of vision, conjunctival injection and chemosis, poor visibility of intraocular structures, and pain suggest infectious endophthalmitis (Fig. 11.45). B-scan ultrasonography demonstrates vitreous echoes. A diagnostic vitreous aspirate for cytology and culture should be expeditiously performed (Fig. 11.46). Although the definitive role of vitrectomy in the management of infectious endophthalmitis is still under study, the vitreous specimens should be placed on appropriate culture media for a variety of bacteria and fungi. Inoculation of blood culture bottles with aliquots of vitrectomy specimens is simple and probably as efficacious as the inoculation of membrane filtering systems.[64] Vitreous specimens must be placed on clean microscope slides and processed in the same fashion as was detailed for infectious keratitis. The information obtained from the cytologic examination guides the selection of antibiotics for intravitreal injections. If bacteria are the causative agents, cultures will not be helpful for approximately 24 hours or longer; for fungi a few days may be required. The known infectious causes of endophthalmitis are listed in Figure 11.2. In cases of endogenous endophthalmitis, the infectious agent at another site (or sites) is very likely the ocular pathogen.

In the United States the incidence of infectious endophthalmitis following intraocular surgery and including cataract extraction, secondary intraocular lens implantation, pars plana vitrectomy, penetrating keratoplasty, and glaucoma filtering surgery is approximately 0.1 percent.[65,65] If an anterior segment procedure requires a vitrectomy, the risk of endophthalmitis increases significantly and may be as much as four times greater.[66,67] The most common causes of postoperative bacterial endophthalmitis are *Staphylococcus epidermidis*, *S. aureus*, *Streptococcus* and *Pseudomonas*. In cases occurring following glaucoma filtering surgery, *Haemophilus* and *Streptococcus* are the most commonly isolated bacteria. Delayed postoperative endophthalmitis is often caused by *Staphylococcus epidermidis* or *Propionibacterium acnes*.[68] These cases

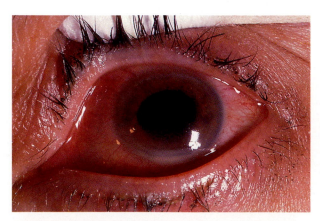

**11.44** | Endogenous endophthalmitis associated with meningococcemia (Waterhouse–Friedrickson syndrome). Elevated intraocular pressure, hypopyon, and other inflammation were noted. (Courtesy of Dr. Vincent Deluise.)

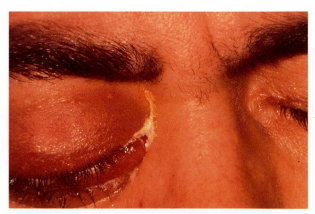

**11.45** | External signs of endophthalmitis with eyelid erythema and edema and conjunctival chemosis.

of endophthalmitis become clinically evident weeks to months following intraocular surgery, are more mild, and the onset is more gradual. Almost all cases of infectious postoperative endophthalmitis are of bacterial origin.

Traumatic endophthalmitis comprises approximately 25 percent of all infectious endophthalmitis cases and occurs in approximately 5 percent of patients with penetrating ocular injuries. Patients with retained intraocular foreign bodies have a greater incidence. In addition to the bacteria mentioned previously, *Bacillus* species cause approximately 30 percent of traumatic endophthalmitis and often have a poor outcome. Additionally, retinal breaks or detachments are associated with bad outcomes. The successful treatment of patients with traumatic endophthalmitis requires prompt and thorough laboratory workup as well as medical and surgical management.

Endogenous endophthalmitis is uncommon. Micro-organisms including bacteria and fungi spread to the eye from other infected sites in the body.[69-73] The situations that predispose people to endogenous endophthalmitis include immunosuppression, intravenous drug abuse, and prolonged use of intravenous devices such as intra-arterial lines, hemodialysis, and parenteral hyperalimentation. Healthy people may also develop acute endophthalmitis as part of an infectious process. For example, a healthy person may develop septicemia and endophthalmitis due to *Neisseria meningitidis*.

The optimal management of infectious endophthalmitis is yet to be determined. There seems to be reasonable agreement that severe cases of endophthalmitis are best managed with vitrectomy and intravitreal injections of two antibiotics. However, specific indications for vitrectomy as well as its extent and timing have not been elucidated. Most vitrectomies are performed as part of the procedure for the diagnostic vitreous aspirate or within a day of obtaining it. The selection of antibiotics is still not completely settled, but good spectrum of coverage and reasonably low retinal toxicity are possible with initial injections of vancomycin, 1 mg in 0.1 ml, and amikacin, 0.4 mg, in 0.1 ml. Intravenous antibiotics are also administered: vancomycin or cefazolin, 1 g intravenously every 6 hours in combination with gentamicin or tobramycin, 1 mg/kg every 8 hours. The added value of topical or subconjunctival antibiotics is uncertain except when there is evidence of infec-

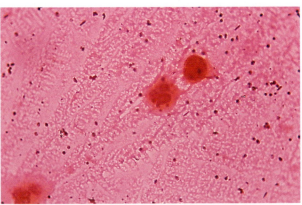
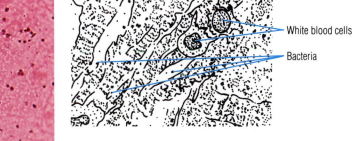

White blood cells

Bacteria

**11.46** | Gram stain of vitreous aspirate from patient with endophthalmitis reveals a few bacteria in addition to two adjacent polymorphonuclear leukocytes and considerable extraneous staining debris.

tious keratitis and their usage is essential. In some cases subsequent intravitreal injections may be useful; their selection is best based on the causative organism, its antibiotic sensitivities, and the relative retinal toxicities of candidate antibiotics. These data are rapidly changing and contemplated antibiotic treatment should rely on the latest information in recent journals. It is obvious that the opportunity to sterilize the infection and salvage useful vision requires a rapid response on the part of the treating ophthalmologist.

Once treatment is initiated, repeated and detailed examinations are required to determine when the process begins to come under control and medications can be tapered. The course of intravenous antibiotics is approximately 5 days in duration. The use of corticosteroids by all routes has been attempted but specific indications are not yet available. Sterilization of the infection is the first priority. Once achieved, the control of inflammation may be beneficial. Topical corticosteroid administration is probably the safest option in antibiotic-treated endophthalmitis. The intravitreal injection of corticosteroids during active infection may potentiate survival of viable micro-organisms.

# 12 | CORNEAL SURGERY

## Sheridan Lam
## John W. Chandler

This chapter will describe various surgical procedures involving the anterior segment, including penetrating keratoplasty, lamellar keratoplasty, superficial keratectomy, conjunctival flap, epikeratoplasty, and keratorefractive surgery.

Although the important steps of each procedure are described with the aid of illustrations, this chapter is not intended to serve as a comprehensive surgical atlas. Because there are many excellent ways to perform a given surgical procedure, this presentation cannot be comprehensive. Surgeons should learn each procedure through formal training (e.g., courses or fellowships) and should practice in a microsurgical laboratory before performing surgery on patients.

## PHAKIC/PSEUDOPHAKIC PENETRATING KERATOPLASTY

### ANESTHESIA

Penetrating keratoplasty is usually performed under local anesthesia. However, general anesthesia is required for infants and children and may be necessary in uncooperative adult patients. Mild sedatives can be used in anxious patients. No specific nerve blocks are preferred, but all blocks must be performed safely and effectively, such that there is no pressure from lids and no extraocular movement except minimal rotation associated with the superior oblique muscle.

### SOFTENING THE GLOBE

Preoperative reduction of intraocular pressure by digital massage or with some mechanical device (e.g., Honan Balloon or Super Pinky) reduces the potential for excessive vitreous pressure, protrusion of intraocular contents, and choroidal hemorrhage during surgery. The eye should be softened such that it is easily indented with the heel of a muscle hook. Acetazolamide and mannitol are not routinely used because of their significant side effects.

Hyperventilation is useful to decrease intraocular pressure during general anesthesia. Intraoperatively, aspiration of liquid vitreous through the pars plana with a 22-gauge needle is effective in rapidly lowering intraocular pressure (Figure 12.1).

## HEAD POSITIONING

The head must be positioned such that the tangential plane through the corneal apex is horizontal and allows the trephine to stand vertically by itself on the host cornea (Fig. 12.2). A roll of sheets or towels placed under the neck is helpful in maintaining the head in proper position. A wrist rest is useful for some surgeons, and its height is set at the level of the lateral canthus.

## PREPARATION

The periorbital region is scrubbed with Betadine® solution and the conjunctival fornices are gently swept with cotton-tipped applicators soaked with a 50:50 mixture of sterile saline and Betadine®.

## GLOBE STABILIZATION

The globe can be stabilized with traction sutures placed through superior and inferior rectus muscles and anchored onto the drapes (Fig. 12.3A). Alternatively, a scleral (Flieringa) ring can be sutured onto the globe over the region of the pars plana, about 3–4 mm from the limbus, with one of the ends of the sutures (5-0 Vicryl® or Dacron®) left long so that they can be anchored to the drape (Fig. 12.3B). A McNeill–Goldman double ring (blepharostat) is useful and serves simultaneously as a supporting ring and a lid retractor. Muscle traction sutures (4-0 silk) are used by us only in phakic cases, whereas scleral rings must be used when the eye becomes aphakic or pseudophakic intra- or postoperatively. To secure a scleral ring, the sutures are passed through superficial sclera with the needle directed towards the limbus in an uphill fashion (Fig. 12.3C).

## RECIPIENT CORNEA TREPHINATION

We almost always use freehanded trephines, which have been shown to create uniform openings.[1] Suction trephines (e.g., Hessburg–Barron) are advocated by some in cases when the globe is perforated and excessive pressure from a hand-held trephine may lead to protrusion of intraocular contents. The sizes of the trephines routinely used are 8 mm and 8.25 mm in diameter. The smaller trephine is used to dissect the host cornea, and the larger trephine is used to punch the donor button. Oversizing of the donor tissue is necessary because trephination from the epithelial surface creates a cornea button with a larger diameter than trephination from the endothelial side.[2] However, oversizing is not necessary if the graft size is 9 mm or greater. Equal-sized donor and recipient or donor graft smaller than the host trephination opening can be used to reduce myopia in keratoconus patients.[3] The size of the graft may need to be reduced for infant eyes or enlarged for keratoconus, pellucid degeneration, or eccentric corneal scars.

If there is no iris abnormality, the trephine is centered over the pupillary center (constriction of pupil with topical pilocarpine preoperatively is helpful in centering the trephine). If the pupil is distorted, the trephine is placed slightly nasal to the geometric center of the host cornea. An epithelial impression is made by gently pressing down on the trephine and is used to

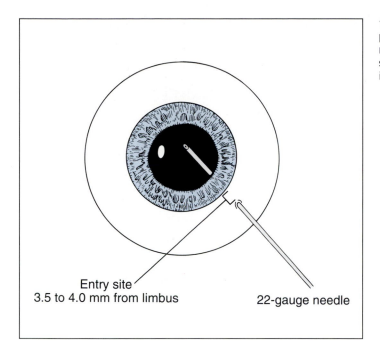

**12.1** | Aspiration of liquid vitreous through the pars plana. The tip of the needle is placed in mid-vitreous and visualized at all times. The entry site is located 3.5 to 4.0 mm from the limbus and is sutured at the end of the procedure.

Entry site
3.5 to 4.0 mm from limbus

22-gauge needle

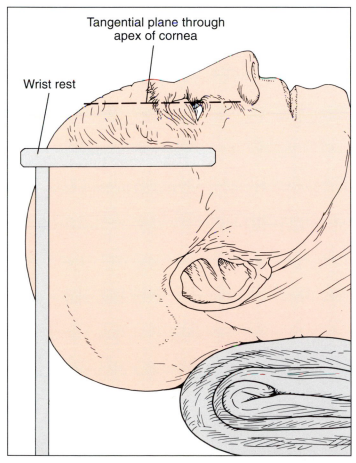

**12.2** | Proper positioning for penetrating kerato-plasty. The tangential plane through the corneal apex should be horizontal. A roll of towels is helpful to keep the head properly tilted.

Tangential plane through apex of cornea

Wrist rest

**12.3** | *A:* Setup for phakic penetrating keratoplasty.

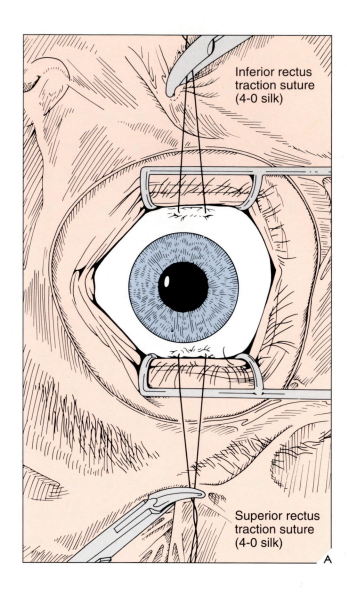

Inferior rectus
traction suture
(4-0 silk)

Superior rectus
traction suture
(4-0 silk)

A

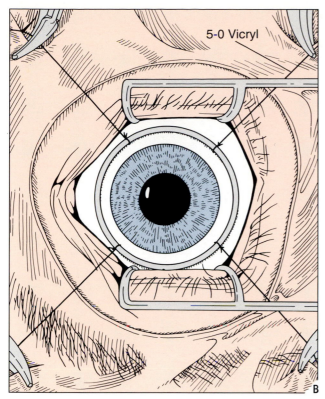

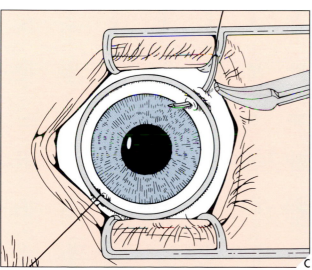

**12.3** | cont. *B*: Setup for aphakic or pseudophakic penetrating keratoplasty. Note that sutures are passed under the speculum. *C*: The scleral ring is secured. The needle is passed through the sclera under the scleral ring and towards the limbus.

**12.4 |** Epithelial impression from the trephine.

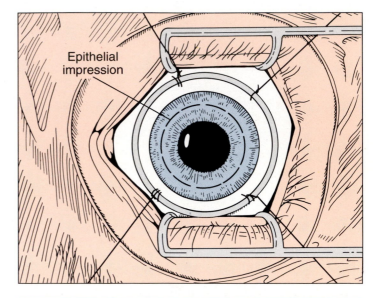

**12.5 |** *A*: The trephine is tilted nasally to deepen the depth of the nasal wound. *B*: The trephine is tilted temporally if the temporal portion of the wound is shallow after the initial trephination.

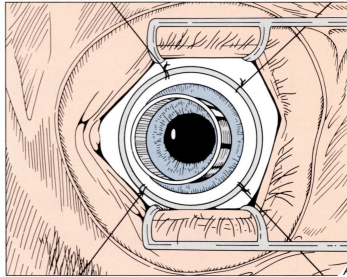

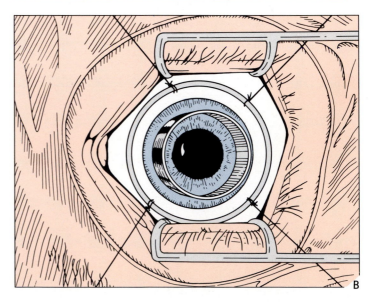

check for the proper centering of the trephine (Fig. 12.4). Adjustments are made before dissecting the cornea.

The host cornea is trephined down to 50%–75% of the stromal thickness. The trephine is held with just enough downward pressure to keep it from sliding and is turned with even pressure to dissect the host cornea evenly in the entire circumference of the groove. The depth of the wound is inspected by using straight tying forceps to spread the wound edges open. If the wound depth is not even, the shallow portion of the wound is deepened with further trephination, with the trephine tilted toward the shallow portion of the wound (Fig. 12.5). Trephination must be stopped immediately if the anterior chamber is entered. If there is excessive corneal neovascularization, conjunctival resection is performed before trephination to reduce intraoperative bleeding and later neovascularization of the corneal graft. Excessive bleeding at the wound is reduced with cellulose sponges soaked in 10% phenylephrine hydrochloride (Neo-Synephrine®).

Several corneal punches are available, and the surgeon should be familiar with the one selected (e.g., the Iowa PK Press and Lieberman Punch). Centering of the donor corneal button is important, especially in large grafts. If the donor button does not drop from the inside of the trephine, it is gently flushed out with balanced salt solution. The donor corneal button is kept in the storage solution or viscoelastic material and covered until it is needed.

PUNCHING THE DONOR
CORNEAL BUTTON

The anterior chamber is entered with a sharp-pointed blade placed in the groove (Fig. 12.6). The anterior chamber should be decompressed slowly, and care must be taken not to damage the lens and iris. The angle of the blade is held such that no or little posterior wound bevel remains.

ENTERING THE
ANTERIOR CHAMBER

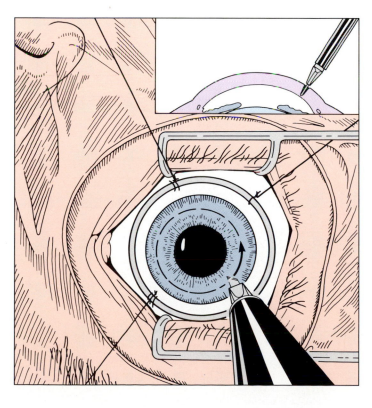

**12.6** | Entering the anterior chamber with a sharp-pointed blade, make sure that the cut follows the groove. *Inset:* The blade should be angled to minimize or prevent a posterior wound bevel.

### REMOVAL OF HOST CORNEAL BUTTON

The surgeon must be light-handed, and the bottom blade of the scissors should be held against the endothelium with a slight upward lift. The internal blade of the scissors should never touch the endothelium peripheral to the cut, because that portion of the host cornea is not replaced by the donor graft. The cut follows the groove created by previous trephination (Fig. 12.7). The scissors are held such that little or no posterior bevel remains. Too much or positive wound bevel leads to excessive irregular astigmatism and should be removed, whereas a negative bevel can make wound closure more difficult (Figs. 12.8 and 12.9). Forceps are used to stabilize the host corneal button dur-

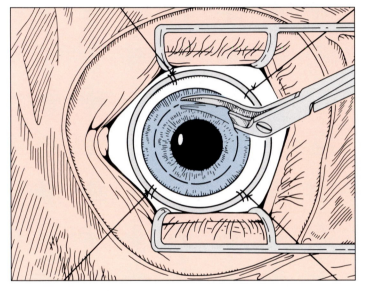

**12.7** | Removal of host corneal button. The top blade must fall into the groove and the corneal scissors should be held with a slight lift.

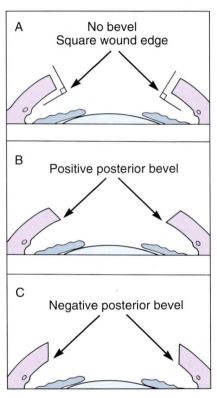

A  No bevel
Square wound edge

B  Positive posterior bevel

C  Negative posterior bevel

**12.8** | Wound bevels.

**12.9** | An excessive posterior bevel must be removed.

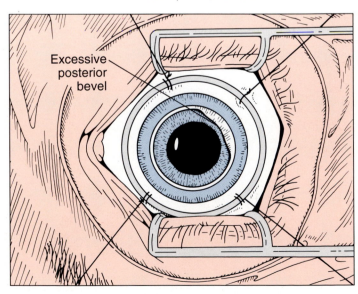

Excessive posterior bevel

ing its removal but are usually not needed if the cutting is done in one continuous direction. However, this necessitates the use of the nondominant hand.

With a small irrigation cannula, a small amount of viscoelastic material is placed over the crystalline lens or intraocular lens implant. Large amounts of viscoelastic material are not necessary and, if left in the anterior chamber, may lead to excessively elevated intraocular pressure postoperatively.

## PLACEMENT OF VISCOELASTIC MATERIAL

The donor corneal button is carried with forceps or a spatula. A cupped hand is placed under the corneal button as it is being transferred.

## TRANSFER AND SUTURING OF DONOR CORNEAL BUTTON

Nylon sutures (10-0) are used most often by us, but other types of fine sutures can be substituted depending on the surgeon's preference.[4,5] The donor button is grasped securely with forceps, and the needle enters tissue just behind the tips of the forceps (Fig. 12.10). The depth of the suture is 75%–90%. The needle enters the recipient cornea in the same relationship to the Descemet's membrane as it was in the donor. The needle exits through the host bed just in front of the limbal vessels. In large grafts, the sutures may have to be placed into the conjunctiva. Full-thickness sutures are not recommended. If some limbal tissue is included in the donor button, rotate the portion with the limbal tissue to 12 o'clock so that it is covered by the upper lid and is less conspicuous.

The placement of the four cardinal sutures at 12, 6, 3, and 9 o'clock positions is crucial. The first suture is placed at 12 o'clock, with counter-traction provided at 6 o'clock by the assistant, and is tied. We routinely use 3-1-1 knots for interrupted sutures, although 1-1-1 knots may also be used. When placing the 6 o'clock suture, first stab through the donor button and then move the needle sideways to adjust the position of the donor, if needed, to

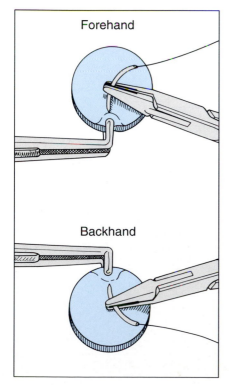

Forehand

Backhand

**12.10** | Passing the needle through the donor cornea.

ensure proper tissue distribution. The 6 o'clock suture should be exactly 180° from the 12 o'clock suture (Fig. 12.11). The sutures at 3 and 9 o'clock require similar relationships. After placing all four cardinal sutures, balanced salt solution is injected to deepen the anterior chamber, and the distribution of the donor graft is inspected (Fig. 12.12). Eight additional sutures are then placed, two for each quadrant. It is important not to compress the wound edges because this can result in irregular astigmatism. Before the running sutures are placed, all the knots of the interrupted sutures are buried and the central topography of the graft is checked with the circular end of a closed safety pin or some other device (e.g., Mandel's ring). Tight sutures in the steep meridian are replaced.

If a running suture is used, a partial-thickness stab incision is made halfway between the 11 and 12 o'clock interrupted sutures. The stabbed incision allows the knot of the running suture to be buried more easily. The first bite of the running suture is placed through the stab incision, and the following bites are passed in a clockwise direction (for a right-handed surgeon)

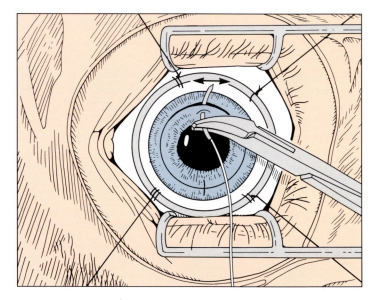

**12.11** | Placement of 6 o'clock interrupted suture. After passing through the donor button, move the needle sideways. Ascertain the proper position of the donor button in relation to the host bed.

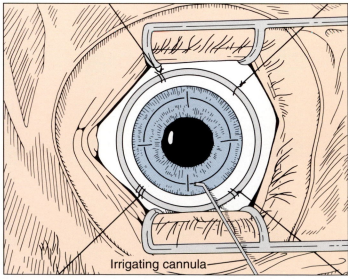

**12.12** | Deepening of the anterior chamber with balanced salt solution. The irrigating cannula should be placed next to a suture to avoid excessive wound gape.

Irrigating cannula

or counterclockwise (for a left-handed surgeon), with each bite placed midway between the interrupted sutures. Before the running suture is tied, the slack of the running suture is removed without excessively compressing the wound. After the running suture (1-1-1) is tied, the knot is rotated into the stab incision by bringing some slack to the knot.

If the running suture is accidentally broken and the suture is double-armed, the other needle is used to complete the running suture in the opposite direction. A separate suture must be used if the original suture is single-armed. This results in two knots in the running suture, and the relative positions of the knots are about the same so that both knots can be buried (Fig. 12.13).

The suture schemes we most often use are 16 interrupted sutures without running or 12-interrupted sutures with a 12-bite running (Fig. 12.14). Running suture is not ordinarily used when there is excessive neovascularization. There are also many other effective schemes to suture the donor cornea. Some surgeons prefer to use 11-0 nylon sutures, and some use Mersilene® or Prolene® sutures.[4,5]

The wound edge is dried with cellulose sponges and gently pushed on the host side to check for leakage of anterior chamber fluid. Additional interrupted sutures may be necessary if there is leakage. The surgeon must be careful not to cut the running suture with the needle.

## INTRAOPERATIVE MEDICATIONS

After removal of the scleral rings or traction bridle sutures, topical atropine and subconjunctival injections of gentamicin and dexamethasone can be given. The eye is patched.

## POSTOPERATIVE FOLLOW-UP

The patient is followed closely for clarity of the corneal graft, elevated intraocular pressure, and epithelial defect. The patient is instructed in the signs and symptoms of corneal graft rejection (e.g., decreased vision, redness, and photophobia).

## SUTURE REMOVAL

When interrupted and running sutures are both used in adult patients, the removal of the interrupted sutures begins 3 months after surgery. Sutures are removed at the steep meridian, according to keratometry and manifest refraction (computerized corneal topography also is a useful adjunct). Antibiotic drops are prescribed and used four times a day. The patient is examined 1 month later, and additional interrupted sutures are removed as indicated. Running sutures can be removed 4 months postoperatively if there is too much irregular astigmatism.

When only interrupted sutures are used in adult patients, it is typical to wait 6–12 months before suture removal begins. A suture can be removed earlier if there is a full-thickness scar, if there is neovascularization at the suture site, or if the suture is loose. The sutures are removed as mentioned above.

In infants and children, sutures are removed earlier, usually within the first 6 weeks after surgery, because of faster wound healing and greater likelihood of neovascularization.

Other effective schemes of suture adjustment are also used by other surgeons. Adjustment of the running suture to correct postoperative astigmatism has been advocated.[6]

**12.13** | Running suture with two knots. The relative position of the knots should be approximately the same.

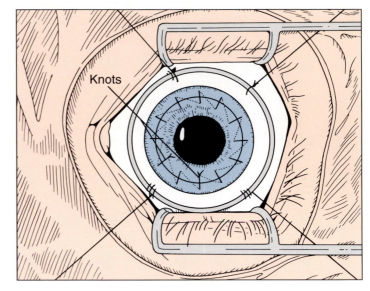

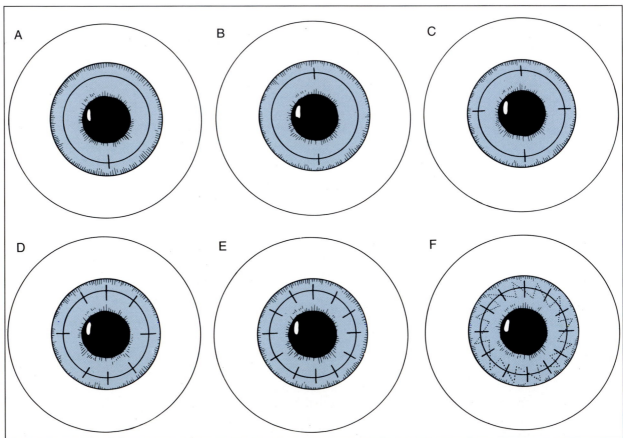

**12.14** | Twelve interrupted sutures are combined with a 12-bite running suture.

Several steps in this section are identical to those described in the section on phakic/pseudophakic penetrating keratoplasty. Only the additional steps that involve cataract extraction and implantation of an intraocular lens (IOL) are described.

## PENETRATING KERATOPLASTY WITH CATARACT EXTRACTION AND INTRAOCULAR LENS IMPLANTATION

### CALCULATION OF IOL POWER

We use the SRK (Sanders–Retzlaff–Kraff) formula [power of the IOL = (A-constant) – 2.5 (axial length) – 0.9 (average postoperative keratometric reading)] in the calculation of the power of the IOL. There are three variables: the average keratometric reading, the axial length, and the A-constant. Other methods of IOL power calculation include the Binkhorst formula and regression formulas which are based on the surgeon's previous postoperative K-readings of the corneal grafts.[7] At present, no particular method of calculation has been shown to be superior.[7]

The keratometric parameter (K-reading) in the SRK formula is the average of surgeon's previous postoperative K-readings or is based on the K-readings of other surgeons who use similar techniques. The average postoperative keratometric reading that we use is 45 diopters. The axial length should be measured carefully and cross-checked with the axial length of the contralateral eye. The value of the A-constant can be obtained from the manufacturer of the implant, and later the A-constant is adjusted based on the surgeon's postoperative K-readings and refractions.

### PREOPERATIVE DILATATION OF THE PUPIL

The pupil should be dilated with topical Neo-Synephrine 2.5% and tropicamide 1%, one drop every 5 minutes administered three times, about 30 minutes before surgery. Cyclopentolate 1% can be used in place of tropicamide, and flurbiprofen (Ocufen®) can be added to prolong mydriasis.

### CORNEAL DIAMETER MEASUREMENT

The horizontal "white-to-white" diameter of the cornea is measured before attaching the scleral ring, because the scleral ring can distort the corneal contour. The appropriate length of an anterior chamber lens is usually 1 mm greater than the horizontal diameter.

### CATARACT REMOVAL

After removal of the host corneal button, the anterior capsulotomy is performed in a can-opener fashion with a sharp-point blade. Alternatively, the anterior capsule can be removed with scissors or by capsulorrhexis. However, with capsulorrhexis, the anterior capsular opening must be at least 7 mm to accommodate the lens nucleus. During the capsulotomy, the assistant can retract the iris gently with a cellulose sponge to provide a better exposure of the lens periphery (Figs. 12.15 and 12.16).

The lens nucleus is loosened by gently rocking with a 25-gauge needle or with hydrodissection by injecting balanced salt solution under the anterior capsule. The lens nucleus is removed by gently pushing near the limbus with the heel of a muscle hook (placed at 6 o'clock) and a lens loop (placed at 12 o'clock). The pressure at 12 o'clock is directed downward, and the pressure at 6 o'clock is directed towards the optic nerve. As the lens nucleus comes forward, the assistant stabs the nucleus with a 25-gauge needle and lifts it from the eye (Fig. 12.17).

**12.15** | Can-opener capsulotomy with a sharp-point blade. Note the direction of the cut.

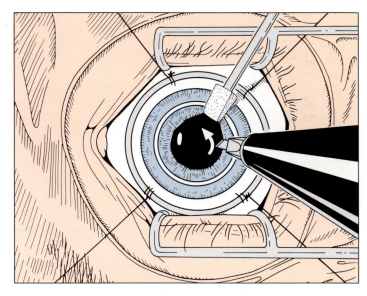

**12.16** | Capsulorrhexis. Note the direction of the forceps.

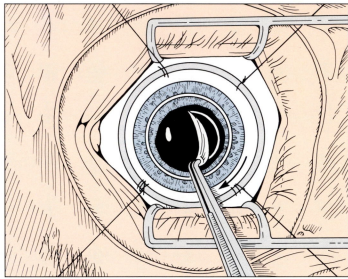

**12.17** | Lens nucleus expression. The arrows at the 12 and 6 o'clock positions indicate the directions of pressure. The lens is impaled with a 25-gauge needle and lifted from the eye.

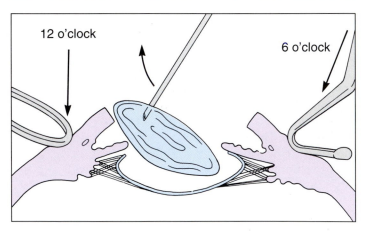

A manual or automated irrigation–aspiration unit is used to remove the residual cortical material. The rate of irrigation is kept low because the eye is open. The posterior capsule is polished if residual lens cortical material or opacities are noted on retroillumination. The iris is retracted at all clock hours to make certain that all cortical material is removed.

A small amount of viscoelastic material is used to inflate the capsular bag. The posterior chamber lens is grasped lengthwise with a long-angled forceps (Kelman–McPherson), and the inferior haptic is placed into the capsular bag. The tip of the superior haptic is then grasped with forceps and pushed inferiorly. With pronation of the wrist and gentle pressure on the optic provided through the tip of a straight forceps held in the other hand, the superior haptic is placed into the capsular bag. The IOL is centered by using a Sinsky hook (Fig. 12.18). A one-piece IOL tends to center itself when placed in the bag.

If there is a break in the posterior capsule with vitreous prolapse, anterior vitrectomy is performed. If enough capsule remains, a posterior chamber lens is placed. The integrity of the posterior capsular bag is carefully inspected by retracting the iris at all clock hours. It is important to make certain that no vitreous encroaches into the anterior chamber, because vitreous–endothelial touch may lead to graft failure. If there is not enough capsular support, an anterior chamber lens is used or, alternatively, a posterior chamber lens is sutured into the posterior chamber. At present, the surgical outcomes between these two techniques are approximately the same.[8] When the anterior chamber IOL is placed, the foot plates of the haptics should not touch the iris. A peripheral iridotomy is performed with implantation of an anterior chamber IOL.

A sutured-in posterior chamber lens is definitely indicated if there is not enough angle support for an anterior chamber IOL. In suturing a posterior chamber IOL, two limbal scleral flaps, 180° apart, are first prepared so that they can cover the sutures. It is perhaps easiest to use IOLs with holes

## IMPLANTATION OF IOL

**12.18** | Placement of posterior chamber lens (right-handed operation). Note the direction of pronation as the optic is pushed down.

on the haptics that are specially designed for this maneuver. A double-armed Prolene suture is threaded through each hole and the two needles are passed under the iris leaflet until they exit through one of the sclera flaps about 1 mm from the limbus (Fig. 12.19). The ends of the suture are tied and the knot is buried. It is advantageous to use 10-0 Prolene with long needles in performing this maneuver. After the IOL is well positioned, the scleral flap is sutured with 10-O nylon or Prolene. This last step can be performed after the donor corneal button has been sutured in place.

If the haptics of the IOL do not have holes, the suture is tied to the elbow of the haptic, leaving the sutures double-armed (Fig. 12.20). The disadvantage of using an IOL with haptics without holes is that the knots cannot be buried and must be covered with scleral flaps. There is also the risk that the knots may slip off the haptics and lead to dislocation of the IOL.

After the IOL is placed, the pupil is constricted with acetylcholine or carbachol. When a posterior chamber IOL is used, the pupil can also be constricted by gently pulling on the iris towards the pupillary center with tying forceps or a dry cellulose sponge.

PENETRATING
KERATOPLASTY

After placement of a small amount of viscoelastic on the optic of the intraocular lens, the corneal button is sutured as described earlier.

## REMOVAL/EXCHANGE OF IOLs AND PENETRATING KERATOPLASTY

One of the most frequent indications for penetrating keratoplasty is pseudophakic bullous keratopathy, which often must be treated with penetrating keratoplasty and removal or exchange of the intraocular lens. The offending lens is frequently an anterior chamber lens with closed-loop haptics.

The patient is prepared in the usually sterile fashion, and because the eye is pseudophakic, a scleral ring is used.

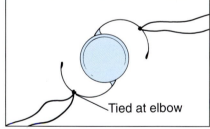

**12.20** | Preparation of posterior chamber IOL without holes for suture. Double-armed 10-0 Prolene sutures are tied at the elbows of the IOL.

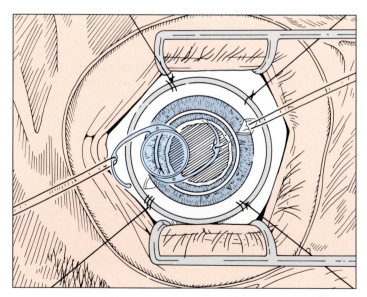

**12.19** | Suturing of the posterior chamber lens. A double-armed 10-0 Prolene suture is threaded through each haptic hole and is passed through the sclera.

Trephination and removal of the host corneal button are carried out. For details of this procedure see the description of penetrating keratoplasty earlier in this chapter.

If the haptics of the anterior chamber lens are not scarred into the iris, the IOL is removed simply by grasping it with tying forceps. However, if one of the haptics is scarred into the iris, the involved haptic is first severed from the rest of the intraocular lens with scissors and gently rotated free with a pair of tying forceps (Fig. 12.21A,B). The assistant can expose the haptic better by grasping the edge of the host cornea with a pair of forceps and retracting the iris at the same time with a dry cellulose sponge. If there is excessive bleeding, cellulose sponges soaked in liquid thrombin can be used. Removal of the haptics must be done gently to prevent iridodialysis.

## REMOVAL OF ANTERIOR CHAMBER LENS

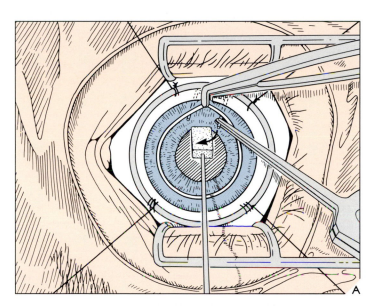

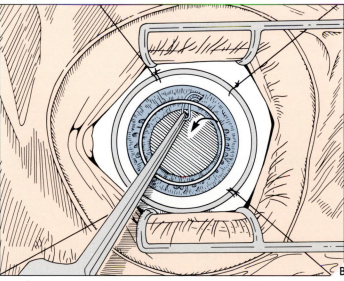

**12.21** | Removal of the anterior chamber lens. *A:* After the haptic is severed from the rest of the IOL, tying forceps grasp the end of the haptic and gently rotate it free (the arrow indicates the direction of rotation, which follows the contour of the haptic). In the meantime, the host corneal edge is grasped with a pair of forceps and a dry cellulose sponge is used to retract the iris. *B:* Removal of a differently shaped haptic. Again, rotation follows the contour of the haptic.

ANTERIOR VITRECTOMY

A central core vitrectomy is performed in an open-sky fashion. A light pipe (in a darkened room) is helpful for visualizing the vitreous strands. The anterior surface of the iris should be free of vitreous, and the presence of vitreous is checked by gently wiping the anterior surface of the iris with a dry cellulose sponge. The iridotomy opening should also be free of vitreous.

IMPLANTATION OF IOL

An anterior chamber intraocular lens can then be placed, or a posterior chamber lens can be sutured in. The pupil is then constricted with acetylcholine or carbachol. Gently pulling on the iris centrally with tying forceps facilitates miosis.

For details of penetrating keratoplasty, see the previous section on this procedure.

## CONJUNCTIVAL (GUNDERSON) FLAP

A conjunctival (Gunderson) flap is usually performed to resolve corneal surface pathology in eyes with limited visual potential or in patients who are not candidates for other surgical interventions (e.g., penetrating keratoplasty).[9,10] Conjunctival flaps can be performed for sterile and nonhealing corneal ulcers, bullous keratopathy, and fungal keratitis. A conjunctival flap is not recommended in cases of active bacterial keratitis until there has been adequate antibiotic therapy.

ANESTHESIA AND PREPARATION

Peribulbar or retrobulbar anesthesia is usually adequate. However, general anesthesia is necessary for children or uncooperative adult patients.

The surgical field is cleaned and draped sterilely. A surgical microscope is set up.

CONJUNCTIVAL PERITOMY

A 360° complete conjunctival peritomy is performed at the limbus with forceps and scissors. Care is taken to avoid creating buttonholes in the conjunctiva.

CORNEAL EPITHELIUM REMOVAL

The corneal epithelium is removed by scraping with the back edge of a scalpel (e.g., 64 Beaver blade). Topical 4% cocaine or absolute alcohol is helpful in loosening the epithelium. The corneal epithelium is completely removed in the area to be covered by the conjunctival flap.

PREPARATION OF FLAP

An incision is made in the superior conjunctiva with scissors, parallel to the superior limbus. The superior conjunctiva is undermined towards the limbus with scissors and forceps. It is preferable to separate Tenon's capsule from the conjunctiva, and the flap should be thin. Care is taken not to buttonhole the conjunctiva. A sufficient amount of conjunctiva is mobilized such that it is not under tension when it covers the cornea. A traction suture (e.g., 6-0 silk suture) placed in the peripheral cornea near the limbus at 12 o'clock helps to provide good exposure for dissection of conjunctiva (Fig. 12.22). Recently, an alternative technique using subconjunctival injections of lidocaine with epinephrine to separate the conjunctiva from Tenon's capsule has been described.[11]

CONJUNCTIVAL FLAP SUTURING

The superior border of the conjunctival flap is sutured to the superior limbus with interrupted absorbable sutures (e.g., 8-0 Vicryl). Depending on the size of the flap, the inferior border of the flap is attached to the cornea or the inferior limbus with sutures (Fig. 12.23A,B). The knots of the sutures are buried. The conjunctival flap should not be under any tension.

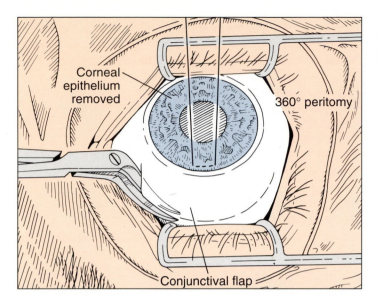

Corneal epithelium removed

360° peritomy

Conjunctival flap

**12.22** | Preparation of the conjunctival flap. With the corneal traction suture anchored at 12 o'clock, a 360° peritomy of conjunctiva is performed at the limbus.

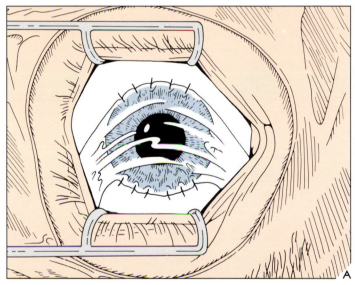

A

**12.23** | Suturing of complete (*A*) or incomplete (*B*) conjunctival flap with 8-0 Vicryl sutures.

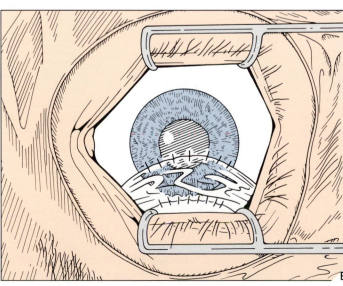

B

POSTOPERATIVE CARE

Immediately after surgery the eye is pressure-patched for 24 hours. An antibiotic/corticosteroid combination ointment is applied 4 times daily for 1 week. With time the conjunctival flap thins, and vision through it may be surprisingly good in some patients.

Alternatively, a vertical bridge flap can be performed by making parallel incisions in the lateral conjunctiva and suturing at the temporal and nasal limbus as described.

## SUPERFICIAL KERATECTOMY

Superficial keratectomy is used to remove lesions on the corneal surface (e.g., superficial vascular membranes and Salzmann's nodular degeneration).

ANESTHESIA AND PREPARATION

Topical anesthesia is usually all that is necessary. However, retrobulbar and peribulbar anesthesia can also be used.

The surgical field is cleaned and sterilely draped, and an operating microscope is set up.

CREATING A CLEAVAGE PLANE

When an elevated corneal lesion is removed (e.g., Salzmann nodular degeneration), a cleavage plane between the lesion and the underlying cornea can be created by pushing the edge of the lesion with a dry cellulose sponge or scraping with the sharp edge of a blade (Fig. 12.24). In cases with superficial vascular membrane, dissection should be begun with a peritomy and carried from the limbus toward the corneal center (Fig. 12.25).

REMOVAL OF LESION

As a cleavage plane is created, the edge of the lesion is held with forceps and can either be peeled off the corneal surface or dissected off with a blade. It is important to remain in the same tissue plane during dissection. After removal of the lesion, the corneal surface can be smoothed with a diamond burr.

POSTOPERATIVE CARE

Immediately after surgery an antibiotic ointment is applied and the eye is patched. The patient is followed closely until the epithelial defect heals.

## LAMELLAR KERATOPLASTY

Lamellar keratoplasty is designed to replace the anterior portion of the host cornea or to reinforce areas of thinning of the host cornea. It is most often used for corneal thinning, anterior stromal scars, and anterior corneal dystrophies, such as Reis–Bückler and granular dystrophies. Lamellar keratoplasty can also be used in cases of anterior infectious keratitis where infection is superficial with well-defined boundaries. The advantage of lamellar keratoplasty is that there is no possibility of endothelial graft rejection, which is a major concern with penetrating keratoplasty.

ANESTHESIA AND PREPARATION

The surgical field is cleaned and draped in a sterile manner. Muscle traction sutures or a scleral supporting ring may be used. It is safer to use the latter in pseudophakic or aphakic eyes, in case of inadvertent perforation of the host corneal bed, which may require conversion to a penetrating keratoplasty. It is advisable to have a donor cornea readily available for penetrating keratoplasty as a precautionary measure.

PREPARATION OF DONOR BUTTON

In cases of deep lamellar keratoplasty where very little host tissue remains, the entire donor button can be used after the donor endothelium is removed. If thinner donor tissue is preferred, it is preferable to use whole donor globes when partial-thickness donor tissue is needed. This requires the globes to be frozen previously or freshly enucleated. The globe is wrapped in gauze for easier handling. A partial-thickness stab incision is made with a blade in the corneal periphery near the limbus, and the anterior portion of the cornea is carefully dissected with a blade using side-to-side motions (Fig. 12.26). It is important to stay in the same lamellar plane during dissection. The donor tissue can be shaped with a trephine or cut with a scissors in a freehand fashion. It is preferable to make the donor tissue slightly thicker and about 0.5 mm larger than the recipient bed.

If part of the host cornea must be removed, trephination with a hand-held or a suction trephine can be done. The dissection is usually made about one half to two thirds of stromal thickness; however, the depth can be varied. A blade is then used to remove the host tissue in a similar fashion as the donor button was prepared (Fig. 12.27). It is important to keep the blade in the same lamellar plane to provide a smooth host bed and to avoid penetrating into the anterior chamber. If the anterior chamber is entered, conversion to penetrating keratoplasty may be necessary. In cases of corneal thinning the host bed does not need to be deepened. The trephination is carried out gen-

## PREPARATION OF HOST CORNEAL BED

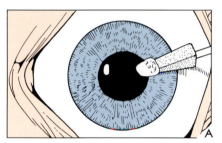
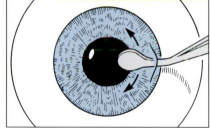

**12.24** | In superficial keratectomy, a cleavage plane is created either by pushing the edge of the lesion with a dry cellulose sponge (*A*) or scraping with the sharp edge of a blade (*B*).

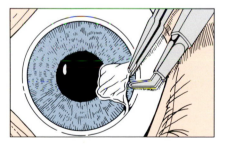
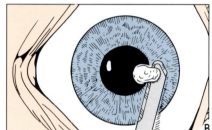

**12.25** | Removal of a superficial vascular membrane requires use of an angled blade.

**12.26** | Dissection of the donor cornea is carried out with a partial-thickness stab incision in the corneal periphery near the limbus and dissection of the anterior portion of the cornea with side-to-side motions (arrows).

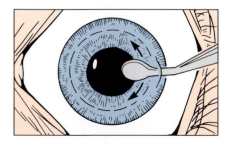

**12.27** | Dissection of the host cornea requires a partial-thickness groove made with a trephine. The blade is moved side to side as in donor cornea dissection.

tly around the area of thinning to provide a solid wound edge for suturing. The host epithelium is first removed in the area where the donor tissue is to be placed, and the host bed should be free of debris before the donor tissue is placed. A limited lamellar dissection (about 1 mm) of host stroma at the wound edge may faciliate suturing of the donor tissue (Fig. 12.28).

### SUTURING OF DONOR TISSUE

The donor tissue is sutured in place in a similar fashion as in penetrating keratoplasty. Cardinal sutures are placed first to ensure an even distribution of tissue. Interrrupted 10-0 nylon sutures are most often used, and because there is no concern about anterior chamber fluid leakage, the sutures do not need to be excessively tight and should be placed with just enough pressure so they can hold the donor tissue in place. The knots of the sutures are buried.

### POSTOPERATIVE CARE

Immediately after surgery, subconjunctival injections of antibiotic and corticosteroids are given and the eye is patched and shielded. As needed, removal of sutures can start about 6 weeks to 2 months after surgery.

# KERATOREFRACTIVE SURGERY

Keratorefractive surgery is intended to correct refractive errors by altering the topography or the configuration of the cornea. Keratorefractive procedures include epikeratophakia, relaxing incisions with or without augmentation sutures, radial keratotomy, keratophakia, keratomileusis, hyperopic keratotomy, and excimer laser. Only the first three will be discussed in detail here.

### EPIKERATOPHAKIA

Epikeratophakia is a surgical procedure to correct refractive error by attaching a lenticule, consisting of donor stromal corneal tissue, on the anterior surface of the host cornea. Epikeratophakia is performed in monocularly aphakic patients and keratoconus patients who are intolerant to contact lenses and have no corneal scarring.[12,13] The lenticule with the proper power is ordered from the manufacturer preoperatively.

Epikeratophakia is not recommended in patients with dry eye, blepharitis, or lagophthalmos. Epikeratophakia should not be performed on children under 1 year of age because of frequent undercorrection in this group of patients.[14,15]

### MARKING THE VISUAL AXIS

It is helpful to make the pupil miotic with topical pilocarpine preoperatively. The patient is asked to fixate on a mark placed in the center of one of the

**12.28** | Suturing of lamellar keratoplasty. Placement of sutures is facilitated by limited peripheral lamellar dissection of the host cornea.

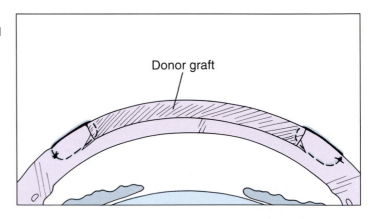

Donor graft

viewing tubes of the microscope, and the surgeon looking monocularly through the same viewing tube marks the corneal epithelium at the mark with a Sinsky hook or a 25-gauge needle.[16] Alternatively, this can also be performed at the slit lamp. Devices (e.g., Aximeter) attachable to the operating microscope can be helpful in locating the visual axis.

## PREPARATION AND ANESTHESIA

The surgical field is cleaned and draped in a sterile manner. General anesthesia or retrobulbar anesthesia with lid block can be used. Muscle traction sutures are useful to stabilize the globe.

## PREPARATION OF HOST CORNEA

After traction sutures through the superior and inferior rectus muscles are anchored, the host cornea is trephined with a Barron twin-blade suction trephine. The trephine is centered on the visual axis. Three quarter turns are made, resulting in two concentric partial-thickness cuts. The depth of the inner circle is 0.3 mm. The central corneal epithelium is removed with the back side of a blade. Topical cocaine 4% is helpful in loosening the epithelium. A partial-thickness strip of corneal tissue between the circular cuts is removed with scissors and forceps (Fig. 12.29). Alternatively, the host cornea can be trephined with a Hessburg–Barron single-blade suction trephine to a depth of about 0.3 mm (three quarter turns) and followed by removal of a 0.5 mm thin strip of corneal tissue from the inner wall of the incision. A limited lamellar dissection, about 1 mm, is performed from the corneal groove towards the limbus with an angled blade (Fig. 12.30).

## SUTURING THE LENTICULE

After the host bed is throughly cleaned and irrigated with balanced salt solution, the lenticule is sutured onto the host cornea with interrupted 10-0 nylon sutures. The suture is initially passed through the peripheral flange of the lenticule, exiting through the side of the flange. The bite in the recipient tissue is passed into the stromal space in the host cornea created by previous

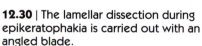

**12.29** | Keratectomy during epikeratophakia. A thin strip of tissue is removed between the double trephine cuts made by a Barron twin-blade suction trephine.

**12.30** | The lamellar dissection during epikeratophakia is carried out with an angled blade.

lamellar dissection (Fig. 12.31). The needle is pushed through the host cornea anterior to the limbal vessels. Four cardinal sutures are first placed, and four additional sutures are placed between the cardinal sutures. After all eight sutures have been placed, the entire flange of the lenticule is pushed into the host cornea (Fig. 12. 32). Eight additional sutures are placed and the knots are buried. Additional sutures are placed if needed. The tension of the sutures should not be excessive, but enough to hold the lenticule in place. The knots are buried.

POSTOPERATIVE CARE

Subconjunctival injections of antibiotics and corticosteroids are given immediately postoperatively. The eye is patched until the lenticule epithelializes. Alternatively, a bandage contact lens can be used. Sutures are removed in about 8 weeks for adults and about 3–4 weeks for children. Epikeratophakia can be repeated if the postoperative refractive error is unacceptable or if there is scarring.

## RELAXING INCISIONS

Relaxing incisions, with or without augmentation sutures, are made to correct postkeratoplasty astigmatism.[17,18] The amount of astigmatism that can be corrected with relaxing incisions alone is about 8.50 diopters or less. If greater correction is desired, additional augmentation (compression) sutures are necessary.[17]

PREOPERATIVE PREPARATION

Careful refraction and keratometric readings are performed. Computerized corneal topography may also be useful. Relaxing incisions are usually made under topical anesthesia at the slit lamp, although the surgical microscope can also be used.

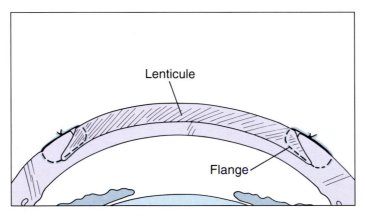

12.31 | Suture placement in epikeratiphakia.

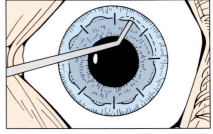

12.32 | After all eight sutures have been placed, the entire flange of the lenticule is pushed into the intrastromal space created by previous lamellar dissection.

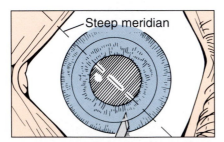

12.33 | Relaxing incisions. A steel blade is used, bevel up, to cut into the surgical wound of penetrating keratoplasty.

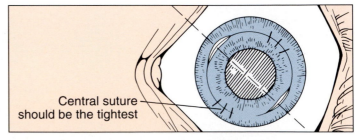

12.34 | Compresion sutures are placed along the meridian 90° from the steep meridian. In all, six sutures are placed, three on each side.

Two incisions are made in the steep meridian, 180° apart, at the surgical wound of the keratoplasty about one half to two thirds depth. The incisions are extended about one clock hour to each side of the steep meridian (Fig. 12.33). Steel blades are ordinarily used because they give the surgeon better control than diamond blades, which are too sharp for this procedure and can easily lead to perforation. If the cornea is perforated during the procedure and the anterior chamber becomes shallow, interrupted sutures are placed to seal the perforation.

   If necessary, augmentation (compression) sutures are placed. A surgical microscope and an operating room setup are necessary in such cases. The augmentation sutures are placed along the meridian 90° from the steep meridian. Six sutures are placed, three on each side. The sutures are made tight such that they create a new steep meridian 90° to the previous one. Usually the side sutures are placed first and the central suture is placed in last so that it is the tightest suture and causes the greatest steepening at the desired meridian (Fig. 12.34).

MAKING THE INCISIONS

A topical antibiotic eyedrop is placed immediately postoperatively. Topical corticosteroids are used 3 to 4 times daily to reduce postoperative inflammation and to delay healing of the relaxing incisions. If the patient had augmentation sutures, they can be removed selectively 1 week after the initial surgery, starting with the ones along the steepest meridian.

POSTOPERATIVE CARE

Radial keratotomy (RK) is a surgical procedure in which the surgeon reduces myopia by making deep radial cuts into the cornea, which flattens the central cornea. The effect of RK is dependent on the length and number of the cuts and the age of the patient. More cuts and longer cuts result in more flattening of the central cornea. Older corneas respond more dramatically to RK than younger ones, (i.e., with same amount of surgery, older corneas flatten more than younger ones). RK should be performed on healthy corneas, the patient should be at least 18 years of age, and the patient's refraction should be stable for the past 18 months.

   Contraindications for RK include collagen–vascular or other autoimmune disorders (e.g., rheumatoid arthritis), corneal scarring, corneal degenerations (e.g., keratoconus, Terrien's, and pellucid), and history of *Herpes simplex* or *Herpes zoster* keratitis. It is probably best not to perform RK on patients with diabetes mellitus, because some diabetics have unstable refractions due to poorly controlled blood glucose levels, and corneal scars from RK may interfere with retinal photocoagulation for diabetic retinopathy.

RADIAL
KERATOTOMY

A detailed medical and occupational history must be taken and careful eye examination must be performed, including a cycloplegic refraction, which is important to prevent overcorrection (i.e., making the patient hyperopic postoperatively). The patient must be made aware that RK may be a disqualification for certain occupations (e.g., military pilot). It is imperative to obtain the patient's exact age; some patients may not readily admit to their correct ages.

PREOPERATIVE
EVALUATION

Depending on the surgeon's techniques and preference, RK can be performed under topical, peribulbar, or retrobulbar anesthesia. In general, patients undergoing RK are cooperative enough such that only topical anesthesia is needed.

   The eye is prepared and draped in a sterile fashion. Topical pilocarpine is used to constrict the pupil, which aids the surgeon in determining the

ANESTHESIA
AND PREPARATION

visual axis. Muscle traction sutures or a scleral support ring are not used. The visual axis is marked (see the section on epikeratophakia).

### MEASURING CENTRAL CORNEAL THICKNESS

The central corneal thickness is measured with an ultrasound pachymeter; this can also be performed preoperatively. We recommend that corneal thickness be measured at the time of surgery, because corneal thickness may vary slightly from time to time. The diamond blade is set according to the thinnest corneal thickness and the surgeon's method. In most cases, the thinnest part of the cornea is located just temporal (about 1.5 mm) to the corneal center.[19] The probe of the pachymeter is held perpendicular to the corneal surface, and consistent readings must be obtained. The blade is usually set at 100% of the pachymetry reading or slightly deeper. Alternatively, some surgeons take pachymetry readings at the edge of the central clear zone (where the radial cuts end centrally) and use the average or the lowest reading as a guide to set the blade.[20] Owing to compression of tissue by the diamond blade, the depth of the cuts is about 90% of the central stromal thickness.

### CHECKING THE NOMOGRAM

The number of radial cuts and the length of cuts to be made are based on nomograms derived either from the surgeon's past results or from results of other surgeons using similar techniques.

### MARKING THE CENTRAL CLEAR ZONE

The radial cuts made in RK are not extended into the optical center of the cornea, so they do not interfere with vision. The area of the clear zone is dependent on the length of the cuts. The longer the cuts, the smaller the central clear zone, and vice versa. A circular marker is used to push on the corneal surface, leaving an epithelial impression. The marker should be centered on the epithelial mark (indicating the visual axis) made previously (Fig. 12.35).

### THE RADIAL CUTS

A radial marker is used to create impressions on the corneal epithelium (Fig. 12.36). The marker is centered on the central epithelial mark. The number of cuts is usually between four and eight at one sitting. In most cases, the maximal number of radial cuts that can be made in a cornea is 16.

The cuts can be made from the limbus towards the corneal center, or vice versa, although recent evidence suggests that the former method may be more effective.[21] The diamond blade is inserted up to the foot plates about 0.5 mm from the limbal vessels and is then directed carefully and deliberately along the radial mark up to the edge of the central clear zone. Conjunctival forceps may be helpful in stabilizing the globe and should be used in patients who have difficulty fixating. The nasal cuts are made first, followed by temporal cuts (Fig. 12.37A–C). Because the temporal cornea is thinner

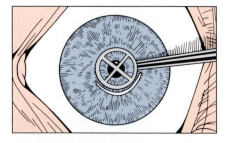

**12.35** | To mark the central optical zone in RK a marker is centered on the visual axis.

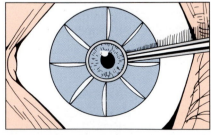

**12.36** | The radial epithelial impressions are marked.

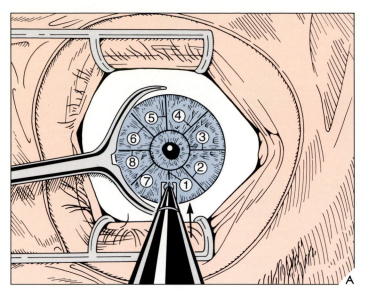

**12.37** | *A*: Nasal cuts in RK. The numbers indicate the sequence of the cuts (the temporal cut is performed last). In the "Russian" technique, the blade is moved from the limbus toward the corneal center (arrow). *B*: Note how the blade is pushed up to the footplates. *C*: Temporal cuts in RK.

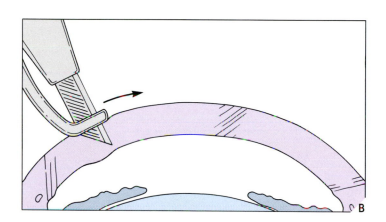

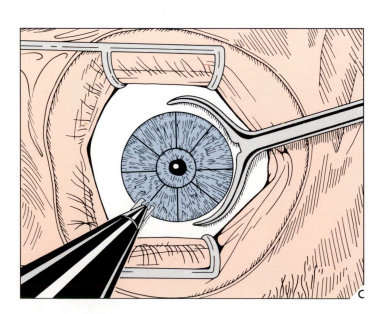

than the nasal portion, perforations are most likely to occur in the temporal cornea, and it is preferable to encounter perforation at the end of the procedure. The corneal surface should be kept dry so that leakage of the anterior chamber can be easily seen. The surgeon must be vigilant in searching for leakage of aqueous humor, which would indicate that corneal perforation has occurred, and the blade must be immediately withdrawn (Fig. 12.38). If the anterior chamber is well maintained, a small perforation is treated with pressure patching only. However, sutures are required if the anterior chamber is shallow and the perforation is large.

POSTOPERATIVE CARE    The eye is immediately patched after surgery, and an antibiotic/steroid combination eye drop is started the following day for 1 week. The patient will experience fluctuations in vision which typically subside within 6 weeks after surgery. Additional surgery (e.g., deepening of previous cuts or making additional cuts) may be necessary if the eye is undercorrected. According to the Prospective Evaluation of Radial Keratotomy (PERK) study, 76% of patients achieve vision of 20/40 or better without correction and 55% of patients have

**12.38** | Perforation of the cornea during RK.

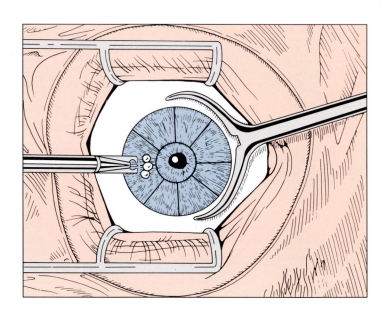

**12.39** | Keratophakia. The donor lenticule is interposed between the host's anterior and posterior stroma.

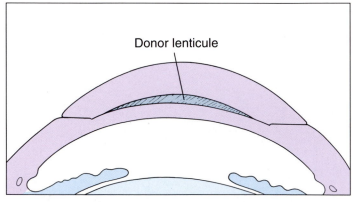

Donor lenticule

refractive errors between +l and -1 diopter.[22] Bacterial keratitis, fluctuation of vision, glare, and overcorrection are some of the risks associated with RK.

## KERATOPHAKIA

This procedure is designed to steepen the anterior corneal curvature by placing a lenticule (consisting of donor cornea) into the host cornea. This procedure requires removal of anterior stroma of the host cornea, placing the donor lenticule on the host bed, and reattaching the anterior host stromal tissue. Because of the complex instrumentation required for this procedure and long recovery time, keratophakia is not frequently performed (Fig. 12.39).

## KERATOMILEUSIS

Keratomileusis is designed to steepen or flatten the anterior corneal curvature, but unlike keratophakia, no donor lenticule is used in this procedure. The anterior stromal tissue is removed and reshaped to a steeper or flatter configuration on a cryolathe and then reattached to the host bed. Like keratophakia, keratomileusis is now infrequently performed because of the complexity of instrumentation (Fig. 12.40).

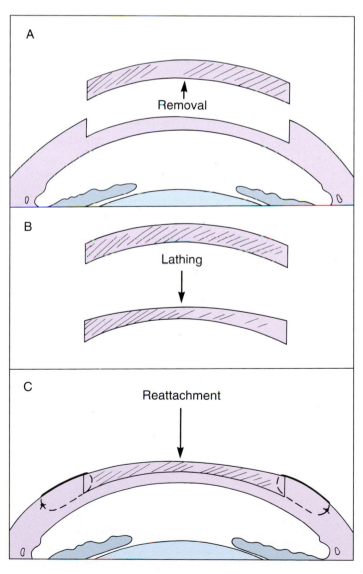

**12.40** | Keratomileusis for correction of myopia. The anterior corneal stroma is removed (*A*), lathed (*B*), and sutured back into place (*C*) Note: Curvature of cornea is made flatter.

### HYPEROPIC KERATOTOMY

Hyperopic keratotomy (HK) is designed to correct hyperopia by steepening the central corneal curvature, which is accomplished by making cuts, usually in the shape of a hexagon, in the corneal midperiphery (Fig. 12.41). The greatest amount of hyperopia that can be corrected with HK is about 4 diopters. The smaller the hexagon, the greater the effect of HK.[19] The indications and contraindications for HK are similar to those of RK. Although HK is not yet as popular as RK, it is presently under study. Instability of the central cornea and induced postoperative astigmatism are some of the problems associated with HK. The holmium-YAG laser shows early promise in the treatment of hyperopia.

### EXCIMER LASER

The excimer laser emits ultraviolet radiation that is produced by excitation of argon fluoride gas. The excimer laser is useful in keratorefractive surgery because of its capability to reshape anterior corneal curvature by ablating corneal tissue. It's usefulness in the ablation of superficial corneal scars has been demonstrated. This device is presently under intense study for its application in correction of myopia. The criteria for patient selection are similar to those of radial keratotomy.

Preoperatively, the patient is sedated, and the central corneal epithelium is removed before treatment. The treatment time is less than 30 seconds. The healing period after excimer laser treatment is 3–6 months, and central subepithelial corneal haze develops in almost all of the eyes postoperatively. Topical corticosteroids are helpful in treating the postoperative corneal haze and are also used to modulate the wound healing and postoperative refraction. With proper postoperative compliance, the preliminary results of excimer laser in the treatment of myopia showed that postoperative refractive errors in 90% of eyes were between +1.00 diopter and -1.00 diopter after 9 months.[23]

## KERATOEPITHELIOPLASTY

Keratoepithelioplasty is a surgical technique designed to replace the epithelium of the ocular surface in patients with bilateral ocular surface disease (e.g., bilateral chemical burns).[24]

### DONOR LENTICULE PREPARATION

A whole globe, enucleated shortly after death and refrigerated for only few hours, is used. The globe is held with gauze and lenticules are shaved off the cornea with a blade. The lenticules consist of the epithelium and a very thin underlying stroma. Multiple lenticules can be obtained from each globe (Fig. 12.42). It is preferable to obtain lenticules near the limbus so that donor epithelial stem cells are included.

### CONJUNCTIVAL RESECTION OF THE RECIPIENT EYE

A complete conjunctival peritomy is performed 5 mm from the limbus. The remnant ring of conjunctival tissue is dissected towards the limbus, and the dissection is carried onto the cornea to include scars and vascular tissues on

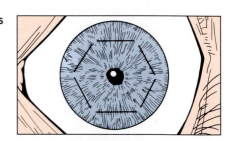

**12.41** | Hyperopic keratotomy. The cuts usually are in the shape of a hexagon.

the cornea. A superficial keratectomy may be necessary. The entire host corneal epithelium is removed.

Four donor lenticules are sutured onto the host sclera, abutting the limbus, with 10-0 nylon sutures (Fig. 12.43). After the knots are buried, a soft bandage contact lens is placed to cover the host cornea to prevent the eyelid from displacing the lenticules.

Immediately after surgery, topical antibiotic and cycloplegic eyedrops are administered. A topical steroid is used to decrease postoperative inflammation and also to prevent epithelial graft rejection. The host cornea usually becomes epithelialized in about one week.

Preoperatively, the most common complication of corneal surgery is retrobulbar (orbital) hemorrhage, which can occur with retrobulbar injection of anesthetics. The signs of retrobulbar hemorrhage include progressive proptosis, bloody chemosis, and elevated intraocular pressure (IOP). Once retrobulbar hemorrhage is recognized, pressure should be placed over the eye to tamponade the source of orbital bleeding. The IOP should be checked either with Schiotz tonometer or with digital palpation. If there is excessive IOP elevation, temporal canthotomy or cantholysis may be performed to relieve it as well as the orbital pressure. Once the orbital hemorrhage is under control, the patient should be followed carefully for decreased color and Snellen visual acuity and elevated IOP, which may require treatment (e.g., topical

## SUTURING OF DONOR LENTICULES

## POSTOPERATIVE CARE

# COMPLICATIONS OF CORNEAL SURGERY
## PREOPERATIVE COMPLICATIONS

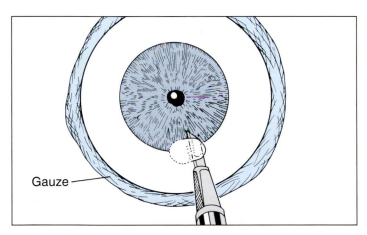

Gauze

**12.42** | Preparation of donor lenticule in keratoepithelioplasty.

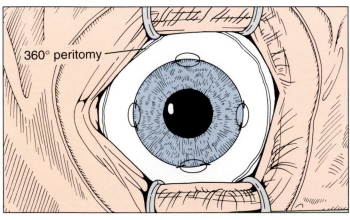

360° peritomy

**12.43** | Keratoepithelioplasty with lenticules in place. The sutures holding the lenticules down are 10-0 nylon.

beta-blockers or oral carbonic anhydrase inhibitors). In mild cases of retrobulbar hemorrhage it may be possible to continue with surgery after the retrobulbar hemorrhage is under control.

INTRAOPERATIVE

Although choroidal hemorrhage occurs rarely, it can be a devastating complication in cases in which the globe is open. Risk factors include glaucoma, increased axial length, elevated IOP, generalized atherosclerosis, and elevated intraoperative pulse.[25] Signs of choroidal hemorrhage include sudden IOP increase, loss of red reflex with elevation of the choroid, and, in severe cases, extrusion of intraocular contents. The immediate treatment for choroidal hemorrhage demands expeditious wound suturing. Silk sutures are preferable because they can be easily handled and made into tight knots. The choroidal hemorrhage can be drained immediately after closure of the wound or a few days later, when the clots have undergone autolysis. In some cases the choroidal hemorrhage may resolve spontaneously. Patients with choroidal hemorrhage should be followed closely for elevated IOP and retinal detachment.

POSTOPERATIVE

After anterior segment surgery some patients may develop uveitis, glaucoma, or endophthalmitis. Uveitis and glaucoma usually respond to medical regimen, whereas endophthalmitis often requires diagnostic vitrectomy and invitreal injection of antibiotics.

In cases of penetrating keratoplasty patients may develop corneal graft rejection involving the epithelium, stroma, or endothelium.[26] Epithelial rejection typically presents as an elevated epithelial line that usually responds to a short course of topical corticosteroids. Subepithelial infiltrates are also signs of corneal graft rejection, and they mimic subepithelial infiltrates that occur with adenovirus keratoconjunctivitis. Subepithelial infiltrates in corneal graft rejection also respond to a short course of topical corticosteroids. Endothelial rejection presents as stromal thickening with keratic precipitates. These precipitates may be diffuse or arranged linearly, in which case they are called Khodadoust line. Endothelial rejection is serious because, if left untreated, it may lead to graft failure. Treatment of endothelial corneal graft rejection involves frequent administration of topical corticosteroids and cycloplegics. In severe cases oral and intravenous corticosteroids are sometimes also recommended.

Wound healing is variable, and suture removal is dependent on numerous factors including astigmatism, vascularization, suture looseness, and so on. Postoperative high astigmatism is dealt with as discussed earlier. Persistent epithelial defects may be treated with lubrication, patching, soft contact lenses, or temporary tarsorrhaphy.

## CONCLUSION

We hope that this chapter will serve as a useful synopsis of corneal surgery, which is in rapid evolution. New techniques and instrumentations are constantly being developed. Anterior segment surgeons should continue to seek improvements in their surgical skills to provide better patient care.

# 13

# THE SCLERA
## John W. Chandler

The sclera, which is a largely avascular tissue contiguous with the cornea, is composed of collagen fibers oriented generally parallel with the surface of the globe but with many fibers more randomly arrayed, creating a dense, tough, opaque structure. The collagen fibers are primarily type I, with III, IV, V, and VI also present.[1] The collagen fibers are surrounded predominantly by dermatan sulfate glycosaminoglycan ground substance. The sclera is approximately 1 mm thick posteriorly, 0.6 mm thick at the equator, and 0.3 mm behind the muscle insertions.[2] Together, the sclera and cornea provide the tough structural elements of the eye, with five-sixths of the outer coat being the sclera. Although it is less well studied than the cornea, the sclera is not an inert tissue. Perforations through the sclera allow the passage of blood vessels, uveal tissue, and nerves, including the optic nerve, and are sites at which a number of abnormal conditions can occur (e.g., staphyloma, external scleral extension of a choroidal melanoma, and sympathetic ophthalmia after evisceration). Although its relative avascularity, as well as the less regular array of collagen fibers than that seen in the cornea, account for the white color of the sclera, the sclera can become discolored in certain conditions (Fig. 13.1).

## EMBRYOLOGY, ANATOMY, AND PHYSIOLOGY

The cranial neural crest contributes most of the ectomesenchyme elements of the eye and adnexa, including the sclera. During embryogenesis, the cellular mass of the neural crest is located on each side of the invaginating neural folds. The sclera is formed from anterior to posterior by neural crest cells which initially are located near the future limbus.[3] The process reaches the posterior pole by 12 gestational weeks, and the sclera is well differentiated by 20 weeks.[4]

The relationship of the sclera and other adjacent structures is shown in Figure 13.2. Sclera is divided into three layers: the episclera, the stroma, and the lamina fusca. The episclera is a loose arrangement of collagen, fibroblasts, glycosaminoglycans, and some melanocytes. It lies in close proximity to subconjunctival tissues, rectus muscle insertions, and Tenon's capsule. Blood vessels derived from the anterior and posterior ciliary arteries supply the episclera. The stroma is composed of collagen lamellae and glycosaminoglycans, with occasional scleral fibroblasts. The lamina fusca is closely related to the uveal tract and is composed of loose collagen lamellae as well as cells from the uvea, including melanocytes. Blood vessels and nerves penetrate through the sclera. In the ciliary body region, small pigmented spots are sometimes seen that represent loops of the long posterior ciliary nerve (intrascleral nerve loop of Axenfeld) (Fig. 13.3). It is important to distinguish these from nevi, foreign bodies, and tumors. The tissue appears inert and largely avascular. However, scleral fibroblasts can pro-

## Figure 13.1. Discolorations of the Sclera and Associated Findings and Diseases

| COLOR | CONDITIONS |
|---|---|
| Blue | Osteogenesis imperfecta |
| Yellow | Elevated bilirubin or hemolysis |
| Yellow to dark brown (triangular deposit) | Ochronosis (alkaptonuria) |
| Dark brown to black | Melanocytoma, extensions of intraocular melanoma |
| Focal blue-gray | Anterior scleral staphyloma, scleral dellen |
| Focal slate gray to black | Nerve loop of Axenfeld |
| Slate gray to brown anterior to horizontal recti | Scleral plaques |
| Brown (especially at limbus) | Acquired melanosis |
| Silver–gray | Melanosis oculi, nevus of Ota, congenital melanosis |

**13.2** | Anatomy of the sclera. (From Hunter PA, Watson PG: Allergic eye diseases: Episcleritis and scleritis, in Spalton DJ, Hitchings RA, Hunter PA (eds): *Atlas of Clinical Ophthalmology*. London: Gower Medical Publishing, 1984, 5.16.)

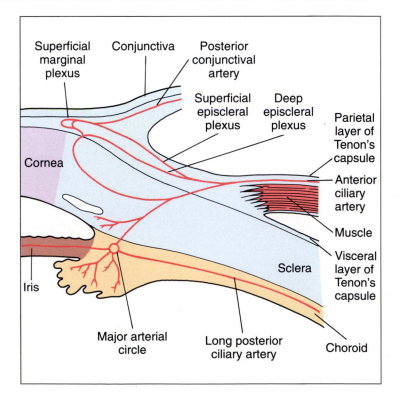

duce functional components involved in the classic pathway of allograft rejection,[5] can express class I HLA antigens on their surfaces, and can respond to cytokines such as gamma-interferon by increasing class I and initiating class II HLA antigen expression. These observations suggest that the sclera is a dynamic tissue. Although it is structurally tough, water-soluble materials (e.g., antibiotics or corticosteroids) readily pass through it to the interior of the eye, and it is probable that there is also fluid outflow from the interior of the eye through the sclera.

The sclera is difficult to examine in detail because of the covering of conjunctival and episcleral tissue anteriorly and lack of visualization throughout most of its extent. The slit lamp is useful for visualizing the anterior portion unless conjunctival edema, blood, or both obscure the view. Transillumination can also be used to determine the integrity of the anterior sclera. Computed tomography and magnetic resonance imaging are useful in examining the more posterior aspects of the sclera.

The sclera is a participant in a variety of conditions that, among other abnormalities, cause changes in its thickness (Fig. 13.4).

Congenital anomalies of the sclera are uncommon. Scleral cysts have been described and are usually seen located at the limbus in children. They may occur in conjunction with conjunctival epithelial inclusions or as a portion of other choristomas (e.g., osseous choristomas of the sclera) (Fig. 13.5). A more severe and rare anomaly that is associated with lethal anomalies in multiple other organs is partial (synophthalmia) or total (cyclopia) union of the elements of the two eyes into one.[6] In this condition the brain is rudimentary and contains mainly midline abnormalities. The anomaly may be associated with a chromosomal defect, most commonly trisomy 13. Most affected infants are stillborn or die soon after birth.

Microphthalmos (an eye less than 15 mm in greatest dimension at birth) (Fig. 13.6) may occur with a number of ocular abnormalities, including failure of proper closure of the fetal fissure, which causes colobomas (Fig. 13.7) and, in some patients, a cystic out-pouching of posterior inferior sclera (microphthalmos with cyst). In other situations the eye seems otherwise normal, except for its smaller size and thickened sclera (nanophthalmos).[7] Patients with nanophthalmos are prone to develop angle-closure glaucoma as well as uveal effusion, especially after ocular surgery. Uveal effusion occurs because of thickened sclera which inhibits fluid transport out of the eye through the sclera and/or obstruction of venous outflow by compression of the vortex veins leading to fluid transudation within the eye. The creation of surgical windows in the sclera, with or without unroofing of the vortex veins, appears to ameliorate greatly this condition.[7]

## DIAGNOSTIC TECHNIQUES

## DISEASES AFFECTING THE SCLERA

### CONGENITAL ABNORMALITIES AND CHANGES IN SCLERAL THICKNESS

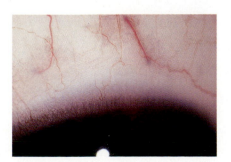

**13.3** | Nerve loop of Axenfeld. Note the pigmentation where the nerve loops and vessels penetrate the sclera. Fine silvery surrounding scleral pigmentation can also be seen in this patient.

## Figure 13.4. Embryologic Abnormalities and Disorders Affecting Scleral Thickness

| **EMBRYOLOGIC ABNORMALITIES** | **THICKNESS DISORDERS** |
|---|---|
| Cyclopia–synophthalmia (often trisomy 13) | Thin sclera |
| |    Axial myopia |
| Microphthalmos |    Keratoglobus |
| Scleral cysts |    Osteogenesis imperfecta |
| | |
| | Thick sclera |
| |    Nanophthalmos |
| |    Atrophy of eye (phthisis bulbi) |

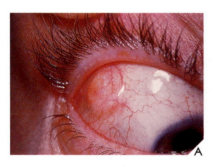 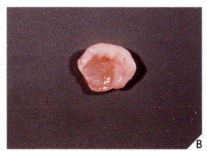 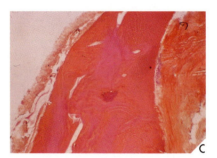

**13.5** | Episcleral osseous choristoma. *A:* Clinical appearance. *B:* Excised lesion. *C:* Histopathology. (Courtesy of Dr. H. Saul Sugar.)

**13.6** | Microphthalmia. (From Kirkness CM: *Ophthalmology.* London: Gower Medical Publishing, 1985, 42.)

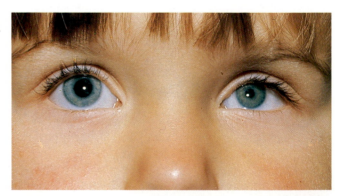

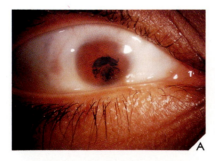 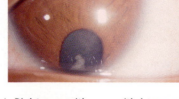 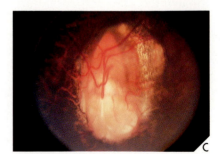

**13.7** | Colobomatous microphthalmos. *A:* Right eye with small cornea and globe and iris coloboma. *B:* Left eye with larger cornea and globe and iris coloboma. *C:* Disc coloboma in eye shown in *B.*

Axial myopia with scleral thinning and elongation of the eye occurs in various degrees and is common. Usually the elongation ceases at the time the general body-growth spurt ceases. In some, the axial myopia progresses and significant scleral thinning, sometimes with equatorial or peripapillary staphyloma, occurs. A continuum in the spectrum of keratoconus may occur so that all the cornea and sclera (keratoglobus) are significantly thinned. The sclera is also thinned and allows the choroidal color to be visualized (blue sclera) in the systemic condition called osteogenesis imperfecta. Recent observations in osteogenesis imperfecta, however, suggest that more uniform size and narrower collagen fibers account for the increased scleral translucency that yields the blue color.[8] Two major forms exist. One is an autosomal recessive form which is obvious at birth and is characterized by several other findings including brittle bones, otosclerotic deafness, dental abnormalities, thin skin, capillary fragility, and joint hyperextendibility. This is usually fatal in early life. Milder forms, transmitted as an autosomal dominant trait with variable penetrance, do not become manifest until early childhood.

Changes in scleral thickness also can occur at later ages in life. Scleral thinning may be noted after inflammatory reactions, such as scleromalacia perforans or contact hypersensitivity following the subconjunctival injection of drugs. In diffuse degeneration of an eye, which may stem from a variety of causes as part of the typical findings in atrophy of the eye or phthisis bulbi (Fig. 13.8), an increase in scleral thickness can also occur. Senile scleral plaques are areas of hyalinization over the insertions of the horizontal rectus muscles and are seen in later life. This is a normal finding that is sometimes confused with postinflammatory scleral thinning or scleral tumor.

Scleral pigmentations are commonly seen as silvery patches or more diffuse blue gray areas as in melanosis oculi. Dendritic melanocytes are present in the superficial (Figs 13.9 and 13.10) sclera or surrounding the exits from the interior of the eye through the sclera.

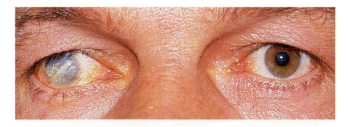

**13.8** | Phthisis bulbi. (From Kirkness CM: *Ophthalmology.* London: Gower Medical Publishing, 1985, 43.)

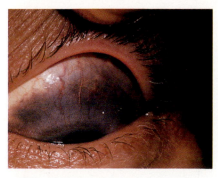

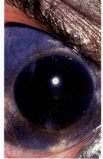

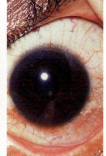

**13.9** | Melanosis oculi. Note denser pigmentation than that seen in Fig. 13.3.

**13.10** | Nevus of Ota. Involved side has increased pigmentation of eyelid skin, sclera, and iris.

## INFLAMMATION OF THE SCLERA

Scleral inflammations are clinically diverse, have varied implications, and must be promptly recognized and treated. Episcleritis and scleritis are rather common, and accurate diagnosis is important to ensure correct treatment and to ascertain the likelihood of associated systemic diseases.[9] The depth of involvement distinguishes episcleritis with inflammation restricted to episcleral structures from involvement that includes scleral inflammation (scleritis). Watson[9] has developed a clinical classification of these inflammations that uses the slit-lamp examination findings (Fig. 13.11). Because of tissue destruction and the association of scleritis with significant systemic diseases, it is mandatory to distinguish pure episcleritis from scleritis. In addition, the treatments for episcleritis and scleritis are vastly different. The characteristics of the three layers of blood vessels on the surface of the sclera and the presence or absence of scleral edema give important diagnostic clues (Fig. 13.12).

### EPISCLERITIS

Both nodular and diffuse types of episcleritis are seen in Figure 13.13. Diagnosis can be aided by the ready blanching of episcleral vessels after application of 10% phenylephrine, whereas in deeper scleritis the vessels fail to blanch. In addition, use of the red-free green light at the slit-lamp examination enhances contrast between vessels and surrounding tissues, making localization of vascular dilatation easier. Episcleritis, although it may be painful, is usually self limited (2–6 weeks) and usually responds to vasoconstrictors or can be left untreated. In some cases, topical mild corticosteroids or oral or topical nonsteroidal anti-inflammatory drugs are helpful. Pure episcleritis is not typically an invariable sign of an underlying systemic disease, although *Herpes zoster*, gout, rosacea, syphilis, and collagen vascular disease have been found in a minority of cases.

### SCLERITIS

Scleritis may be manifest in a number of different patterns (Fig. 13.14) and can be associated with a variety of infectious and noninfectious conditions (Fig. 13.15). Life-threatening systemic disease may be heralded by scleritis, and therefore careful evaluation of these patients is mandatory. Scleritis is usually more gradual in onset, involves more severe and "deeper" pain, and is profoundly more important in its systemic implications than is episcleritis. Deep scleral inflammation and edema are present and deep vascular dilatation usually persists after the instillation of 10% phenylephrine. Tenderness

### Figure 13.11. Classification of Episcleritis and Scleritis*

| **EPISCLERITIS** | **SCLERITIS** |
|---|---|
| Simple | Anterior |
| Nodular |    Diffuse |
| |    Nodular |
| |    Necrotizing |
| |       With inflammation |
| |       Without inflammation |
| |         (scleromalacia |
| |         perforans) |
| | Posterior |

*Adapted from Watson PG: The diagnosis and management of scleritis. *Ophthalmology 1980;87:716–720.*

over the involved area may be extreme. Watson's classification[10] (see Fig. 13.11) is useful in approaching these patients. Anterior scleritis involves the readily visible sclera and is classified clinically into diffuse, nodular, and necrotizing forms. Diffuse anterior scleritis is the least severe although the most frequent. Nodular scleritis presents with more focal scleral thickening and greater tenderness. Necrotizing scleritis may present with severe inflammation and pain or, in the scleromalacia perforans form, may present with

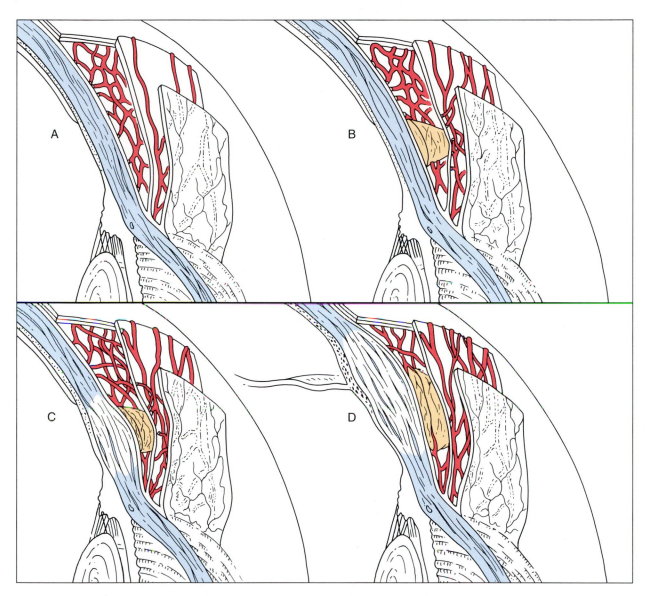

**13.12** | *A:* Diagram of a transected eye. Three vascular layers cover the anterior segment, the conjunctival vessels, the superficial episcleral vessels within Tenon's capsule, and the deep crisscrossing vessels in the episclera closely adherent to sclera itself. *B:* Episcleritis. Maximal congestion is within the superficial episcleral vascular plexus. Tenon's capsule and the episclera are infiltrated with inflammatory cells but the sclera is not involved and is not swollen. *C:* Anterior scleritis. Maximal congestion is in the deep vascular plexus adjacent to the sclera, which is swollen. There is always some accompanying episcleritis but this should be ignored in trying to make the diagnosis. Vessels of superficial episcleral plexus are often distorted and new vessels may form. *D:* Posterior scleritis. When inflammation in the sclera progresses behind the equator, inflammation induces an exudative retinal detachment and a subretinal mass can be seen. If inflammation extends outward, proptosis and extraocular muscle limitation are induced. (Adapted from Watson PG: The diagnosis and management of scleritis. *Ophthalmology 1980;87:716–720.*)

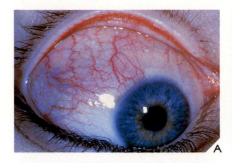
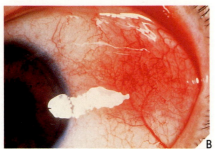

**13.13** | Episcleritis. *A:* Diffuse. *B:* Nodular.

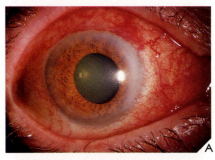
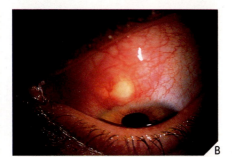

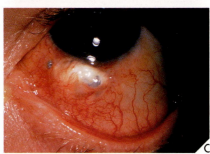
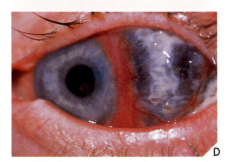

**13.14** | Scleritis. *A:* Diffuse. *B:* Nodular. *C:* Necrotizing. *D:* Scleromalacia perforans.

## Figure 13.15. Systemic Diseases and Infections Associated with Scleritis

| | |
|---|---|
| Rheumatoid arthritis | Gout |
| Wegener's granulomatosis | *Pseudomonas* |
| Systemic lupus erythematosis | *Acanthamoeba* |
| Periarteritis nodosum | Tuberculosis |
| Relapsing polychondritis | Syphilis |
| Ankylosing spondylitis | *Herpes zoster* |
| Crohn's disease | *Herpes simplex* |

## Figure 13.16. Findings Associated with Posterior Scleritis

| | |
|---|---|
| Proptosis | Papilledema |
| Exudative retinal detachment | Thickened sclera (ultrasonography |
| Motility disorders | or CT scan) |
| Macular edema | |

scleral necrosis with minimal inflammation. Posterior scleritis may present with exudative retinal detachment and other retinal findings, as well as proptosis and orbital pain[11] (Fig. 13.16). Because of these associated systemic conditions, patients with scleritis should have a complete physical examination and a diagnostic laboratory work-up (Fig. 13.17). Similarly, treatment is more aggressive for scleritis (Fig. 13.18). Subconjunctival corticosteroids should not be used. In cases of infectious scleritis, it may be necessary to supplement topical antibiotics with systemic antibiotics. Subconjunctival antibiotics may be contraindicated because of the danger of perforation. It is not unusual for both the sclera and cornea to be involved (Fig. 13.19).

Posterior scleritis is sometimes overlooked because of the number and degree of intraocular findings (Fig. 13.20). In this condition, the intraocular abnormalities (see Fig. 13.16) and motility disorders give false leads and correct diagnosis is often delayed. A computed tomographic scan (Fig. 13.21) or ultrasonography can be diagnostic.

Rheumatoid arthritis is the most common systemic condition associated with scleritis. Although the scleritis may take any form, the most characteristic is scleromalacia perforans (Fig. 13.22). Wegener's granulomatosis is a disorder characterized by the presence of necrotizing granulomatous vasculitis. Pulmonary, paranasal sinus, and kidney involvement are common, and a significant number of patients also have ocular involvement. Peripheral keratitis and necrotizing scleritis are the most common manifestations (Fig. 13.23). The antineutrophil cytoplasmic antibody (ANCA) is usually elevated in the sera of these patients and this can be used to monitor response of the disease to treatment.[12] The collagen vascular diseases and Crohn's disease may cause similar corneal and scleral changes (Figs. 13.19 and 13.24). Infectious diseases involving the cornea may spread to the sclera, or the sclera may itself become infected after trauma or surgery, or scleritis may occur after surgery in patients with underlying systemic disease or for unknown cause (Fig. 13.25). Bacterial, protozoal, and viral infections from the cornea can extend into the sclera, most commonly *Pseudomonas*, Acanthamoeba, and the *Herpes* viruses (Fig. 13.26). Syphilis can also cause gummatous necrosis of the sclera or less focal scleral inflammation (Fig. 13.27).

## SCLERAL TRAUMA

Both sharp and blunt trauma can disrupt the sclera. Chemical injuries may also involve the sclera. At the time of blunt injury, the sclera can rupture at the site of injury, at the equator, beneath the insertions of the rectus muscles or at the optic nerve. The extent of any break in the sclera must be visualized by surgical exploration if necessary, because scleral ruptures are often larger

### Figure 13.17. Laboratory Work-up for a Patient with Scleritis

| | |
|---|---|
| Sedimentation rate | Sinus x-ray |
| WBC with differential | In posterior scleritis |
| Urinalysis |   Ultrasonography |
| VDRL/FTA-ABS |   CT scan (with infusion) |
| Rheumatoid factor |   Antineutrophil cytoplasmic |
| Antinuclear antibody |     antibody (ANCA) |
| PPD |   Scrapings and cultures |
| Chest x-ray |     when indicated |

## Figure 13.18. Treatment of Scleritis Based on Type of Clinical Involvement and Coexisting Conditions

**NON-NECROTIZING SCLERITIS**
1% prednisolone acetate hourly
Avoid subconjunctival steroids
Nonsteroidal antiinflammatory
   drugs, oral
Systemic prednisone 60–100
   mg/day for 5 days, then taper

**NECROTIZING**
Systemic prednisone
± cyclophosphamide or azathio-
   prine
Cyclosporin-A[13]

**INFECTIOUS CAUSES**
Syphilis; penicillin
Tuberculosis; antituberculosis
   drugs
*Pseudomonas;* aminoglycosides
*Acanthamoeba;* brolene,
   neomycin, etc.
*Herpes zoster;* acyclovir

**SURGICAL INTERVENTION—SCLERAL
REINFORCEMENT MATERIALS**
Donor sclera
Fascia lata
Autologous periosteum

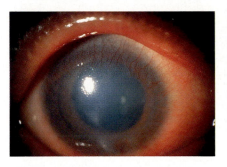

**13.19** | Sclerokeratitis in patient with Crohn's disease. Note diffuse scleritis as well as corneal infiltration and vascularization.

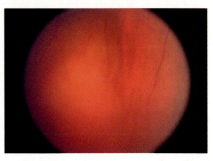

**13.20** | Posterior scleritis with exudative retinal detachment.

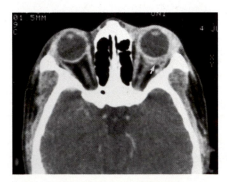

**13.21** | CT scan in posterior scleritis. Note diffuse enhancement along the posterior left side, with fluid and infiltration seen in Tenon's capsule (arrow). (Courtesy of Dr. M. Mafee.)

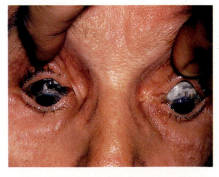

**13.22** | Bilateral scleromalacia perforans in patient with rheumatoid arthritis and no ocular complaints.

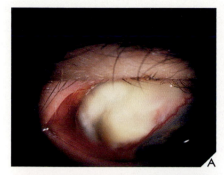

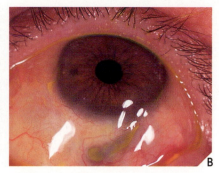

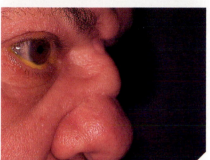

**13.23** | Wegener's granulomatosis. *A:* Necrotizing scleritis in patient with Wegener's granulomatosis. *B:* Scleral thinning in another patient with Wegener's. *C:* Nasal deformity in patient shown in *B.*

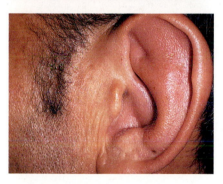

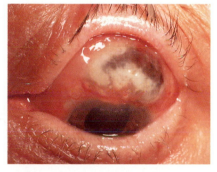

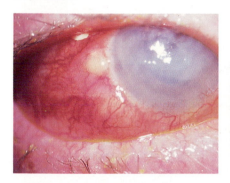

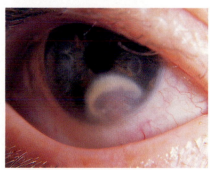

**13.24** | Auricular pinna inflammation in patient with relapsing polychondritis and scleritis.

**13.25** | Necrotizing scleritis along superior limbus subsequent to cataract surgery.

**13.26** | Nodular scleritis and necrotizing keratitis in patient with *Herpes simplex* recurrent ocular disease.

**13.27** | Syphilitic gumma in sclera and cornea in patient with tertiary syphilis.

than initially suspected on clinical examination. Penetrating injuries may be deceptive because an anterior penetration that is readily recognized may be only part of a double penetration. In some situations repair of the more posterior damage is not feasible. With scleral trauma there is commonly involvement of the uveal tract and there may also be retinal and vitreous involvement, requiring more complex surgical repair than just simple suturing of the laceration. In repairing scleral lacerations it is important to approximate cleanly the scleral edges, avoiding incarceration of other tissues. Healing is preceded by healing of the episclera and is achieved by ingrowth of fibroblasts from the episclera and uveal tissues. Chemical injuries may damage the sclera by causing direct toxic melting or by necrosing the surrounding vessels and tissues, leading to subsequent scleral necrosis. Acute injuries may also cause acute shrinkage of scleral collagen, resulting in an acute elevation of intraocular pressure.

## TUMORS OF THE SCLERA

Scleral tumors are uncommon; most are secondary to extension from either the conjunctiva or the inside of the eye. The vascular and nerve channels are the common locations for these extensions. Figure 13.28 lists the tumors of the sclera.

## METABOLIC DISEASES INVOLVING SCLERA

The appearance of the sclera may be altered in persons with systemic metabolic diseases. This can be seen in ochronosis (alkaptonuria), which produces a yellow to dark-brown scleral discoloration, most marked at the insertions of the rectus muscles. The blue discoloration seen in osteogenesis imperfecta has been discussed earlier. The yellow color of jaundice is characteristic of diseases producing elevated bilirubin.

### Figure 13.28. Tumors Involving the Sclera

| | |
|---|---|
| Fibrous | Episcleral osseous choristoma |
| Nodular fasciitis | Ectopic lacrimal gland |
| Hemangioma | Spread of contiguous tumors |
| Neurofibroma | |

# 14 | LACRIMAL SYSTEM: DRY-EYE STATES AND OTHER CONDITIONS

Antonio R. de Toledo

John W. Chandler

Frank V. Buffam

## EMBRYOLOGY

Precursors of the lacrimal excretory system first appear during the sixth week of gestation along the cleft between the lateral nasal and maxillary processes. The excretory system appears as a cord of epithelial cells. The solid cord extends downward into the mesenchyme to form the naso-optic fissure and detaches from the surface (Fig. 14.1). The sequestered epithelial cord lies between precursors of the medial canthus and the nose. During the 6–12-week gestation period, the lacrimal ectodermal bud proliferates to extend towards the inner canthus and the nasal cavity. As the epithelial cord approaches the medial canthus, it splits, conforming to the medial canthal angle. The precursors of the canalicular system are thereby established. Canalization of the duct begins at around 12 weeks of gestation and is completed by 6 months. The lacrimal punctum opens onto the lid margin just before the lids separate during the seventh month.[1] The lower end of the nasolacrimal duct frequently remains occluded until birth or later and is separated from the cavity of the inferior meatus by a membrane. This membrane consists of the opposed mucosal linings of the nasal fossa and the lower end of the duct (valve of Hasner).[2] The lacrimal gland similarly derives from ectodermal cords, growing into the orbit from the upper temporal conjunctiva (Fig. 14.2).[3]

## ANATOMY OF THE LACRIMAL SYSTEM

The lacrimal system is divided into secretory and excretory components. The secretory portion is composed of the main lacrimal gland and the accessory lacrimal glands of Krause (forniceal) and Wolfring (tarsal edge), and those in the caruncle and the plica (Fig. 14.3).

The main lacrimal gland is in the anterosuperolateral portion of the orbit in between the lateral angular process of the frontal bone and the eye (Fig. 14.4). It is held in place by fibrous septae extending from the upper surface of the gland to

**14.1** | Embryology of the lacrimal excretory system. By 5–6 weeks, tissue grows towards the midline, compressing and burying surface ectoderm in the nasolacrimal groove between the lateral nasal swelling and the maxillary swelling. By 12 weeks canalization is beginning in the nasolacrimal duct. By 24 weeks canalization is almost complete but remains imperforate at the lower end of the nasolacrimal duct (valve of Hasner).

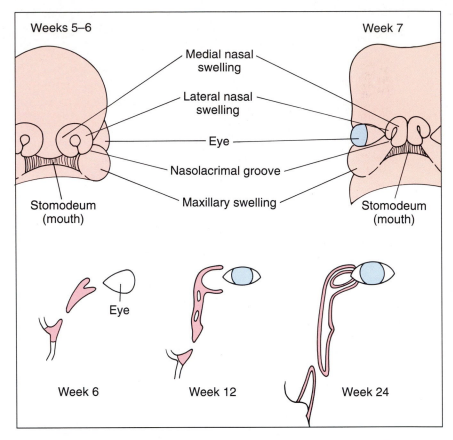

**14.2** | Embryology of the lacrimal gland. By week 8 the epithelial cords grow from surface conjunctiva in the upper fornix into the orbit. Mesoderm condenses and proliferates around the epithelial cords. By week 12 lumen appears in the cords. Around the fifth month the levator aponeurosis indents the gland, producing the orbital and palpebral lobes. The gland is fully developed by 3–4 years postpartum.

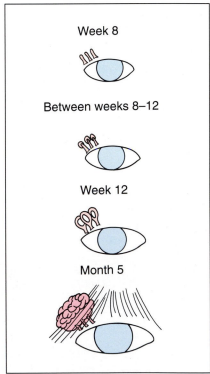

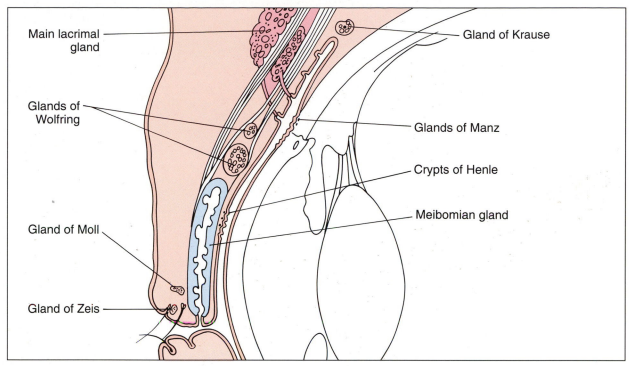

Main lacrimal gland

Glands of Wolfring

Gland of Moll

Gland of Zeis

Gland of Krause

Glands of Manz

Crypts of Henle

Meibomian gland

**14.3** | Secretory components of the lacrimal system include the main and accessory lacrimal glands. These glands have similar microscopic anatomy.

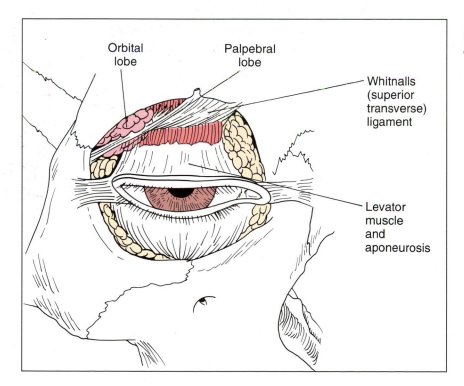

Orbital lobe

Palpebral lobe

Whitnalls (superior transverse) ligament

Levator muscle and aponeurosis

**14.4** | Relationship of the main lacrimal gland to the orbit, other adnexal structures, and eyeball.

the periosteum of the orbital roof. The lateral extension of the aponeurosis of the levator muscle and Whitnall's (superior transverse) ligament separates the lacrimal gland into two lobes (a larger superior or orbital lobe and a smaller inferior or palpebral lobe). These lobes, however, are continuous posteriorly by a bridge of glandular tissue.[4] There are approximately 12 excretory ducts of the lacrimal gland; 2 to 5 of them originate from the superior lobe and 6 to 8 from the inferior lobe. Most of them open into the superotemporal portion of the forniceal conjunctiva 4–5 mm above the upper border of the tarsus. Since all ducts from the superior lobe pass through the inferior lobe, extirpation of the latter is functionally equivalent to excision of the entire gland.[5]

The arteries enter the gland posteriorly as branches of the lacrimal artery, a division of the ophthalmic artery. Sometimes branches of the infraorbital artery (a branch of the maxillary artery from the external carotid artery) supply the gland. The lacrimal vein may join the superior ophthalmic (orbital) vein or enter the cavernous sinus separately. The lymphatics join the conjunctival and palpebral lymphatic systems and pass to the preauricular lymph nodes.

The nerve supply of the lacrimal gland is not yet completely elucidated. Innervation is derived from three sources: the trigeminal, the facial, and the sympathetic (Fig. 14.5); however, some of their functions are disputed.[6]

## THE TRIGEMINAL NERVE

The primary innervation of the lacrimal gland is through the lacrimal nerve, which is a branch of the ophthalmic division (V-1) of the trigeminal nerve. A few fibers may also reach the gland from the zygomatic nerve, which is a branch of the maxillary division (V-2), through the lacrimal nerve.

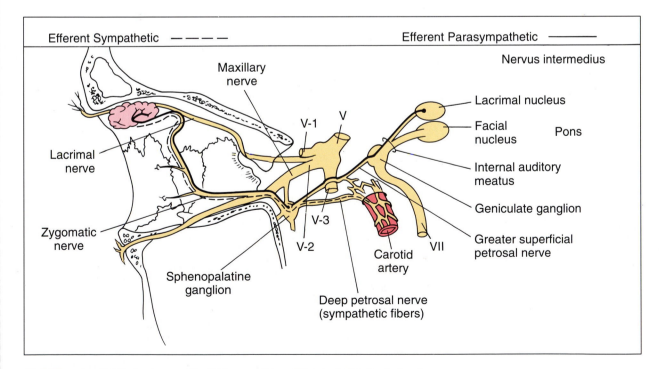

Efferent Sympathetic  – – – –          Efferent Parasympathetic  ———

Nervus intermedius

Maxillary nerve

Lacrimal nucleus

Facial nucleus          Pons

V-1      V

Internal auditory meatus

Lacrimal nerve

Geniculate ganglion

V-3

Zygomatic nerve

Greater superficial petrosal nerve

V-2          VII

Sphenopalatine ganglion

Carotid artery

Deep petrosal nerve (sympathetic fibers)

**14.5** | Parasypathetic and sympathetic innervation of the main lacrimal gland.

The nerve fibers going through the facial nerve are parasympathetic in nature. They are believed to start from the lacrimal nucleus (near the facial nucleus at the pons) and then travel through the nervus intermedius (of the facial nerve), the greater superficial petrosal nerve, the nerve of the pterygoid canal (vidian nerve), the sphenopalatine ganglion, and then either through the zygomatic branch of the maxillary nerve, which anastomoses with the lacrimal nerve, or perhaps by small twigs of the ganglion to the lacrimal gland.

## THE FACIAL NERVE

The postganglionic cervical sympathetic fibers, after traveling through the internal carotid artery (carotid plexus), may reach the lacrimal gland by way of the deep petrosal nerve, the nerve of the pterygoid canal, the sphenopalatine ganglion, and then the zygomatic nerve, or else along the lacrimal artery.

## THE SYMPATHETIC NERVES

The accessory lacrimal glands have the same structure as the main lacrimal gland, although smaller in scale. The glands of Krause are located deep in the substantia propria of the conjunctiva. They number about 20 in the upper fornix and 8 in the lower fornix, particularly on the lateral side. Near the upper border of the tarsal plate, a few glands of Wolfring are found. Rudimentary accessory lacrimal glands also occur in the plica and the caruncle (Fig. 14.6). Autonomic innervation of the accessory lacrimal glands has not yet been demonstrated.

The excretory portion of the lacrimal system consists of the canaliculi (upper and lower), common canaliculus, lacrimal sac, and nasolacrimal duct. Tears pool toward the medial canthus at the lacus lacrimalis. Tears then enter the lacrimal puncta that lie near the nasal end of each eyelid. The lower

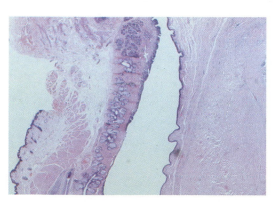

**14.6** | Accessory lacrimal glands and surrounding eyelid structures. Histologic section shows the accessory lacrimal glands deep in the substantia propria of the conjunctiva. (From Yanoff M, Fine BS: *Ocular Pathology: A Color Atlas*. New York, Gower Medical Publishing, 1992, 6.2, with permission.)

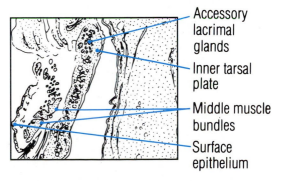

Accessory lacrimal glands

Inner tarsal plate

Middle muscle bundles

Surface epithelium

punctum lies slightly lateral to the upper (Fig. 14.7). Normally, both are turned inward to receive tears and are therefore not visible to direct inspection. Each punctum is surrounded by a ring of relatively dense fibrous tissue which serves to keep it patent. The puncta vary from 0.5 to 1.5 mm in diameter. The canaliculi are collapsed in vivo but dilate easily to 2 mm in transverse diameter. They are lined with stratified , nonkeratinized squamous epithelium. The lacrimal sac also is lined with nonkeratinized squamous epithelium but, unlike the canaliculi, contains many goblet cells and foci of columnar ciliated (respiratory type) epithelium. This epithelium becomes more prevalent lower in the nasolacrimal duct. The duct itself occupies roughly 75% of the 3–4 mm wide bony nasolacrimal canal. The remainer of the canal is filled with a rich vascular plexus resembling that covering the inferior turbinate.[7] Many so-called "valves" have been described in the duct. These represent folds of the mucosa rather than true valves, but presumably retard flow in some individuals. (See Volume IV, Chapter 7, for further discussion of the lacrimal system.)

## PHYSIOLOGY OF THE LACRIMAL SYSTEM

The lacrimal glands (main and accessory) make important contributions to the aqueous layer of the tear film, which is approximately 7 μm thick. Their secretion is regulated, and the relative contribution of the main and accessory lacrimal glands appears to vary with the level of stimulation. However, neuronal control of baseline secretion has not been proven.[8] The parasympathetic innervation clearly plays an important role in several lacrimation reflexes, regulating lacrimal gland fluid secretion rates.[9] Stimulation of the sphenopalatine ganglion elicits lacrimal gland fluid secretion, as does administration of parasympathomimetics.[10,11] In contrast, parasympatholytic drugs and blocking of the sphenopalatine ganglion reduce tear flow.[12,13] The gland becomes hypersensitized to parasympathomimetics such as topical or systemic pilocarpine, after parasympathetic denervation.[14] The role of sympathetic innervation is contradictory. It is possible that general vasomotor function of the sympathetic system regulates tear flow by changes in lacrimal blood flow.[10]

The secreted tears pass outward from the excretory ducts over the surface of the conjunctiva to reach the tear meniscus along the eyelid margins of the open eye. Under normal conditions there is 7–9 μl of preocular tears in

**14.7** | Functional anatomy of the lacrimal excretory system.

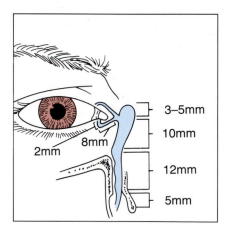

each tear film.[15] Blinking spreads the tear film, producing a vertical distribution of tears, while horizontal tear flow occurs in the tear meniscus at the lid margin. With each blink the entire precorneal and conjunctival tear film is renewed and reconstituted. The oily layer forms a hydrophobic barrier along the lid margin, preventing the tear strip from overflowing onto the skin.

Under normal conditions, human tear flow is approximately 0.6–1.2 µl/min. About 10% to 25% of tears are lost by evaporation, although under dry atmospheric conditions evaporation can be much more significant. Impaired oily layer secretion may increase evaporation from the cornea 10- to 20-fold.[16]

When the lacrimal fluid reaches the puncta, the capillary attraction created by the opening phase of the blink cycle is sufficient to draw the fluid from the marginal tear strips into the canaliculi. Doane[17] has proposed the lacrimal pump theory on the basis of high speed movies (Fig. 14.8). He noted that early in the blinking cycle, the nasal portion of the eyelids approximate to effectively occlude the puncta, which is followed by compression of the canaliculi and lacrimal sac. At the time of maximal eyelid closure, the volume of fluid within the lacrimal system is at its minimum. He estimates that this system can handle 14–18 µl/min of tear.[18] As the eyelid opens, the ampulla and canaliculi revert to their normal size and position. Elasticity of the tear sac results in saccular collapse and the expulsion of fluids through the nasolacrimal duct.

## TEAR FILM

The precorneal tear film (PCTF) is essential for maintaining the health of the underlying cornea and conjunctiva. It offers protection to the eyes while providing a smooth optical surface. The precorneal tear film consists of three layers: a lipid outer layer, an aqueous middle layer and mucous inner layer (Fig. 14.9). These three layers must be in perfect homeostasis in order to maintain the effective and unique characteristics of the PCTF.

## THE LIPID LAYER

The lipid layer is produced primarily by the Meibomian glands in the superior and inferior tarsus and, to a lesser extent, by the glands of Zeis in the palpebral margin, and by the glands of Moll at the roots of cilia. The layer is composed of low-polarity lipids, such as waxy and cholesterol esters; in addition, negligible amounts of triglyceride, free fatty acids, and phospholipids are found.[19] The average thickness of the lipid layer is estimated at 0.1 µm; it helps to maintain the integrity of the PCTF by creating a low surface tension between the liquid–solid interface.[20] It retards evaporation and provides a limiting hydrophobic barrier, preventing tears from running over the edge of the eyelid.

## THE AQUEOUS LAYER

In physiologic conditions the aqueous layer is produced by accessory lacrimal glands of Krause in the upper and lower fornix, by the accessory glands of Wolfring, and by an occasional gland in the plica and caruncle. These accessory lacrimal glands are responsible for the basic secretion of the

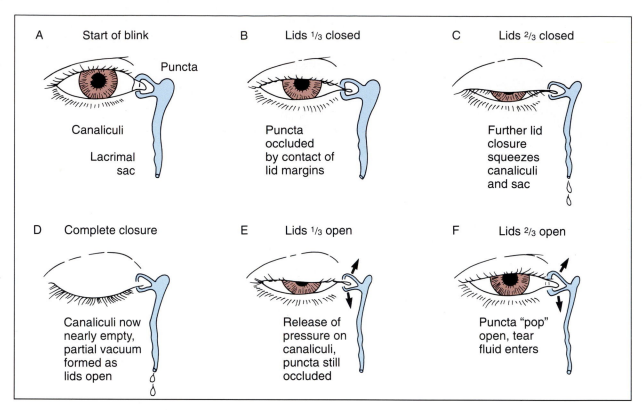

A   Start of blink

Puncta

Canaliculi

Lacrimal sac

B   Lids ⅓ closed

Puncta occluded by contact of lid margins

C   Lids ⅔ closed

Further lid closure squeezes canaliculi and sac

D   Complete closure

Canaliculi now nearly empty, partial vacuum formed as lids open

E   Lids ⅓ open

Release of pressure on canaliculi, puncta still occluded

F   Lids ⅔ open

Puncta "pop" open, tear fluid enters

**14.8** | Mechanism of lacrimal drainage. *A:* At the start of the blink, the lacrimal drainage passages already contain tear fluid that has entered after the previous blink. *B:* As upper lid descends, the papillae containing the punctal openings elevate from the medial lid margin. By the time the upper lid has descended halfway, the papillae forcefully meet the opposing lid margin, effectively occluding the puncta and preventing fluid regurgitation. *C:* The remaining portion of lid closure acts to squeeze the canaliculi and sac through the action of the orbicularis oculi, forcing out the contained fluid by way of the nasal lacrimal duct. *D:* At complete lid closure, the system is compressed and largely empty of fluid. *E:* During beginning of opening phase of blink, puncta are still occluded, and valving action at inner end of canaliculi (and perhaps nasolacrimal duct) act to prevent reentry of fluid or air. Compressive action ends and elastic walls of passages try to expand to their normal shape. This elastic force causes a partial vacuum or suction to form within the canaliculi and sac. *F:* Suction force holding the punctal region of the lid margin together is released when lid separation is sufficient, about two thirds fully opened. Punctal papillae suddenly "pop" apart at this point, opening the canaliculi for fluid entry, occurring during the first few seconds after the blink. (Modified and published courtesy of *Ophthalmology 1981; 88:844–851.*)

aqueous layer of the PCTF. The main lacrimal gland is primarily involved in reflex tearing. The aqueous layer is composed of approximately 98% water and about 1.2% solid content and represents the bulk of the precorneal tear film, with an average thickness of 6–7 μm.

### TEAR pH

Human tear pH varies from 6.5 to 7.6 under normal conditions.[21] Inflammatory conditions of the cornea or conjunctiva tend to shift to a more acid tear film. The tear film is also more acid on awakening, owing to prolonged closure of the eyelid.[22]

### TEAR OSMOLARITY

The osmotic pressure of the tears under normal conditions averages 302 mOsm/L. Tear secretion and tear evaporation influence the osmotic pressure of the tear film. Prolonged closure of the lids tends to decrease tear osmotic pressure, probably by retarding evaporation.[23]

### GLUCOSE

The average glucose in tears is 2.5 mg/100 ml, which accounts for 40% of the total reducing substance in tears. This amount of glucose is insufficient to provide for the corneal epithelium, which relies on the aqueous for its glucose supply.[24,25]

### PROTEIN COMPONENTS

Many protein components have been isolated from human tears. As many as 10 to 12 different protein fractions have been reported.[26] Major fractions include specific tear albumin or prealbumin, albumin, lysozyme, immuno-

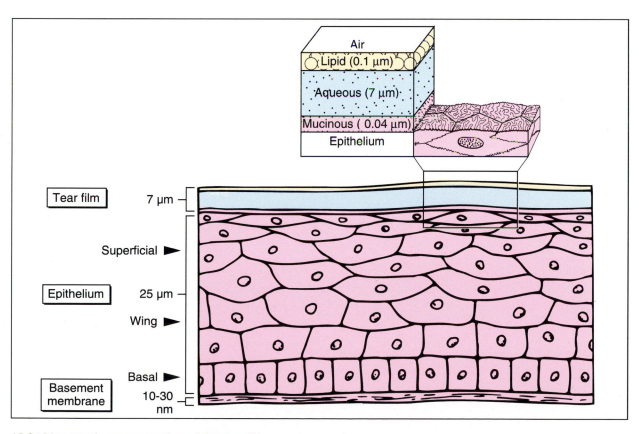

**14.9** | Diagramatic representation of the tear film.

globulin, lactoferrin, and other metal-carrying proteins. The protein in tears serves many functions, including lowering surface tension, metal transport, buffering, and osmotic regulation. It also contains all the components necessary to establish and control inflammatory reactions (Fig. 14.10).

ALBUMIN

Specific tear albumin accounts for 30% of human tear protein content. It is electrophoretically distinct from serum albumin and its function is unknown, but it may provide osmotic balance or buffering.[27] Serum albumin is a minor component of tears.

Lysozyme is one of the most important protein components of the human tear film and accounts for 20% of the tear protein content.[28] It is bactericidal to certain Gram-positive organisms by enzymatically disrupting bacterial cell walls. Lysozyme bacteriolytic activity in tears is much higher than in any other body fluid. Practolol toxicity,[29] Sjögren's disease,[30] malnutrition,[31] and air pollution[32] have all been associated with a decreased level of lysozyme in tears.

IMMUNOGLOBULINS

Globulins account for about one third of the total tear protein. IgA is the most prevalent (about 10%) immunoglobulin found in normal tears.[33] IgA appears to be synthesized by resident interstitial plasma cells in the main and accessory lacrimal gland and, as it enters the intercellular space, is coupled to secretory component and secreted as secretory IgA.[34] IgG is present in very low concentration in normal tears, although after mild trauma to the mucosal surface of the conjunctiva, it can easily be detected. IgE is present in small amounts, whereas little or no IgM or IgD is present.

LACTOFERRIN

Lactoferrin is an iron-binding protein that accounts for up to 25% of human tear protein. It has both bacteriostatic and bactericidal properties. Its affinity for binding iron probably accounts for its bacteriostatic activity by making essential metal ions unavailable to microbial metabolism.[35]

THE MUCIN LAYER

The mucin layer is produced by the conjunctival goblet cells, and it is composed mainly of N-acetylneuraminic acid (sialic acid). The mucous layer is only 0.02–0.05 μm thick and converts the hydrophobic corneal epithelium to a wettable surface.[36]

## Figure 14.10. Immune Components of Human Tears

| | |
|---|---|
| Lysozyme | β-lysin |
| Immunoglobulin A | Interferon |
| Immunoglobulin G | Histamine |
| Immunoglobulin E | Lymphocytes and neutrophils present |
| Complement | Peroxidase–thiocyanate–peroxidase system |
| Lactoferrin | Antibiotic-producing commensal organisms |
| Transferrin | |

Modified from reference 86.

Congenital disorders of the lacrimal gland and excretory ductules are rare and include such abnormalities as congenital alacrima, lacrimal gland cysts, lacrimal gland fistulas, and ectopic lacrimal gland tissue.

Absence of the lacrimal gland is an extremely rare condition and is often associated with other congenital ocular anomalies, such as anophthalmos and cryptophthalmos.[37] Another condition in which congenital absence of the lacrimal gland may be seen is in anhidrotic hereditary ectodermal dysplasia, an X-linked recessive syndrome characterized by deficient tear production, reduced sweating and salivation causing heat intolerance, hypotrichosis, partial or complete anodontia, prominent frontal ridge, and a saddle nose. Vestigial remnants of the lacrimal gland and ducts may be present but nonfunctional.[38]

Congenital alacrima can be due to disorders of the lacrimal gland itself or to the neuronal pathway responsible for reflex tearing. Symptoms are those of keratoconjunctivitis sicca with irritation, photophobia, conjunctival injection with mucoid discharge, and predisposition to corneal erosion and infection.[39]

Innervational dysgenesis abnormalities of the lacrimal gland may occur with congenital aplasia of the facial nerve nuclei, as well as with congenital trigeminal dysfunction.

Familial dysautonomia (Riley–Day syndrome) is an autosomal recessive disorder that mainly affects people of Jewish descent.[40] It is characterized by excessive salivation and sweating, skin blotching with excitement, transient hypertension, poor motor coordination, and decreased life expectancy. Ophthalmic findings include absent or deficient tearing, corneal anesthesia (which may be accompanied by indolent corneal ulcers) and often strabismus. The lacrimal gland is supersensitive to cholinergic agents.[41,42] Histology shows a normal lacrimal gland.

Congenital alacrima can also occur in individuals with no ocular or systemic abnormalities. These patients usually have symptoms of bilateral keratoconjunctivitis sicca and a history of having never shed any tears. Schirmer's test is abnormal. The lacrimal gland has a normal histological pattern.

Congenital lacrimal gland cysts are rare. They are often present at birth as a fluctuant cystic mass on the temporal half of the upper lid, and may cause significant proptosis with inferior displacement of the globe. Because of their early presentation, congenital lacrimal gland cysts are difficult to distinguish from solid orbital tumors. Aspiration of the cyst is often not curative and cysts tend to recur. Surgical excision is usually required.[37]

Lacrimal gland fistula is also a rare condition that presents during childhood and may be associated with tearing from the fistula orifice, localized irritation, and purulent discharge. The fistulas can be divided into two groups on the basis of the location of their orifices. The tarsal group has its orifice at the upper border of the tarsal plate of the upper eyelid, and the lateral group has

## CONGENITAL AND EMBRYOLOGIC DISORDERS
### LACRIMAL GLAND AND SECRETORY DUCTULES
#### ABSENCE OF LACRIMAL GLAND

#### CONGENITAL ALACRIMA

#### LACRIMAL GLAND CYSTS

#### LACRIMAL GLAND FISTULAS

its orifice at variable distances from the lateral canthus.[43] These fistulas are often associated with the palpebral portion of the lacrimal gland. Probing of the fistula and delineation by x-ray contrast photography should be employed if surgical correction is contemplated. Treatment consists of conservative excision of the fistula, the involved palpebral portion of the lacrimal gland, or transplantation of the fistula to the upper fornix.

### ECTOPIC LACRIMAL GLAND TISSUE

Ectopic lacrimal gland tissue may be found anywhere under palpebral or bulbar conjunctival tissue. It may also be present at the corneal limbus, in the plica, or in any of the external ocular structures. Most often the ectopic tissue is in an epibulbar location, and less often in the orbit, the outer canthal area, the lower lid, and the eye itself (Fig. 14.11).[44] Clinical manifestations are usually dependent on the location of the ectopic tissue. Epibulbar lesions may manifest as early as the neonatal period, whereas orbital lesions may remain undetected until adulthood.

Epibulbar lesions are usually located in the superotemporal area and are generally unilateral, although 4% to 11% are bilateral. Differential diagnosis includes dermoids and lipodermoids and can be confirmed only by histologic examination.

Orbital lesions may remain clinically undetected until adulthood, at which time they may become acutely inflamed, giving rise to painful unilateral proptosis, diplopia, and visual loss. Ectopic lacrimal gland tissue may undergo malignant transformation, and the patient, therefore, must be closely followed once initial surgery establishes the diagnosis.[45]

### LACRIMAL DRAINAGE SYSTEM

The lacrimal excretory passages are often divided into upper (proximal) and lower (distal) excretory passages. An upper system block is an obstruction along the drainage pathway that includes external lacrimal puncta and canaliculi, internal common canaliculi, and internal common punctum to the lacrimal sac. The lower system consists of the lacrimal sac, nasolacrimal duct, and the inferior meatus of the nose.

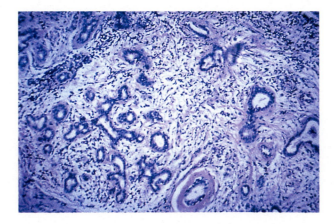

**14.11** | Biopsy of ectopic lacrimal gland tissue in the orbit.

Complete absence of punctae and canaliculi is rare, but imperforate punctum is less rare.[37] The lacrimal punctum can usually be identified by a shallow depression in the papilla or by a thin membrane occluding the punctal orifice. The treatment for imperforate punctum consists of gentle puncture with a dilator, followed by dilation and then irrigation. A punctoplasty is sometimes necessary. Correction for atresia of the canaliculi usually requires more complex surgical intervention, such as silastic intubation, anastomosis of the canaliculi to the sac, or conjunctivodacryocystorhinostomy. The latter is indicated if the former two have failed or when there is a true congenital atresia of the canaliculi, as well as for obstructions of more than 2 mm in length.

**UPPER EXCRETORY SYSTEM BLOCKAGE**
Congenital Absence of Punctae and Canaliculi

There is often a hereditary component to this type of congenital deformity. They are usually found 2–10 mm inferior to the medial canthus and are usually asymptomatic, although they may cause maceration of the surrounding skin owing to chronic excretion of tears. Treatment consists of excision and closure of the anomalous passageway.[46]

Supernumerary Puncta and Canaliculi

The most common nasolacrimal congenital abnormality is obstruction low in the nasolacrimal duct at the nasal mucosal entrance (valve of Hasner). It accounts for about 85% of congenital epiphora. The presenting symptoms include mucous discharge and epiphora, with no signs of conjunctival infection. Digital pressure over the lacrimal sac may result in reflux of sterile mucous material. Conservative treatment is indicated and consists of massage over the lacrimal sac 2 to 4 times a day to minimize stagnation. Topical antibiotics (drops or ointment) are also indicated before massaging. If massage is done daily, epiphora will disappear in 96% to 98% of infants by the age of 1 year.[47] About 80% of congenital lacrimal duct obstructions improve during the first 6 to 8 months of life, and by 13 months 90% of the obstructions resolve without surgical intervention.[48] The nasolacrimal duct may open spontaneously or may yield to probing. There is no consensus on the best time for probing the nasolacrimal duct, although best results are obtained when it is performed within the first 13 months of life.[49] Probing is indicated if obstruction persists after 6 months of age despite treatment, when the infant experiences recurrent episodes of conjunctivitis, and after an acute episode of dacryocystitis. Congenital obstruction may also be due to a more extensive atresia of the duct or a failure of canalization of the bony nasolacrimal canal.

**LOWER EXCRETORY SYSTEM BLOCKAGE**
Atresia of the Nasolacrimal Duct (Dacryostenosis)

Mucocele is believed to be caused by an obstruction below the tear sac, combined with a blockage at the opening of the canaliculi into the tear sac. This condition presents at birth with unilateral epiphora. The mucocele contains a sterile accumulation of mucous or amniotic fluid entrapped in the lacrimal sac. Treatment consists of early probing of the nasolacrimal duct, which is usually curative.[50] This is one of the few indications for probing the nasolacrimal duct before the age of 2 or 3 months. In the absence of secondary infection, the differential diagnosis should include congenital glaucoma.

Congenital Lacrimal Amniotocele (Mucocele)

## INFECTIOUS AND INFLAMMATORY CONDITIONS
### SECRETORY SYSTEM

Infection and inflammation of the lacrimal gland (dacryoadenitis) are rare and can have an acute or chronic presentation. Despite their rarity, it is believed that 50% to 75% of all enlargements of the lacrimal gland are of inflammatory origin. Acute bacterial infection of the gland is usually secondary to systemic infection but may be due to contiguous spread of a local infection such as conjunctivitis, hordeola, or orbital cellulitis. Primary bacterial infection of the gland is rare. Chronic bacterial infection of the lacrimal gland is usually due to granulomatous diseases such as tuberculosis, syphilis, or Hansen's disease (leprosy).

### ACUTE DACRYOADENITIS

Acute primary dacryoadenitis is usually unilateral. At onset there is a swelling in the outer part of the upper lid or orbit. A tender ipsilateral preauricular node may be palpable, and pain and tearing may be present (Fig. 14.12). Both the palpebral and the orbital lobe of the lacrimal gland can be affected. However, more severe symptoms, such as proptosis and globe displacement, are most often seen when the orbital lobe is involved. The process is often self-limited, and conservative treatment with warm compresses and oral analgesics is indicated.[51]

Secondary acute dacryoadenitis is more common than primary dacryoadenitis and is usually secondary to systemic infection. The presentation is similar to that of primary acute dacryoadenitis, except that it is usually bilateral. Acute endemic parotitis (mumps) and gonorrhea are the most commonly associated systemic infections. Others include *Staphylococcus aureus*, infectious mononucleosis, herpes zoster ophthalmicus, and histoplasmosis. Treatment consists of determination of the causative agent and appropriate antibiotic therapy when indicated.

---

### Figure 14.12. Inflammatory and Infectious Conditions of the Lacrimal Gland

| ACUTE DACRYOADENITIS | CHRONIC DACRYOADENITIS |
| --- | --- |
| **Infectious** | **Infectious** |
| Primary (usually unilateral) | Tuberculosis |
| Secondary (usually bilateral) | Syphilis |
| **Inflammatory** | Hansen's disease (Leprosy) |
| Pseudotumor | Trachoma |
| Graves' disease | **Inflammatory** |
| | Pseudotumor |
| | Graves' disease |
| | Sarcoidosis |
| | Sjögren syndrome |

Modified from Weiss RA, Hurwitz JJ: Lacrimal gland infections and inflamations, in Hornblass A (ed): *Oculoplastic, Orbital and Reconstructive Surgery*, Vol 2. Baltimore, Williams & Wilkins, 1990, 1508.

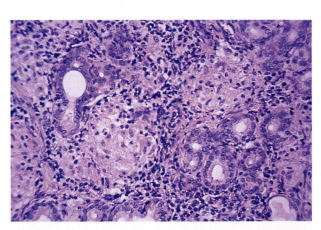

14.13 | Sarcoidosis of the lacrimal gland with noncaseating granulomatous tubercles and lymphocyte infiltration.

Chronic dacryoadenitis is more common than acute dacryoadenitis. The involvement of the lacrimal gland is usually bilateral but not necessarily symmetrical. The gland may be tender on palpation, and a hard, mobile, lobulated mass can be felt under the upper outer orbital rim in the lacrimal gland area. Pain is not usual with chronic dacryoadenitis and its presence may be an indication of malignancy. Chronic inflammatory disorders such as sarcoidosis, Sjögren syndrome, Graves' disease, and pseudotumor account for most cases of chronic dacryoadenitis. The chronicity of the process and the physical characteristics of the compromised lacrimal gland often make it difficult to determine whether the clinical findings are inflammatory in origin or are due to malignancy. Open biopsy of the lacrimal gland is usually necessary to establish the diagnosis.

Infectious causes of chronic dacryoadenitis are rare. In tuberculosis, syphilis, and Hansen's disease, involvement of the lacrimal gland is usually secondary to systemic dissemination of the infectious process, whereas in trachoma involvement is probably due to the contiguous conjunctival infection.[51]

**CHRONIC DACRYOADENITIS**

When affected, the lacrimal gland in Graves' disease shows infiltrative changes identical to those seen in the orbit and extraocular muscles. The infiltrative adenitis consists of a lymphocytic infiltrate, edematous fibrous tissue, and glandular degeneration. These changes may cause enlargement of the gland, occasional prolapse, and disturbance in lacrimal secretion.

Graves' Disease

In the orbit, the lacrimal gland is the most common locus of sarcoidosis. Approximately 7% of patients with sarcoidosis have either unilateral or bilateral lacrimal gland enlargement (Fig. 14.13).[52] The disease is more common in women and blacks. The patient may have dry-eye symptoms and, as a rule, involvement of the lacrimal gland is only one manifestation of generalized sarcoidosis with involvement of the lymph nodes of the mediastinum, lungs, and other organs.[53] Histology shows noncaseating granulomatous tubercles, lymphocyte infiltration, giant-cell nests, and replacement of the secretory acini by fibrous tissue. A variant of sarcoidosis is uveoparotid fever or Heerfordt's disease, which includes uveitis, fever, parotid swelling, and a subclinical enlargement of the lacrimal gland. Topical steroids are not usually adequate and systemic steroids are necessary to treat the condition.

Sarcoidosis

The lacrimal gland is not usually enlarged in Sjögren syndrome, but significant decrease in tear production may occur due to infiltration of the lacrimal gland tissue by lymphocytes and plasma cells, leading to progressive atrophy of the gland (Fig. 14.14). Sjögren syndrome will be discussed in detail under dry-eye states in this chapter.

Sjögren Syndrome

Mikulicz syndrome is an antiquated term. The syndrome has been shown to be caused mainly by granulomatous diseases, and the appropriate name, e.g., sarcoidosis, of the disease should be used. Mikulicz's disease is an even more confusing term and should not be used. Probably, Godwin's benign lymphoepithelial lesion is the entity most people refer to when using the term Mikulicz's disease.

Mikulicz Syndrome and Disease

Dacryocystitis in infants is usually secondary to congenital obstruction of the nasolacrimal duct and can be classified as acute, chronic, or recurrent. The

DRAINAGE SYSTEM

symptoms include epiphora and chronic or recurrent conjunctivitis. When redness, tenderness, and swelling of the inner canthus are present, acute dacryocystitis should be suspected (Fig. 14.15). The most common organisms in children with acute or chronic dacryocystitis are *Haemophilus influenza, S. aureus, Pneumococcus,* and ß-hemolytic *Streptococcus.*[54]

Conjunctivitis of the newborn may have a similar presentation and must be excluded in the differential diagnosis. Tearing without either discharge or reflux from the nasolacrimal sac may be an indication of congenital glaucoma.

CANALICULITIS
Infection of the canaliculus is uncommon. When present it is usually unilateral, and the lower canaliculus is most often affected. Epiphora, itching, and persistent conjunctivitis, marked most around the inner canthus, are usually present. This picture is pertinent to canaliculitis secondary to *Actinomyces israelii*, the most common organism that infects the canaliculi.

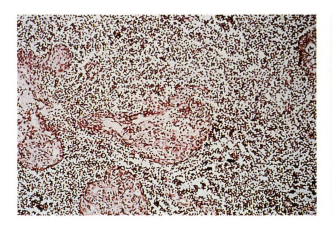

**14.14** | Lymphoepithelial infiltration of the main lacrimal gland in Sjögren syndrome.

**14.16** | Acute dacryocystitis with external fistulization.

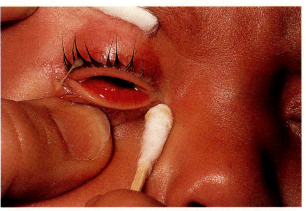

**14.15** | Acute dacryocystitis in infant, with acute signs of inflammation and reflux of purulent material on compression of the lacrimal sac.

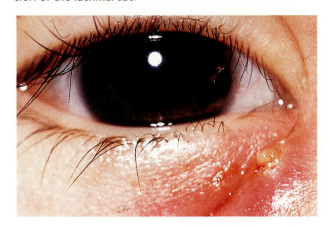

Other causes are trachoma, tuberculosis, syphilis, and herpes simplex and zoster.[51]

Acute dacryocystitis occurs more often in women and in whites over 40 years of age. Patients often complain of tearing and pain that is usually out of proportion to the clinical presentation. The pain may radiate to the upper teeth, to the ear, or to the temple. Exuberant signs of inflammation are usually present, and cellulitis of the surrounding area is a common finding (Fig. 14.16). Gentle palpation reveals a firm mass on the lacrimal sac area, and regurgitation can not usually be demonstrated owing to a closure of the valve of Rosenmuller in the entrance of the sac. The most common organism isolated in acute dacryocystitis is *S. aureus*, although streptococci and pneumococci have also been isolated.[54]

Older debilitated patients or the immunocompromised are at a greater risk for orbital cellulitis as a complication of acute dacryocystitis. Cavernous sinus thrombosis, optic atrophy, and blindness are other potential complications.[51]

Treatment consists of systemic antibiotics, analgesics, and warm compresses. Topical antibiotics are indicated in the presence of concurrent conjunctival infection. Careful probing of the sac can be performed if the area is not too tender. After remission of the acute process, many patients experience recurrent acute dacryocystitis, and chronic dacryocystitis may develop. Dacryocystorhinostomy is the treatment of choice for these patients.

Chronic dacryocystitis may present with a variety of symptoms, including unilateral tearing and intermittent milky discharge that accumulates in the inner canthus. A nontender mass in the medial canthus that is reducible by finger pressure is a common complaint. The patient may describe a past history of acute dacryocystitis and discharge on awakening. This chronic discharge is a potential source of infection, and intraocular surgery is therefore contraindicated. The most common organisms cultured in chronic dacrocystitis include *S. aureus*, *Pneumococcus*, ß-hemolytic *Streptococcus*, *Pseudomonas*, *Klebsiella*, enterobacteria, and *actinomyces*.[55] Fungal infection may also occur, with *Candida* and *Aspergillus* being the most common agents.

Definitive treatment of chronic dacryocystitis is achieved with dacryocystorhinostomy.

The saccharin test described by Hornblass[56] is performed with the patient erect. One drop of topical anesthetic is instilled in the inferior conjunctival cul de sac and 0.4 ml of 2% saccharin solution in distilled water is instilled in the inferior cul de sac. If the patient can taste the saccharin solution after 20 min, this is supportive evidence of system patency. A minimum of 30 min should elapse before the second eye is tested. For some individuals the test must be performed on two separate occasions, as the taste can be so intense that a positive test on one side precludes effective evaluation of the other.

If the saccharin test is negative, irrigation of the lower canaliculus with normal saline is the next step. The procedure is performed by anesthetizing the lacrimal punctum area with a cocaine pledget. A lacrimal needle on a 2-ml

## ACUTE DACRYOCYSTITIS

## CHRONIC DACRYOCYSTITIS

## THE WORK-UP FOR EPIPHORA (FIG. 14.17)
### SACCHARIN TEST

### IRRIGATION OF THE LOWER CANALICULUS

syringe is inserted in the lower canaliculus and the solution is injected. Interpretation of results is shown in Figure 14.18.

JONES' PRIMARY DYE TEST    Jones' #1 test is performed to differentiate partial obstruction of the nasolacrimal duct from lacrimal gland hypersecretion. The test is done by placing a drop of 2% fluorescein in the patient's inferior conjunctival cul de sac. In the normally patent lacrimal drainage system, the dye will be retrieved in the

**14.17** | The work-up for epiphora.

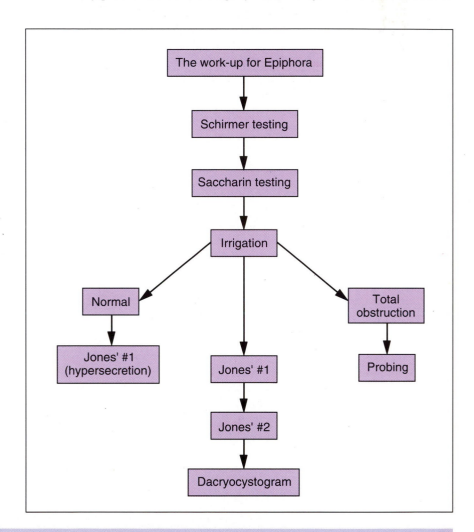

**Figure 14.18 Interpretation of Irrigation of Nasolacrimal Drainage System Through Lower Canaliculus**

| TO PHARYNX | REGURGITATION | INTERPRETATION |
|---|---|---|
| Yes | None | Normal |
| Yes | Upper | Partial obstruction distal to common canaliculus |
| No | Upper | Obstruction distal to common canaliculus |
| No | Lower | Obstruction proximal to common canaliculus |

nose after 5 min. Inspection for patency should be done with a nasal speculum after anesthetizing the inferior turbinate and meatus with lidocaine spray. A head-light is essential to provide adequate illumination for correct placement of a cotton-tipped applicator in the inferior meatus. The applicator is then examined under cobalt blue illumination for the presence of fluorescein. Blowing of the nose usually enhances test results, and dye can be detected on a tissue. Subsequent reexamination of the inferior meatus under cobalt blue filter illumination may show the presence of fluorescein. If dye is recovered, Jones' #1 test is positive, meaning that the lacrimal drainage system is normal. If no fluorescein is recovered, an obstruction (either anatomic or functional) exists, although the exact location cannot be determined and Jones' #2 test is required.

Excess fluorescein is washed out of the conjunctival cul de sac, and topical anesthetic is instilled. The head of the patient is tilted 60° over a kidney basin and clear irrigation fluid is flushed through the inferior canaliculus. Evidence of fluorescein dye in the basin is a positive test result, and indicates a partial obstruction distal to the lacrimal sac. If fluid was retrieved but unstained, the obstruction is between the punctum and the lacrimal sac and may indicate punctal stenosis, punctal ectropion, partial canalicular obstruction, or an orbicularis pump weakness.

JONES' SECONDARY DYE TEST

After completion of the Jones' test, most causes of tearing are diagnosed.

For the few patients who remain with unexplained tearing or in whom surgery is contemplated, intubation dacrocystography should be performed. Obstruction in the common canaliculus or evidence of a shrunken sac indicates the need for silicone tubing at surgery, whereas obstruction lateral to the common canaliculus indicates the need for a permanent Pyrex® (Jones) tube. Obstruction due to tumors or dacryoliths will also be evident.

DACROCYSTOGRAPHY

Dacryocystorhinostomy can be performed under local anesthesia. The region of the involved anterior lacrimal crest is infiltrated with 0.5 ml of lidocaine plus epinephrine 1:200,000, and the nostril adjacent to the middle turbinate is packed with a 4% cocaine pack. A cornea protector is placed in the conjunctival fornix. A straight incision, roughly 1.5 cm long, is made through the skin anterior to the lacrimal crest (Fig. 14.19). Two periosteal elevators are used to separate the orbicularis muscle in the direction of its fibers and to reflect the angular vein from the field. The periosteum is incised and a Tenzel periosteal elevator is used to elevate the periosteum towards the bridge of the nose and laterally, elevating the lacrimal sac from its fossa. The rhinostomy opening can be made with any of a number of instruments, our preference being the microsurgical air drill with an appropriate-sized bit. The drill is readily controlled, the ball of the hand resting on the cheek and the drill moving back and forth much as if one were writing. In this way the hole can be made quickly to the appropriate size. We remove the nasal packing before drilling. Ethmoid air cells are often encountered in the posterior superior portion of the rhinostomy. They have a thin mucosal lining, unlike the thick nasal mucosa, and should be deflected from the surgical field. The hole

## DACRYOCYSTORHINOS-TOMY

should be made roughly 12–15 mm in the vertical and anteroposterior diameter, straddling the anterior lacrimal crest with roughly one third before and two thirds posterior to it. The exact size of the hole is less important than ensuring that the bone lies within 5 mm of the internal common punctum. The upper portion of the medial wall of the nasolacrimal duct should be removed to permit complete opening of the sac into the nasolacrimal duct, preventing postoperative development of a "sump" in the lacrimal sac outlet. Anterior and posterior nasal flaps are made and are anastomosed to simi-

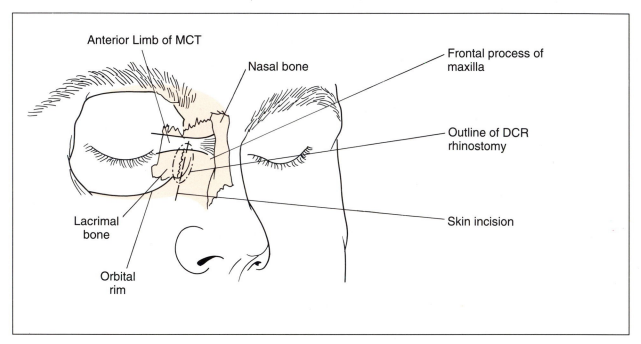

**14.19** | Skin incision and site of DCR rhinostomy in relation to bony anatomy. Bone medial to upper end of nasolacrimal duct is removed, leaving orbital rim anteriorly intact. (MCT=medial canthal tendon.)

**14.20** | Rhinostomy created; nasal mucosa incised, making anterior and posterior flaps.

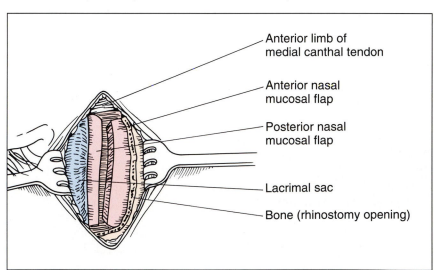

lar flaps in the medial wall of the lacrimal sac (Fig 14.20). A No. 0 Bowman probe slid along the upper canaliculus can be used as a guide in making the sac flaps (Fig. 14.21). Obstructions in the region of the internal punctum or canaliculus can be excised after opening the sac. Silastic tubing should be inserted through both canaliculi and tied in the rhinostomy in this instance (Fig. 14.22). The tubing is left in place for 6 months before removal. Vaseline packing can be placed in the rhinostomy opening before the end of surgery to hold the flaps apart and reduce the risk of immediate postoperative hemorrhage.

If the canaliculi are obliterated, a conjunctival rhinostomy is required.

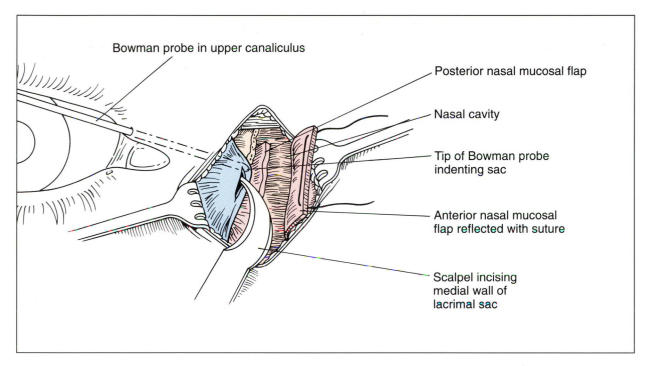

Bowman probe in upper canaliculus

Posterior nasal mucosal flap

Nasal cavity

Tip of Bowman probe indenting sac

Anterior nasal mucosal flap reflected with suture

Scalpel incising medial wall of lacrimal sac

**14.21** | Lacrimal sac indented by Bowman probe through upper canaliculus. Sac flaps being created by #12 scalpel blade.

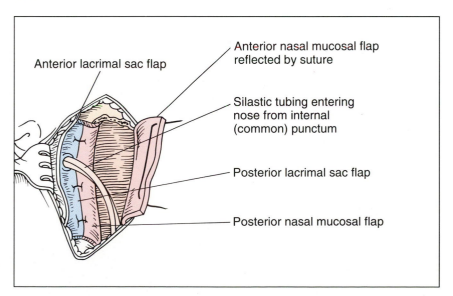

Anterior lacrimal sac flap

Anterior nasal mucosal flap reflected by suture

Silastic tubing entering nose from internal (common) punctum

Posterior lacrimal sac flap

Posterior nasal mucosal flap

**14.22** | Posterior flaps sutured together. Silastic tubing entering nose through internal (common) punctum. Anterior flaps reflected.

A Jones' Pyrex® tube is inserted after the dacryocystorhinostomy has been performed and the flaps prepared. The eyelids are held apart with a Guyton–Park speculum. The apex of the caruncle is excised and a 1.5-inch 25-gauge needle is used as a trocar to determine the appropriate path of the tube. Ideally, it should have a slightly dependent position and be angled so that the flange does not push on the globe. Once this track has been determined, it can be enlarged with a No. 52 Beaver blade. The appropriate length of the Pyrex® tube is determined by trial and error. Because the most commonly used size is 15 mm, we take that as a starting point and routinely use one that has a 4-mm flange, reducing it as the postoperative swelling decreases. The tube is inserted by placing it on a Bowman probe, inserting the probe through the track, and gently pushing the nonflanged end of the tube through the tissue with the handle of a cotton-tipped applicator. The flanged end of the tube is sutured to the skin temporarily with a 6-0 silk (Fig. 14.23). Patients are instructed that when they sneeze or cough, the eyes should be closed to prevent extrusion of the tube. Not infrequently the Pyrex® tube becomes crusted with debris after a year or so. Replacement is done easily under topical anesthesia. The lids are held apart with a lid speculum, the tube is removed, and a new one is inserted. If the tube requires sizing the track can be held open or dilated as necessary using the brass-tipped dilator that comes with the Jones tube set.

Complications of dacryocystorhinostomy include failure of the procedure, hemorrhage, infection, and prolapse of the Quickert tube.

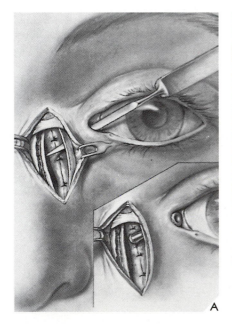

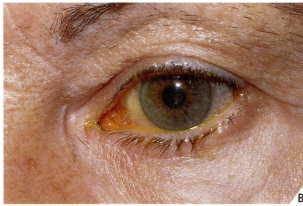

**14.23** | *A:* Creation of conjunctivorhinostomy site and insertion of Jones' tube. *B:* Jones' tube in position in the medial canthus.

Keratoconjunctivitis sicca (KCS) is the most common cause of dry eye. It may manifest as an isolated involvement of the lacrimal glands, decreasing aqueous tear production by lymphocyte infiltration of the gland. Mucous membranes of the mouth, vagina, and respiratory tract may also be affected. Enlargement of the salivary gland is common, and xerostomia is usually pronounced. When KCS manifests in association with connective tissue diseases, it is called Sjögren syndrome. In addition to the symptoms related to the dryness of the mucous membranes, these patients also exhibit symptoms peculiar to the underlining connective tissue disease. Sjögren syndrome reflects an underlying autoimmune disorder and is most commonly associated with rheumatoid arthritis. Other associated connective tissue diseases include progressive systemic sclerosis, systemic lupus erythematosus, and polyarteritis nodosa. Additional disorders associated with Sjögren syndrome include Hashimoto's thyroiditis, chronic hepatobiliary disease, pulmonary fibrosis, and Waldenstrom's hyperglobulinemic purpura (Fig 14.24).[57] Most laboratory findings are related to the immunologic nature of the disease. The degree of lymphocyte infiltration of the lacrimal and salivary gland is usually correlated with the severity of the disease, which can be assessed by biopsy of these glands.[58]

Other causes of KCS include cicatrizing ocular diseases such as trachoma, chemical burns, mucous membrane pemphigoid, and Stevens–Johnson syndrome. The gland may be infiltrated by sarcoid and amyloid cells or by neoplastic cells, particularly leukemia and lymphomas.

Rare congenital lacrimal gland disorders such as congenital alacrima and anhidrotic ectodermal dysplasia have been discussed above.

Dry-eye states can be caused by a multitude of factors described previously and are usually classified into four main categories. The first three are related to abnormalities in one of the three layers of the tear film: abnormalities of

## DRY-EYE STATES
### CAUSES

### CLASSIFICATION

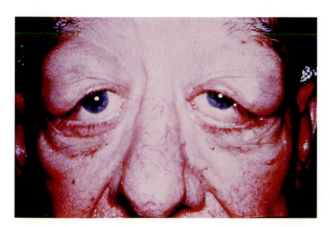

**14.24** | Sjögren syndrome associated with macroglobulinemia.

the lipid layer, abnormalities of the aqueous layer, and abnormalities of the mucous layer. The last category is related to abnormalities of the eyelid (Fig. 14.25).

**ABNORMALITIES OF THE AQUEOUS LAYER**

Abnormalities of the aqueous layer are the most common tear film disorder. Keratoconjunctivitis sicca occurs most often in women in the fifth or sixth decade. Onset is usually gradual, and in the early stages it may go undetected. Common complaints are foreign body sensation, burning, and irritation. Clinical signs include increased debris in the tear film, decreased marginal tear strip, and accumulation of material at the canthi. As the disease progresses, patients may complain of itching, pain, and photophobia, and filamentary keratitis may be present. At this stage the disease is easy to identify, although in the incipient stage a good degree of clinical suspicion and the following tests are necessary to establish correct diagnosis.

**Size of the Lacrimal Tear Strip**

The inferior tear meniscus height in normal individuals is, on average, 0.2 mm.[59] Decreased values may be found in individuals with moderate to severe KCS, along with increased amounts of debris in the tear film.

## Figure 14.25 Classification of Dry-Eye States

| | CAUSES | SYMPTOMS AND SIGNS |
|---|---|---|
| Abnormalities of the aqueous layer | Sjögren syndrome<br>Keratoconjunctivitis sicca<br>Lacrimal gland tumors<br>Alacrima<br>Radiation<br>Cicatricial surface diseases | Foreign body sensation, burning, debris in the tear film<br>+ Rose bengal staining<br>Decreased Schirmer test<br>Decreased tear lysozyme concentration |
| Abnormalities of the lipid layer | Blepharitis<br>Acne rosacea<br>Preservatives | Burning sensation more pronounced in the morning<br>Foamy material in the canthus<br>Collarettes around the eyelashes<br>Inflamed eyelid margin<br>Teleangiectatic vessels around lashes, cheek, nose |
| Abnormalities of the mucin layer | Stevens–Johnson syndrome<br>Mucous membrane pemphigoid<br>Vitamin A deficiency<br>Radiation<br>Chemical burns<br>Trachoma<br>Preservatives | Clinical history, photophobia, irritation<br>Symblepharon<br>Decreased tear break-up time |
| Abnormalities of the lids | Ectropion<br>Entropion<br>Lagophthalmos | Ocular examination |

**Tear Film Break-Up Time**

Tear film break-up time measures the stability of the precorneal tear film and depends on the innermost mucin layer. The test is defined as the time that elapses between the end of the blink and the appearance of the first dry spot in the precorneal tear film.[60] One drop of fluorescein is instilled into the conjunctival sac and the patient is instructed to blink once and then to refrain from blinking until the test is completed. On the slit lamp under cobalt blue illumination, the observer notes the time at which the first dry spot appears. Normal tear film break-up time is 15–30 sec, and the test should be repeated a few times to establish an abnormal low value. Values below 10 sec suggest mucin deficiency.[61]

**Rose Bengal Staining**

Rose bengal stains devitalized epithelial cells and is a very sensitive stain for detection of early alterations in conjunctival epithelium secondary to dry-eye conditions.[62] It is used clinically as a 1% solution, and staining of abnormal conjunctival epithelium is usually more intense in the interpalpebral space (Fig 14.26). Recently, Feenstra and Tseng[63] demonstrated that Rose bengal is not a vital stain, and stains whenever cells are not covered by such components as albumin and mucin.

**Schirmer I Test**

The Schirmer I test is performed by placing a 5-mm-wide strip of Whatman No. 41 filter paper over the lid margin. Although imprecise, less than 5 mm in 5 minutes suggests hyposecretion; more than 5 mm suggests either normal secretion or reflex tearing compensating for deficient basal secretion.

**Schirmer Basal Secretion test**

The basal secretion test differentiates reflex from basal secretion. The conjunctiva is anesthetized with topical anesthetic. Wetting of less than 5 mm at 5 min indicates hyposecretion caused by failure of the basic secretors alone. If the Schirmer I test has shown more than 5 mm of wetting, the difference between the basal secretor and the Schirmer I test gives some indication of the effort of the reflex secretors to compensate for the failure of the basic secretors. This hypothesis, however, has been brought into some question by Jordan and Baum,[64] who suggest that most tearing is reflex in nature.

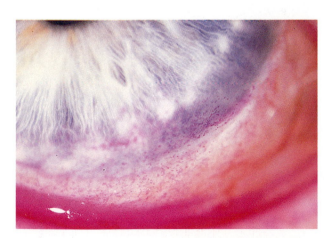

**14.26** | Typical rose bengal stain in patient with keratoconjunctivitis sicca.

Tear Lysozyme and Osmolarity Determination

Patients with KCS usually have decreased lysozyme concentration in their tears. Lysozyme concentration is more sensitive than Schirmer testing in detecting patients with dry-eye conditions.[65] In addition, higher tear osmolarity is a common finding, and values greater than 312 mOsm/L suggest that the patient has or will develop signs of KCS.[66] Despite the higher sensitivity of these tests over the Schirmer test, they are not widely used by clinicians because of the need for specialized and not readily accessible laboratory equipment.

## ABNORMALITIES OF THE LIPID LAYER

Abnormality of the lipid layer is a common cause of dry-eye symptoms and is very often overlooked. The most common cause associated with instability of the lipid layer is Meibomian gland dysfunction, which can be caused by chronic staphylococcal marginal blepharitis, acne rosacea, and seborrheic blepharitis.[67] The patient often complains of a burning sensation, more pronounced in the morning, and accumulation of foamy material in the canthus. Foreign body sensation is not as prominent a complaint as is usual in patients with dry-eye conditions due to deficiency of the aqueous layer, although under dry atmospheric conditions these patients may have significant complaints because of increased evaporation of the tear film.

Signs include crusting and collarettes around the lashes in cases with blepharitis, or a chronic inflamed eye lid margin with plugged Meibomian gland orifices whose contents are often difficult to express (Fig. 14.27). Telangiectatic vessels around the lashes should prompt further examination of the surrounding skin of the cheek and nose for evidence for acne rosacea (Fig. 14.28). The tear breakup time is often decreased, and superficial punctate epitheliopathy may be present.

## ABNORMALITIES OF THE MUCIN LAYER

Abnormalities of the mucin layer are usually related to impairment or destruction of the conjunctival goblet cells. Mucous membrane pemphigoid, chemical burns, Stevens–Johnson syndrome, and drug toxicity account for

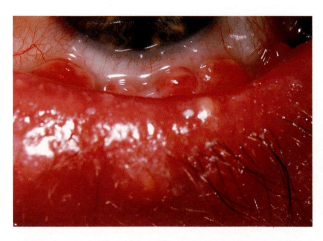

**14.27** | Acute meibomitis with plugged Meibomian gland orifices.

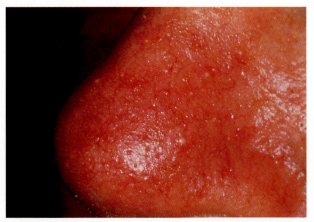

**14.28** | Typical telangiectatic vessels on the nose of a patient with acne rosacea.

most cases of mucin layer deficiency in developed countries, and trachoma and vitamin A deficiency are still major causes in underdeveloped countries (Fig. 14.29).[68] In developed countries, xerophthalmia is seen in association with cystic fibrosis, alcoholism, and eating disorders.[69,70] Burning sensation, irritation, and photophobia are usual complaints. The tear breakup time is often decreased in patients with deficiency in mucin layer production, and values under 10 sec are highly suggestive of primary mucin deficiency.[61]

It has been shown that eyes with KCS exhibit stratification or flattening of the superficial bulbar conjunctival epithelial cells, with decreased numbers of goblet cells.[71] This is a dynamic process that eventually leads to a total loss of conjunctival goblet cells and keratinization of the conjunctival and corneal surface (Fig. 14.30). On the basis of cellulose acetate impression cytology, Nelson[72] has proposed a classification for the severity of conjunctival morphologic alterations secondary to dry-eye conditions. In grade 0 the epithelial cells are small, round, and cohesive, with a nucleocytoplasmic ratio of 1:2. Goblet cells are abundant and have an intensely PAS-positive cytoplasm.

## EFFECTS OF DRY-EYE STATES ON OCULAR TISSUE
### CONJUNCTIVA

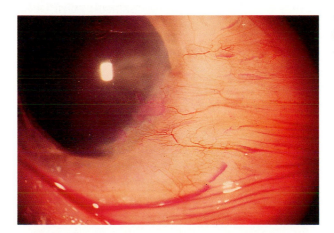

**14.29** | KCS secondary to ocular pemphigoid. Note the presence of pseudopterygium.

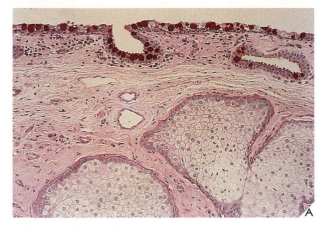
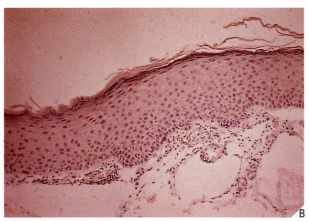

**14.30** | *A:* Normal conjunctiva with abundant PAS-stained goblet cells. *B:* Keratinization of the conjunctiva in advanced stage of KCS.

In grade 1 the epithelial cells are slightly enlarged, with some loss of cohesion and a nucleocytoplasmic ratio of 1:3. Goblet cells are decreased in number and maintain an intensely PAS-positive cytoplasm. Most patients with KCS are in this category. They usually have no symptoms and may present a Rose bengal staining of mild degree along with a Schirmer test below 5 mm. In grade 2 the epithelial cells are enlarged and polygonal, with cohesion disrupted. The nuclei are small, with a nucleocytoplasmic ratio of 1:4 or 1:5. Goblet cells are few, with poorly defined cell borders and decreased PAS staining. In grade 3 the epithelial cells are large and isolated, with pycknotic nuclei that may be absent in many cells. The nucleocytoplasmic ratio is greater than 1:6. Goblet cells are absent. These stages correspond to patients with severe symptoms, Schirmer values below 1 mm, and extensive Rose bengal staining.

CORNEA

The corneal epithelial cells may show a shift of surface cell population to smaller cells that manifest abnormal uptake of Rose bengal dye.[73] Corneal mucous plaques are a common finding in patients with KCS. They are semi-translucent and elevated. They tend to become larger in size and can be easily scraped off although they tend to recur. Corneal filaments consist of a central mucous encased by corneal epithelial cells and are easily detected by Rose bengal staining.[74] These filaments are usually seen in association with corneal mucous plaque (Fig. 14.31). The lacrimal punctae may become atrophic and undergo squamous metaplasia secondary to KCS. Sterile corneal ulceration and perforation may occur in advanced stages of KCS[75] and in severe vitamin A deficiency (Fig. 14.32).[76]

## MANAGEMENT
### MEDICAL

Artificial tears, either preserved or unpreserved, are the mainstay for treatment of KCS. Preserved artificial tears are indicated for patients with mild symptoms requiring tear replacement up to four to five times a day. If, to keep a patient comfortable, it is necessary to augment the frequency of treatment, preserved artificial tears are not recommended. Most preservatives used in artificial tear formulations, particularly benzalkonium chloride,[77] can

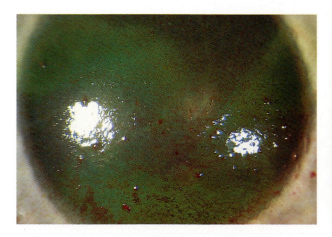

**14.31** | Cornea in advanced stage of keratoconjunctivitis sicca.

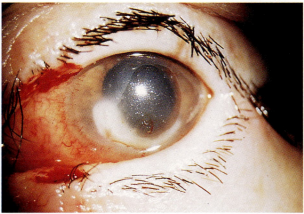

**14.32** | Corneal ulceration and scarring secondary to KCS.

cause deleterious effects on tear film stability and on the superficial epithelium, if used in excess.[78]

Patients with moderate to severe KCS may require artificial tears as often as every hour or less. The introduction of preservative-free solutions has provided great benefits to these patients by avoiding undesirable complications, such as sensitivity reactions to the preservatives and progressive keratitis medicamentosa.[79] Other than patient inconvenience, frequency of treatment is no longer a limiting factor and preservative-free artificial tears can be prescribed as often as necessary. They should also use unpreserved ointment at bedtime.

Some patients develop severe irritation secondary to mucous threads attached to the surface epithelium and may benefit from the use of acetylcysteine, a mucolytic agent.[80] The 20% solution is better tolerated if it is made alkaline by combining with an equal volume of alkaline artificial tear solution.[81]

Patients with KCS are often very vulnerable to wind and to dry atmospheric conditions. They must be made aware that in the winter time, in air-conditioned working environments, and also in long car commutes with the air conditioner on, the need for artificial tears may be increased.

The use of moisture-chamber glasses, swim goggles, or ski goggles helps to protect the eyes from the environment and increases the humidity around the eyes. At work or at home, an ultrasonic vaporizer placed near the patient may be necessary to improve humidity conditions.

## MECHANICAL

Punctal occlusion is used in an attempt to preserve the patient's own tears, and may be temporary or permanent. Temporary occlusion is useful for assessment of the efficacy of punctal occlusion and for identification of patients who will develop epiphora secondary to obliteration of the puncta. It can be achieved by placing a silicone punctal plug[82] in the inferior canaliculus, which can remain in place, or by using collagen intracanalicular inserts, which dissolve over a period of 5–7 days or less.[83] Electrodessication can also be used to achieve temporary punctal occlusion; it can last from 2 days to 2 weeks and can be repeated if necessary. Permanent punctal occlusion is achieved by inserting a fine electrocautery needle within the proximal canaliculus. This may require occlusion of both superior and inferior canaliculus to obtain therapeutic results.[84]

## SURGICAL

Surgical intervention to prevent further deterioration of dry-eye states is usually limited. Earlier procedures, such as parotid duct transplantation, have been abandoned. Lateral tarsorrhaphy is effective in reducing the area of ocular surface exposed, decreasing evaporation of tears and preserving vision. It is indicated for patients who are under maximal topical medication and who have undergone permanent punctal occlusion without amelioration of their symptoms. For the few patients who do not benefit from these measures, total tarsorrhaphy may be required to preserve the globe while sacrificing the vision. If it is the patient's only seeing eye, a keratoprosthesis can be used as a last attempt to preserve vision.

An uncommon but sight-threatening occurrence is sterile corneal perforation in patients with Sjögren syndrome. Small perforations should be managed with therapeutic soft contact lenses, along with umpreserved artificial tears and prophylactic preservative-free topical antibiotics because of increased risk of infection.[85] Isobutylcyanoacrylate can be employed to seal the wound and to restore the anterior chamber.[75] Larger perforations usually require surgical intervention. If Descement's membrane is intact, a lamellar graft is indicated; otherwise, a penetrating keratoplasty may be required.

Surgery is effective in correcting dry-eye conditions secondary to abnormalities of the eyelids such as ectropion, entropion, and irregularities of the lid margin.

In undeveloped countries, xerophthalmia still affects approximately 5 million children a year and about a quarter million are becoming blind due to keratomalacia.[68] Unlike corneal perforations associated with Sjögren syndrome, the devastating effects of vitamin A deficiency are totally preventable by oral administration of 200,000 IU on 2 successive days.

# 15 CORNEAL AND EXTERNAL EYE MANIFESTATIONS OF SYSTEMIC DISEASE

## Joel Sugar

Numerous systemic disorders, congenital or acquired, affect the anterior segment of the eye. Rather than an exhaustive review of such disorders, this chapter presents tabular summaries of various categories of disease. In some circumstances it is more helpful to group them by biochemical (e.g., mucopolysaccharidoses) or causative (congenital) categories and in others by anatomic categories (e.g., hepatocorneal syndromes). Many disorders have been covered earlier in this volume and are not reviewed again here. As some disorders fit into more than one category, some redundancy is inevitable.

## CONGENITAL DISORDERS

This category refers to some nonmetabolic generalized disorders present at birth and affecting the cornea and external eye. Subdivision of these disorders is, again, somewhat arbitrary. Figure 15.1 reviews some craniofacial malformation syndromes that

### Figure 15.1. Craniofacial Malformation Syndromes with Corneal Involvement

| SYNDROME | SYSTEMIC MANIFESTATIONS | OCULAR FINDINGS |
|---|---|---|
| Crouzon and Apert | Craniofacial malformation and syndactyly (Apert) | Shallow orbits, decreased motility, secondary corneal exposure |
| Meyer–Schwickerath (oculo-dentodigital dysplasia) (Fig. 15.2) | Syndactyly, dysplastic tooth enamel | Microphthalmos and microcornea |
| Goldenhar | Facial asymmetry, vertebral anomalies, ear deformities | Limbal dermoids, microphthalmos, anophthalmos, lid notching |
| Hallerman–Streiff | Facial malformation, hypoplastic mandible, short stature, skin atrophy | Microphthalmos, spontaneously resorbing cataracts, macular pigment changes |

have associated corneal involvement (Fig. 15.2). Patients with craniofacial abnormalities commonly have ocular findings, and their treatment requires a multispeciality approach involving at times ophthalmologists, neurosurgeons, facial plastic surgeons, and others.

Categorization of chromosomal disorders is based on the location of the chromosomal abnormality in the genetic material (Fig. 15.3).[1-3] In the future, more sophisticated genetic techniques will further subdivide these

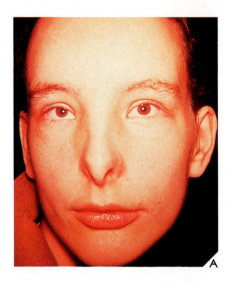

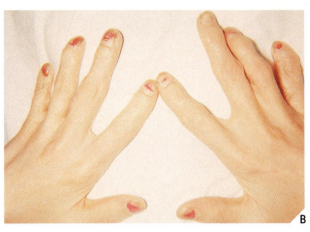

**15.2** | Meyer–Schwickerath syndrome. *A:* Facial appearance and bilateral microphthalmos. *B:* Finger deformities.

## Figure 15.3. Chromosomal Disorders with Corneal Manifestations

| GENETIC FINDINGS | SYSTEMIC MANIFESTATIONS | OCULAR MANIFESTATIONS |
|---|---|---|
| 13q- | MC, FA, absent thumbs | H, P, EF, M, retinoblastoma |
| 18p- | Brachycephaly, GR, MR | P, EF, H, CO, keratoconus, M |
| 18q- | GR, MR, FA, MC | H, EF, nystagmus, CO, M, corneal staphyloma, microcornea |
| 18r | GR, MR, FA, MC | Same as 18p-, 18q- |
| 4p- Wolf–Hirschhorn syndrome | GR, MC, micrognathia, hypotonia, seizures | H, P, M, strabismus, cataract |
| ring D chromosome | MR, MC, FA | P, EF, M, strabismus, nystagmus |
| Turner syndrome (45X0) | Female, short stature, webbed neck | P, EF, strabismus, rarely microcornea, blue sclera, CO |
| Trisomy 13 (Fig. 15.4) (Patau syndrome) | MC, cleft lip and palate, low-set ears | M, CO, Peters anomaly, cataract, retinal dysplasia |
| Trisomy 18 (Edwards syndrome) | Low birth weight, failure to thrive, brain hypoplasia, cardiac, GI, renal, musculoskeletal anomalies | CO, P, EF, M, colobomas, cataract, retinal dysplasia |
| Trisomy 21 (Down syndrome) | Cardiac defects, MR, short stature, characteristic facies | Shortened, slanted palpebral fissure, neonatal ectropion, later trichiasis and entropion, keratoconus, cataract |
| Partial trisomy 22 (Cat eye syndrome) | MR, MC, cardiac anomalies, ear anomalies, anal atresia | M, H, colobomas |

- = deletion; CO = corneal opacity; EF = epicanthal folds; FA = facial malformation; GR = growth retardation; H = hypertelorism; M = microphthalmos; MC = microcephaly; MR = mental retardation; P = ptosis; p = short arm of chromosome; q = long arm; r = ring.

categories into more specific genetic disorders. The striking feature about these disorders is the frequent similarity of ophthalmic findings despite very different chromosomal abnormalities.

A number of inherited connective tissue disorders have corneal manifestations. The best known to the ophthalmologist are listed in Figure 15.5 and are classified by syndrom. All of these have been discussed elsewhere in this volume.

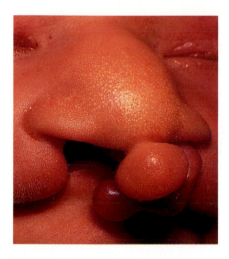

**15.4** | Trisomy 13. Note lip clefting. The globes were very small with corneal opacities and retinal dysplasia.

## Figure 15.5. Inherited Connective Tissue Disorders with Corneal Manifestations

| DISEASE | BIOCHEMICAL DEFECT | SYSTEMIC MANIFESTATIIONS | OCULAR FINDINGS |
|---|---|---|---|
| Marfan | Fibrillin gene mutation[14] | Long extremities, lax joints, aortic/mitral dilation, aortic dissection | Megalocornea, lens subluxation, high myopia, retinal detachment |
| Osteogenesis imperfecta (Fig. 15.6) | Type I procollagen[15] | Bone deformities, otosclerosis, dental anomalies | Blue sclera, keratoconus, megalocornea, optic nerve compression |
| Ehlers–Danlos (Type VI) | Lysyl hydroxylase deficiency | Skin stretching, scarring, joint hypermobility, scoliosis | Blue sclera, keratoconus keratoglobus, lens subluxation, myopia, ocular fragility to trauma |

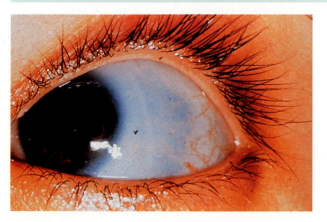

**15.6** | Osteogenesis imperfecta. Note the subtle blue sclera.

## METABOLIC DISORDERS

A number of metabolic disorders, genetic in origin, affect the external eye and the cornea.[4] In general, these disorders are autosomal recessive with a single enzyme deficiency. Chromosomal localization and gene defects have been described in many of these entities. Unlike most of the corneal dystrophies, these usually involve more than one layer of cornea, affect the peripheral as well as the central cornea, and are progressive. This group is subdivided according to the biochemical abnormality found.

### Figure 15.7. Disorders of Protein and Amino Acid Metabolism

| Disorder | Enzyme Deficiency | Metabolite Accumulated | Mode of Inheritance | Ocular Manifestations | Systemic Manifestations |
|---|---|---|---|---|---|
| Cystinosis (Fig. 15.8) | Probably abnormality in transport of cysteine or cystine across lysosomal membranes | Cystine | Autosomal recessive | All forms: conjunctival and corneal cystine crystal deposition (needle-shaped, refractile polychromatic crystals in full thickness of peripheral corneal and anterior central stroma), band keratopathy, photophobia. Infantile and adolescent forms: patchy retinal pigment abnormalities, occasional macular changes | Infantile form, renal failure, death; Adolescent, renal failure; Adult, no renal failure |
| Tyrosinemia type II (tyrosinosis, Richner-Hanhart syndrome) | Tyrosine aminotransferase | Tyrosine | Autosomal recessive | Dendritiform corneal epithelial changes (branches or snowflake opacities), red eye, photophobia | Palmar-plantar hyperkeratosis, mental retardation |
| Alkaptonuria (Fig. 15.9) | Homogentisic acid oxidase | Homogentisic acid | Autosomal recessive | Triangular patches of intrascleral pigmentation near insertion of horizontal rectus muscles, "oil-droplet" opacities in limbal corneal epithelium and Bowman's layer, pigmented pingueculae, irregular pigmented granules in episclera, no functional changes | Joint pain and stiffness |
| Wilson's disease (Fig. 15.10) | Defective excretion of copper from hepatic lysosomes | Copper | Autosomal recessive | Kayser-Fleischer ring, "sunflower" cataract | Liver dysfunction, spasticity, behavior disturbance |
| Lattice dystrophy type II (Meretoja syndrome) | Gelsolin gene defect | Amyloid | Autosomal dominant | Lattice dystrophy, ptosis, glaucoma | Progressive cranial neuropathy, cardiac disease |

Adapted from Sugar J: Metabolic disorders of the cornea, in Kaufman HE, Barron BA, McDonald MB, Waltman SR (eds): *The Cornea.* New York: Churchill Livingstone, 1988.

Disorders of protein and amino acid metabolism are grouped together, although they are actually quite diverse both biochemically and clinically. Figure 15.7 lists a number of them, and they also are covered in Figures 15.8–15.10.

The mucopolysaccharidoses, reviewed in Figure 15.11, are a group of disorders in which glycosaminoglycans or mucopolysaccharides accumulate in lysosomes. Glycosaminoglycans are carbohydrates made up of chains of uronic acids, amino sugars, and neutral sugars. These are linked to protein to form proteoglycans which make up the ground substance of the cornea. Keratan sulfate, chondroitin sulfate, and chondroitin-4-sulfate are found in normal cornea. Dermatan sulfate is not normally found but is present in corneal scars. In the mucopolysaccharidoses, a deficiency in catabolic enzymes leads to accumulation of glycosaminoglycans. Accumulation of

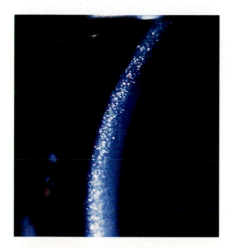

**15.8** | Cystinosis. Numerous corneal crystals are present in photophobic patient with adolescent cystinosis.

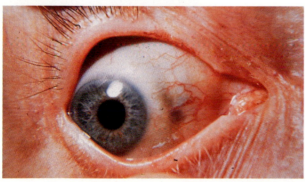

**15.9** | Alkaptonuria. Dark pigmentation can be observed at the medial rectus insertion in patient with ochronosis.

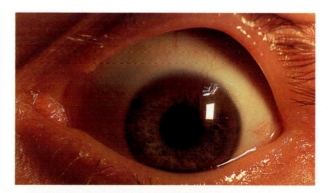

**15.10** | Wilson's disease. Kayser–Fleischer ring in 24-year-old woman with progressive spasticity and dementia.

dermatan sulfate (Fig. 15.12) and keratan sulfate in the cornea leads to corneal clouding, whereas heparan sulfate accumulation leads to dysfunction of the retina and central nervous system.

The sphingolipidoses occur due to decreased activity of enzymes that catabolize sphingolipids. Accumulation of sphingolipids leads to the abnormalities shown in Figures 15.13 and 15.14. Although omitted in our presentation, a number of sphingolipidoses without corneal abnormalities have been described.

## Figure 15.11. The Mucopolysaccharidoses

| DISORDER | ENZYME DEFICIENCY | METABOLITE ACCUMULATED | MODE OF INHERITANCE | OCULAR MANIFESTATIONS | SYSTEMIC MANIFESTATIONS |
|---|---|---|---|---|---|
| MPS I-H (Hurler syndrome) (Fig. 15.12) | α-L-iduronidase | Heparan sulfate Dermatan sulfate | Autosomal recessive | Corneal clouding, pigmentary retinopathy, optic atrophy, trabecular involvement | Gargoyle facies, mental retardation, dwarfism, skeletal dysplasia |
| MPS I-S (Scheie syndrome) | α-L-iduronidase | Heparan sulfate Dermatan sulfate | Autosomal recessive | Corneal clouding, pigmentary retinopathy, optic atrophy, glaucoma | Coarse facies, claw-like hands, aortic valve disease |
| MPS I-H/S (Hurler–Scheie) | α-L-iduronidase | Heparan sulfate Dermatan sulfate | Autosomal recessive | Corneal clouding, pigmentary retinopathy, optic atrophy | More severe than I-S, less than I-H |
| MPS II (Hunter syndrome) | Iduronate sulfate sulfatase (iduronate sulfatase) | Heparan sulfate Dermatan sulfate | X-linked recessive | Rare corneal clouding, pigmentary retinopathy, optic atrophy | Similar to I-H with less bony deformity |
| MPS III (Sanfilippo syndrome) | A: heparan-S-sulfaminidase (heparan sulfate N-sulfatase) | Heparan sulfate | Autosomal recessive | All Forms: clinically clear cornea, occasional slit lamp corneal opacities (mucopolysaccharide accumulation in intracytoplasmic vacuoles in keratocytes, endothelium, and epithelium), pigmentary retinopathy, optic atrophy | All forms: mild dysmorphism, progressive dementia |
| | B: α-N-acetyl-glucosaminidase (N-acetyl——D-glucosaminidase) | Heparan sulfate | Autosomal recessive | | |
| | C: acetyl-CoA——glusosaminidase-N-N-acetyl-transferase | Heparan sulfate | Autosomal recessive | | |
| | D:N-acetylglucosamine-6-sulfate sulfatase | Heparan sulfate | Autosomal recessive | | |
| MPS IV (Morquio syndrome) | A: N-acetyl-galactosamine-6-sulfate sulfatase | Keratan sulfate | Autosomal recessive | Corneal clouding, optic atrophy | Severe bony deformity, aortic valve disease, normal intelligence |
| | B: β-galactosidase | | Autosomal recessive | | |
| MPS V (reclassified as MPS I-S) | — | — | — | — | — |
| MPS VI (Maroteaux–Lamy syndrome) | N-acetylglucosamine-4-sulfate sulfatase (arylsulfatase B) | Dermatan sulfate | Autosomal recessive | Corneal clouding, optic atrophy | Similar to I-H, but normal intellect |
| MPS VII (Sly syndrome) | β-Glucuronidase | Dermatan sulfate Heparan sulfate | Autosomal recessive | Corneal clouding | Similar to I-H |

MPS = mucopolysaccharidosis.
Adapted from Sugar J: Metabolic disorders of the cornea, in Kaufman HE, Barron BA, McDonald MB, Waltman SR (eds): *The Cornea.* New York: Churchill Livingstone, 1988.

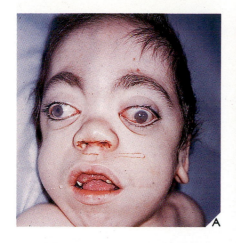

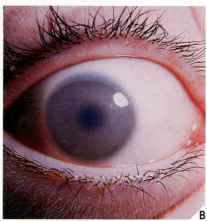

**15.12** | Hurler syndrome (MPS I-H). *A:* Typical facial appearance. *B:* Corneal clouding.

## Figure 15.13. The Sphingolipidoses

| DISORDER | ENZYME DEFICIENCY | METABOLITE ACCUMULATED | MODE OF INHERITANCE | OCULAR MANIFESTATIONS | SYSTEMIC MANIFESTATIONS |
|---|---|---|---|---|---|
| $G_{M2}$ gangliosidosis II (Sandhoff's disease) | Hexosaminidase A and B | $G_{M2}$-ganglioside | Autosomal recessive | Membrane-bound vacuoles within corneal keratocytes, cherry-red macula | Psychomotor retardation, hepatosplenomegaly |
| Metachromatic leukodystrophy (Austin's juvenile form) | Arylsulfatases A, B, and C and other sulfatases | Sulfatide | Autosomal recessive | Corneal clouding | Mental retardation, seizures |
| Fabry's disease (Fig. 15.14) | α-galactosidase | Ceramide trihexoside | X-linked recessive | Conjunctival and retinal vascular tortuosity, white granular anterior subcapsular lens opacities, oculomotor abnormalities, whorl-like corneal epithelial changes (cornea verticillata) | Renal failure, peripheral neuropathy |

Adapted from Sugar J: Metabolic disorders of the cornea, in Kaufman HE, Barron BA, McDonald MB, Waltman SR (eds): *The Cornea.* New York: Churchill Livingstone, 1988.

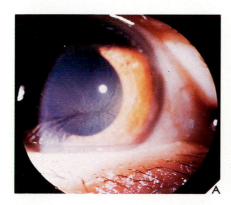

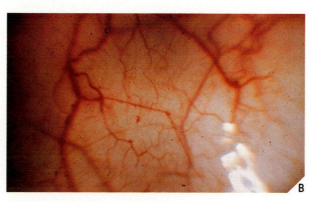

**15.14** | Fabry's disease. *A:* Cornea verticillata. *B:* Conjunctival vascular tortuosity.

## Figure 15.15. The Dyslipoproteinemias

| Disorder | Enzyme Deficiency | Metabolite Accumulated | Mode of Inheritance | Ocular Manifestations | Systemic Manifestations |
|---|---|---|---|---|---|
| LCAT deficiency | Lecithin-cholesterol acyl-transferase | Free cholesterol | Autosomal recessive | Dense peripheral arcus, diffuse greyish dots in central stroma, no visual changes | Atherosclerosis, renal insufficiency |
| Tangier disease | Unknown | Triglycerides (low HDL, cholesterol, and phospholipids) | Autosomal recessive | Fine dot corneal clouding, no visual changes, no arcus | Lymphadenopathy, hepatosplenomegaly, coronary artery disease |
| Fish eye disease | Unknown | Triglycerides, VLDL | Unknown (rare) | Progressive gray-white-yellow dot corneal clouding, increased corneal thickness | None |
| Hyperlipoproteinemia I (Fig. 15.16) (hyperchylomicronemia) | Lipoprotein lipase | Triglycerides, chylomicrons | Autosomal recessive | Lipemia retinalis, palpebral eruptive xanthomata | Xanthomas |
| Hyperlipoproteinemia II | | | | | |
| IIa. Hyper-β-lipoproteinemia | Thought to be defective or absent LDL receptors | LDL, cholesterol | Autosomal dominant | Both forms: corneal arcus, conjunctival xanthomata, xanthelasma | Coronary artery disease |
| IIb. Hyper-β- and hyper-pre-β-lipoproteinemia | Unknown | LDL, VLDL, cholesterol, triglycerides | Autosomal dominant | | |
| Hyperlipoproteinemia III (dys-β-lipoproteinemia) (broad beta disease) | Defective remnant metabolism in the liver caused by an abnormality in apo-E | VLDL remnants, cholesterol, triglycerides | Autosomal recessive | Arcus, xanthelasma, lipemia retinalis | Peripheral vascular disease, diabetes |
| Hyperlipoproteinemia IV (hyperpre-β-lipoproteinemia) | Unknown | Triglycerides, VLDL, cholesterol | Autosomal dominant | Arcus, xanthelasma, lipemia retinalis | Vascular disease, diabetes mellitus |
| Hyperlipoproteinemia V (hyper-pre-β-lipoproteinemia and hyperchylomicronemia) | Unknown | VLDL, cholesterol, triglycerides, chylomicrons | Unknown | Lipemia retinalis, no arcus | Xanthomas, hepatosplenomegaly |

Adapted from Sugar J: Metabolic disorders of the cornea, in Kaufman HE, Barron BA, McDonald MB, Waltman SR (eds): *The Cornea*. New York: Churchill Livingstone, 1988.

## DYSLIPOPROTEINEMIAS

A number of disorders of lipid metabolism have been described. Many of them have ocular manifestations, either with accumulation of lipids in the cornea, in the retinal blood vessels, or in the skin of the eyelids. These are reviewed in Figure 15.15. The categories described here for the hyperlipidemias are the classic types, slowly being replaced by more specific descriptions of the pathophysiologic processes involved.[5]

## MUCOLIPIDOSES

The mucolipidoses are disorders with abnormalities in the carbohydrate moiety of both glycoproteins and glycolipids. Oligosaccharides accumulate and

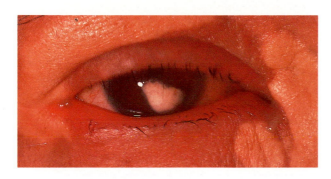

**15.16** I Xanthoma tuberosum involving the eyelids and cornea in a hyperlipoproteinemic patient.

## Figure 15.17. The Mucolipidoses

| DISORDER | ENZYME DEFI-CIENCY | METABOLITE ACCUMULATED | MODE OF INHERITANCE | OCULAR MANIFESTATIONS | SYSTEMIC MANI-FESTATIONS |
|---|---|---|---|---|---|
| MLS I (dysmor-phic sialido-sis, Spranger syndrome) | Glycoprotein sialidase (neu-raminidase) | Unknown | Autosomal recessive | Macular cherry-red spot, tortuous reti-nal and conjuncti-val vessels, spoke-like lens apacities, progressive corneal clouding | Coarse facies, retardation, hearing loss |
| MLS II (I-cell dis-ease) | GluNac-1-phos-photrans-ferase | Unknown | Autosomal recessive | Small orbits, hypoplastic supraorbital ridges and prominent eyes, glaucoma, megalocornea, corneal clouding | Hurler-like facies, mental retar-dation |
| MLS III (pseudo-Hurler's poly-dystrophy) | GluNac-1-phos-photrans-ferase | Unknown | Autosomal recessive | Corneal clouding | Milder growth and mental retardation |
| MLS IV (Berman syndrome) | Ganglioside sialidase | Sialogangglio-sides, mucopolys accharides | Autosomal recessive | Corneal clouding, reti-nal degeneration | Slowed psy-chomotor development |
| Goldberg syndrome (galactosiali-dosis) | Sialidase, β-D-galactosidase | Unknown | Autosomal recessive | Macular cherry-red spot, diffuse mild corneal clouding | Seizures, mental retardation |
| Mannosidosis and fucosi-dosis | α-D-mannosi-dase, α-D-fucosidase | Unknown | Autosomal recessive | No corneal abnormal-ities, or mild corneal clouding | Coarse facies, mental retardation, hearing loss |

MLS = mucolipidosis (oligosaccharidosis).
Adapted from Sugar J: Metabolic disorders of the cornea, in Kaufman HE, Barron BA, McDonald MB, Waltman SR (eds): *The Cornea*. New York: Churchill Livingstone, 1988.

the patients develop changes similar to those seen in the mucopolysacchari-doses and sphingolipidoses. These are reviewed in Figure 15.17.

## OCULAR ANATOMIC DISORDERS

As mentioned at the beginning of this chapter, it is often useful to group dis-orders that involve a nonocular organ and the eye for purposes of defining a group of potential causes of such an association. For example, the patient with renal disease or with multiple skin tumors referred for ocular evaluation.

The corneorenal syndromes grouped in this section (Fig. 15.18) are

### Figure 15.18. Corneorenal Syndromes

| SYNDROME | SYSTEMIC MANIFESTATIONS | OCULAR FINDINGS |
|---|---|---|
| Alport | Renal failure, hearing loss | Posterior polymorphous corneal dystrophy, juvenile arcus, pigment dispersion, lenticonus, retinal pigmentary changes |
| Cystinosis | Infantile form—renal failure, death. Intermediate form—renal failure. Adult—no renal failure | See Figure 15.7 |
| Fabry | Renal failure, peripheral neuropathy | See Figure 15.13 |
| Lowe (Fig. 15.19) | Mental retardation, amino acid uria, renal tubular acidosis, angiokeratomas | Corneal keloids, glaucoma, cataracts |
| Wegener's granulomatosis | Granulomatous vasculitis of lungs, kidneys, nasopharynx | Marginal keratitis, scleritis, episcleritis |
| Wilm's tumor-aniridia (Miller syndrome) | Wilm's tumor, mental retardation, craniofacial anomalies, growth retardation | Superficial corneal opacity and vascularization, aniridia, glaucoma, foveal hypoplasia, optic nerve hypoplasia |
| Zellweger | Craniofacial anomalies, hypotonia, seizures, severe retardation, hepatic degeneration, cystic kidneys, cardiac defects, early death | Axenfeld's anomaly, corneal clouding, glaucoma, retinal degeneration |

**15.19** | Lowe syndrome. Corneal keloid is present in aphakic eye of patient.

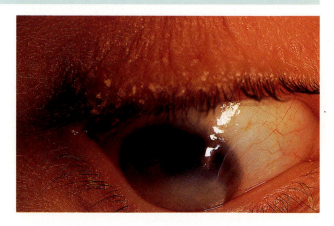

very disparate, but have the combined presence of both corneal abnormalities and significant renal disease.[6–8]

The hepatocorneal syndromes[8,9] are significantly less common. Figure 15.20 covers only three, including Gaucher syndrome (Fig. 15.21).

Cutaneous disorders associated with anterior segment ocular disease

### Figure 15.20. Hepatocorneal Syndromes

| DISORDER | SYSTEMIC MANIFESTATIONS | OCULAR MANIFESTATIONS |
| --- | --- | --- |
| Gaucher (Fig. 15.21) | Hepatosplenomegaly, bone pain, accumulation of glucocerebroside | Prominent pinguecu-lae, white deposits in corneal epithelium, vitreous opacities, paramacular gray ring |
| Wilson's disease | Liver dysfunction, neurologic dysfunction with dysarthria, spasticity, behavior disturbances | Kayser–Fleischer ring See Figure 15.7 |
| Zellweger | See Figure 15.18 | See Figure 15.18 |

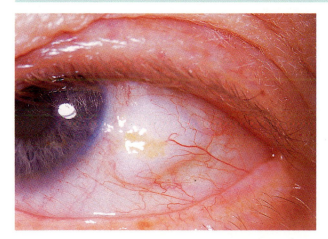

**15.21** | Gaucher syndrome. Prominent pingueculum is visible, presumably caused by accumulation of lipid-laden histiocytes.

are numerous. Many of these are discussed in Chapters 1 and 2. Some additional syndromes are mentioned in Figures 15.22 and 15.23 as well.

This nonencyclopedic and extremely brief review highlights just some of the many systemic conditions that affect the cornea and external eye.

## Figure 15.22. Cutaneous Disorders

| DISORDER | CUTANEOUS/SYSTEMIC FINDINGS | OCULAR MANIFESTATIONS |
|---|---|---|
| Basal cell nevus syndrome | Multiple basal cell carcinomas, jaw cysts, bony anomalies | Multiple basal cell carcinomas of the eyelids, hypertelorism |
| Xeroderma pigmentosum | Basal cell carcinoma, squamous cell carcinomas, and malignant melanomas develop in sun-exposed areas | Lid neoplasms, conjunctival and corneal neoplasia, corneal exposure, drying |
| Ichthyosis (multiple types) (Fig. 15.23) | Scaly skin | Eyelid and lash scaling (all types) Ectropion with corneal exposure (lamellar ichthyosis) |
| KID syndrome (keratitis-ichthyosis-deafness) | Ichthyosis, deafness | Keratoconjunctivits with corneal pannus formation |
| Epidermolysis bullosa (numerous types) | Skin blistering, in severe dystrophic type, contractures | Corneal epithelial cysts, blebs, corneal erosions, corneal scarring, conjunctival bullae, eyelid deformities |
| EEC (ectrodactyly-ectodermal dysplasia-clefting) | Lobster claw deformity of hands and feet, ectodermal dysplasia, cleft lip and palate | Dysplastic meibomian glands, blepharitis, corneal pannus formation, corneal scarring |
| Porphyria (numerous types) | Photosensitivity of skin | Corneal, conjunctival, and eyelid scarring, scleral necrosis |
| Richner-Hanhart syndrome (tyrosinemia Type II) | See Figure 15.7 | See Figure 15.7 |

**15.23** | Ichthyosis. Secondary corneal involvement is shown along with significant eyelid skin scaling.

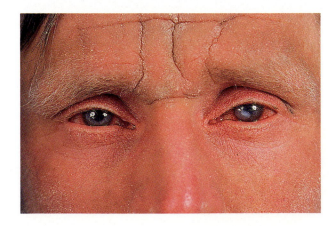

# REFERENCES

1. Sevel D: A reappraisal of the development of the eyelids. *Eye 1988;2:123–129.*
2. Wulc AE, Dryden RM, Khatchaturian T: Where is the gray line? *Arch Ophthalmol 1987;105:1092–1098.*
3. Gioia VM, Linberg JV, McCormick SA: The anatomy of the lateral canthal tendon. *Arch Ophthalmol 1987;105:529–532.*
4. Robin JB, Jester JV, Nobe J, et al: In vivo transillumination biomicroscopy and photography of meibomian gland dysfunction. *Ophthalmology 1985;92:1423–1426.*
5. Straus SE: Clinical and biological differences between recurrent herpes simplex virus and varicella-zoster virus infections. *JAMA 1989;262:3455–3458.*
6. Cobo LM, Foulks GN, Liesegang T, et al: Oral acyclovir in the treatment of acute herpes zoster ophthalmicus. *Ophthalmology 1986;93:763–770.*
7. Gonnering RS, Kronish GW: Treatment of periorbital molluscum contagiosum by incision and curettage. *Ophthal Surg 1988;19:325–327.*
8. Barr CC, Gamel JW: Blastomycosis of the eyelid. *Arch Ophthalmol 1986;104:96–97.*
9. Kincaid MC: Pediculosis and phthiriasis, in Fraunfelder FT, Roy FH (eds): *Current Ocular Therapy 3.* Philadelphia: WB Saunders, 1990, 115–117.
10. English FP, Cohn D, Groeneveld ER: Demodetic mites and chalazia. *Am J Ophthalmol 1985;100:482–483.*
11. McCulley JP, Dougherty JM, Deneau DG: Chronic blepharitis: classification and mechanisms, in Suran A, Gery I, Nussenblatt RB (eds): *Immunology of the Eye. Workshop III.* 1981, 55–72.
12. Robin JB, Nobe JR, Suarez E, et al: Meibomian gland evaluation in patients with extended wear soft contact lens deposits. *CLAO J 1986;12:95–98.*
13. Mathers WD, Jester JV, Shields WJ: Differentiation of chronic blepharitis by meibomian function: A new classification system. *Ophthalmology 1990;(suppl 97):138.*
14. Osgood J, Dougherty J, McCulley JP: Meibum sterol and wax ester fatty acids in chronic blepharitis. *Invest Ophthalmol Vis Sci 1990;(suppl 31):299.*
15. Epstein GA, Putterman AM: Combined excision and drainage with intralesional corticosteroid injection in the treatment of chronic chalazia. *Arch Ophthalmol 1988;106:514–516.*
16. Foster CS, Calonge M: Atopic keratoconjunctivitis. *Ophthalmology 1990;97:992–1000.*
17. Bergin DJ, McCord CD, Berger T, et al: Blepharochalasis. *Br J Ophthalmol 1988;72:863–867.*
18. van Bijsterveld OP: Bacterial proteases in moraxella angular conjunctivitis. *Am J Ophthalmol 1971;72:181–184.*
19. Tames SM, Goldenring JM: Madarosis from cocaine use. *N Engl J Med 1986;314:1324.*
20. Nerad JA, Whitaker DC: Periocular basal cell carcinoma in adults 35 years of age and younger. *Am J Ophthalmol 1988;106:723–729.*
21. Mohs FE: Micrographic surgery for the microscopically controlled excision of eyelid cancers. *Arch Ophthalmol 1986;104:901–909.*
22. Reifler DM, Hornblass A: Squamous cell carcinoma of the eyelid. *Surv Ophthalmol 1986;30:349–365.*
23. Doxanas MT, Iliff WJ, Iliff NT, Green WR: Squamous cell carcinoma of the eyelids. *Ophthalmology 1987;94:538–541.*
24. Kass LG, Hornblass A: Sebaceous carcinoma of the ocular adnexa. *Surv Ophthalmol 1989;33:477–490.*
25. Lisman RD, Jakobiec FA, Small P: Sebaceous carcinoma of the eyelids. The role of adjunctive cryotherapy in the management of conjunctival pagetoid spread. *Ophthalmology 1989;96:1021–1026.*
26. Weiner JM, Henderson PN, Roche J: Metastatic eyelid carcinoma. *Am J Ophthalmol 1986;101:252–254.*
27. Mansour AM, Hidayat AA: Metastatic eyelid disease. *Ophthalmology 1987;94:667–670.*

**CHAPTER 1**
THE EYELIDS

28. Arnold AC, Bullock JD, Foos RY: Metastatic eyelid carcinoma. *Ophthalmology 1985;92:114–118.*

29. Jakobiec FA, Knowles DM: An overview of ocular adnexal lymphoid tumors. *Trans Am Ophthalmol Soc 1989;87:420–444.*

30. Kivela T, Tarkkanen A: The Merkel cell and associated neoplasms in the eyelids and periocular region. *Surv Ophthalmol 1990;35:171–187.*

## CHAPTER 2
## THE CONJUNCTIVA

1. Lavker RM, Dong G, Schermer A, et al: Limbal involvement of corneal epithelial differentiation: A model (abstr). *Invest Ophthalmol Vis Sci 1986;27(suppl):251.*

2. Thoft RA, Friend J: The X, Y, Z hypothesis of corneal epithelial maintenance (letter). *Invest Ophthalmol Vis Sci 1983;24:1442–1443.*

3. Kessing SV: On the conjunctival papillae and follicles. *Acta Ophthalmol 1966;44:846–852.*

4. Greiner JV, Covington HI, Allansmith MR: Surface morphology of the human upper tarsal conjunctiva. *Am J Ophthalmol 1977;83:892–905.*

5. Kessing SV: Mucous gland system of the conjunctiva: A quantitative normal anatomical study. *Acta Ophthalmol 1968;95(suppl):1–133.*

6. Tseng SCG: Staging of conjunctival squamous metaplasia by impression cytology. *Ophthalmology 1985;92:728–733.*

7. Tseng SCG, Maumenee AE, Stark WJ, et al: Topical retinoid treatment for various dry-eye disorders. *Ophthalmology 1985;92:717–727.*

8. Dilly PN: On the nature and the role of the subsurface vesicles in the outer epithelial cells of the conjunctiva. *Br J Ophthalmol 1985;69:477–481.*

9. Greiner JV, Kenyon KR, Henriquez AS, et al: Mucus secretory vesicles in conjunctival epithelial cells of wearers of contact lenses. *Arch Ophthalmol 1980;98:1843–1846.*

10. Maurice DM: Electrical potential and ion transport across the conjunctiva. *Exp Eye Res 1973;15:527–532.*

11. Baum JL: A histochemical study of corneal respiratory enzymes. *Arch Ophthalmol 1963;70:59–68.*

12. Goldenhar M: Associations malformatives de l'oeil et de l'oreille, en particulier le syndrome dermoide epibulbaire—appendices auriculaires—fistula auris congénita et ses relations avec la dysostose mandibulo-faciale. *J Genet Hum 1952;1:243–282.*

13. Sugar HS: The oculoauriculovertebral dysplasia syndrome of Goldenhar. *Am J Ophthalmol 1966;62:678–682.*

14. Cogan DG, Kuwabara T, Howard J: The nonelastic nature of pingueculas. *Arch Ophthalmol 1959;61:388–389.*

15. Spencer WH: *Ophthalmic Pathology: An Atlas and Textbook,* Vol 1, ed 3. Philadelphia: WB Saunders, 1985, 174–176.

16. Singh G, Wilson MR, Foster CS: Long-term follow-up study of mitomycin eye drops as adjunctive treatment for pterygia and its comparison with conjunctival autograft transplantation. *Cornea 1990;9:331–334.*

17. Hayasaka S, Noda S, Yamamoto Y, et al: Postoperative instillation of mitomycin C in the treatment of recurrent pterygium. *Ophthalmic Surg 1989;20:580–583.*

18. Singh G, Wilson MR, Foster CS: Mitomycin eye drops as treatment for pterygium. *Ophthalmology 1988;95:813–821.*

19. Spencer WH: *Ophthalmic Pathology: An Atlas and Textbook,* Vol 1, ed 3. Philadelphia: WB Saunders, 1985, 176–177.

20. Duke-Elder S (ed): *System of Ophthalmology,* Vol VIII. *Diseases of the Outer Eye.* Part I. *Conjunctiva.* St. Louis: CV Mosby, 1965, 585–586.

21. Duke-Elder S (ed): *System of Ophthalmology.* Vol VIII. *Diseases of the Outer Eye.* Part I. *Conjunctiva.* St. Louis: CV Mosby, 1965, 167–176.

22. Wan WL, Farkas GC, May WN, et al: The clinical characteristics and course of adult gonococcal conjunctivitis. *Am J Ophthalmol 1986;102:575–583.*

23. Ullman S, Roussel TJ, Culbertson WW, et al: *Neisseria gonorrhoeae* keratoconjunctivitis. *Ophthalmology 1987;94:525–531.*

24. Vastine DW, West CE, Yamashiroya H, et al: Simultaneous nosocomial and community outbreak of epidemic keratoconjunctivitis with types 8 and 19 adenovirus. *Trans Am Acad Ophthalmol Otolaryngol 1976;81:Op826–840.*

25. Dawson CR, Sheppard JD: Follicular conjunctivitis, in Tasman W, Jaeger EA (eds): *Duane's Clinical Ophthalmology,* Vol 4. Philadelphia: JB Lippincott, 1990, 10.

26. Anonymous: A technique for rapid epidemiologic assessment—Nevada. *MMWR 1982;31:61–63.*

27. Chandler JW, Alexander ER, Pheiffer TA, et al: Ophthalmia neonatorum associated with maternal chlamydial infections. *Trans Am Acad Ophthalmol Otolaryngol 1977;83:Op302–308.*

28. Arffa RC: *Grayson's Diseases of the Cornea,* ed 3. St. Louis: Mosby–Year Book, 1991, 114–116.

29. Rapoza PA, Chandler JW: Neonatal conjunctivitis: Diagnosis and treatment, in *Focal Points 1988: Clinical Modules for Ophthalmologists,* Vol VI. Module 1. San Francisco: American Academy of Ophthalmology, 1988, 5–6.

30. Chandler JW, Rapoza PA: Ophthalmia neonatorum. *Int Ophthalmol Clin 1990;30:36–38.*

31. Fransen L, Nsanze H, Klauss V, et al: Ophthalmia neonatorum in Nairobi, Kenya: The roles of *Neisseria gonorrhoeae* and *Chlamydia trachomatis. J Infect Dis 1986;153:862–869.*

32. Forbes GB, Forbes GM: Silver nitrate and the eyes of the newborn: Credé's contribution to preventive medicine. *Am J Dis Child 1971;121:1–4.*

33. Credé CSF: Die Verhütung der Augenentzündung der Neugeborenen. *Arch Gynäkol 1881;17:50–53.*

34. Laga M, Plummer FA, Piot P, et al: Prophylaxis of gonococcal and chlamydial ophthalmia neonatorum: A comparison of silver nitrate and tetracycline. *N Engl J Med 1988;318:653–657.*

35. Hammerschlag MR, Cummings C, Roblin PM, et al: Efficacy of neonatal ocular prophylaxis for the prevention of chlamydial and gonococcal conjunctivitis. *N Engl J Med 1989;320:769–772.*

36. Sandström I: Treatment of neonatal conjunctivitis. *Arch Ophthalmol 1987;105:925–928.*

37. Chandler JW: Controversies in ocular prophylaxis of newborns (editorial). *Arch Ophthalmol 1989;107:814–815.*

38. Benevento WJ, Murray P, Reed CA, et al: The sensitivity of *Neisseria gonorrhoeae, Chlamydia trachomatis,* and *Herpes simplex* type II to disinfection with povidone–iodine. *Am J Ophthalmol 1990;109:329–333.*

39. Duke-Elder S (ed): *System of Ophthalmology.* Vol VIII. *Diseases of the Outer Eye.* Part I. *Conjunctiva.* St. Louis: CV Mosby, 1965, 258–299.

40. Wear DJ, Malaty RH, Zimmerman LE, et al: Cat scratch disease bacilli in the conjunctiva of patients with Parinaud's oculoglandular syndrome. *Ophthalmology 1985;92:1282–1287.*

41. Brenner DJ, Hollis DG, Moss CW, et al: Proposal of *Afipia* gen. nov., with *Afipia felis* sp. nov. (formerly the cat scratch disease bacillus), *Afipia clevelandensis* sp. nov. (formerly the Cleveland Clinic Foundation strain), *Afipia broomeae* sp. nov, and three unnamed genospecies. *J Clin Microbiol 1991;29:2450–2460.*

42. Bogue CW, Wise JD, Gray GF, et al: Antibiotic therapy for cat-scratch disease? *JAMA 1989;262:813–816.*

43. Chin GN, Hyndiuk RA: Parinaud's oculoglandular conjunctivitis, in Tasman W, Jaeger EA (eds): *Duane's Clinical Ophthalmology,* Vol 4. Philadelphia: JB Lippincott, 1990, 1–6.

44. Dawson CR, Sheppard JD: Follicular conjunctivitis, in Tasman W, Jaeger EA (eds): *Duane's Clinical Ophthalmology,* Vol 4. Philadelphia: JB Lippincott, 1990, 17–18.

45. Dawson CR, Sheppard JD: Follicular conjunctivitis, in Tasman W, Jaeger EA (eds): *Duane's Clinical Ophthalmology,* Vol 4. Philadelphia: JB Lippincott, 1990, 18.

46. Theodore FH: Superior limbic keratoconjunctivitis. *Eye Ear Nose Throat Mon 1963;42:25–28.*

47. Wright P: Superior limbic keratoconjunctivitis. *Trans Ophthalmol Soc UK 1972;92:555–560.*

48. Udell IJ, Kenyon KR, Sawa M, et al: Treatment of superior limbic keratoconjunctivitis by thermocauterization of the superior bulbar conjunctiva. *Ophthalmology 1986;93:162–166.*

49. Passons GA, Wood TO: Conjunctival resection for superior limbic keratoconjunctivitis. *Ophthalmology 1984;91:966–968.*

50. Hidayat AA, Riddle PJ: Ligneous conjunctivitis: A clinicopathologic study of 17 cases. *Ophthalmology 1987;94:949–959.*

51. Holland EJ, Chan C-C, Kuwabara T, et al: Immunohistologic findings and results of treatment with cyclosporine in ligneous conjunctivitis. *Am J Ophthalmol 1989;107:160–166.*

52. Melikian HE: Treatment of ligneous conjunctivitis. *Ann Ophthalmol 1985;17:763–765.*

53. Holland EJ, Chan C-C, Kuwabara T, et al: Immunohistologic findings and results of treatment with cyclosporine in ligneous conjunctivitis. *Am J Ophthalmol 1989;107:160–166.*

54. Rubin BI, Holland EJ, de Smet MD, et al: Response of reactivated ligneous conjunctivitis to topical cyclosporine (letter). *Am J Ophthalmol 1991;112:95–96.*

55. Wilson FM II: Adverse external ocular effects of topical ophthalmic medications. *Surv Ophthalmol 1979;24:57–88.*

56. Allansmith MR: Vernal conjunctivitis, in Tasman W, Jaeger EA (eds): *Duane's Clinical Ophthalmology,* Vol 4. Philadelphia: JB Lippincott, 1990, 1–8.

57. Allansmith MR, Hahn GS, Simon MA: Tissue, tear and serum IgE concentrations in vernal conjunctivitis. *Am J Ophthalmol 1976;81:506–511.*

58. Abelson MB, Soter NA, Simon MA, et al: Histamine in human tears. *Am J Ophthalmol 1977;85:417–418.*

59. Ballow M, Donshik PC, Mendelson L, et al: IgG specific antibodies to rye grass and ragweed pollen antigens in the tear secretions of patients with vernal conjunctivitis. *Am J Ophthalmol 1983;95:161–168.*

60. Ben Ezra D, Peer J, Brodsky M, et al: Cyclosporine eyedrops for the treatment of severe vernal keratoconjunctivitis. *Am J Ophthalmol 1986;101:278–282.*

61. Allansmith MR, Ross RN: Giant papillary conjunctivitis, in Tasman W, Jaeger EA (eds): *Duane's Clinical Ophthalmology,* Vol 4. Philadelphia: JB Lippincott, 1990, 1.

62. Korb DR, Allansmith MR, Greiner JV, et al: Prevalence of conjunctival changes in wearers of hard contact lenses. *Am J Ophthalmol 1980;90:336–341.*

63. Udell IJ, Gleich GJ, Allansmith MR, et al: Eosinophil granule major basic protein and Charcot–Leyden crystal protein in human tears. *Am J Ophthalmol 1981;92:824–828.*

64. Allansmith MR, Ross RN: Giant papillary conjunctivitis, in Tasman W, Jaeger EA (eds): *Duane's Clinical Ophthalmology,* Vol 4. Philadelphia: JB Lippincott, 1990, 3–4.

65. Mondino BJ, Brown SI: Ocular cicatricial pemphigoid. *Ophthalmology 1981;88:95–100.*

66. Foster CS: Cicatricial pemphigoid. *Trans Am Ophthalmol Soc 1986;84:527–663.*

67. Mondino BJ: Bullous diseases of the skin and mucous membranes, in Tasman W, Jaeger EA (eds): *Duane's Clinical Ophthalmology,* Vol 4. Philadelphia: JB Lippincott, 1990, 5.

68. Jabs DA: Personal communication, 1991.

69. Jabs DA: Personal communication, 1991.

70. Mondino BJ: Bullous diseases of the skin and mucous membranes, in Tasman W, Jaeger EA (eds): *Duane's Clinical Ophthalmology,* Vol 4. Philadelphia: JB Lippincott, 1990, 6.

71. Jabs DA: Personal communication, 1991.

72. Jabs, DA: Personal communication, 1991.

73. Dohlman CH, Doughman DJ: The Stevens-Johnson syndrome, in *Symposium on the Cornea. Transactions of the New Orleans Academy of Ophthalmology*. St. Louis: CV Mosby, 1972, 236–252.

74. Chan LS, Soong HK, Foster CS, et al: Ocular cicatricial pemphigoid occurring as a sequela of Stevens-Johnson syndrome. *JAMA 1991;266:1543–1546.*

75. Rasmussen JE: Erythema multiforme in children: Response to treatment with systemic corticosteroids. *Br J Dermatol 1976; 95:181–186.*

76. Spencer WH: *Ophthalmic Pathology: An Atlas and Textbook,* Vol 1, ed 3. Philadelphia: WB Saunders, 1985, 162.

77. Mondino BJ: Bullous diseases of the skin and mucous membranes, in Tasman W, Jaeger EA (eds): *Duane's Clinical Ophthalmology,* Vol 4. Philadelphia: JB Lippincott, 1990, 13–14.

78. Thoft RA: Conjunctival transplantation. *Arch Ophthalmol 1977;95:1425–1427.*

79. Yanoff M: Hereditary benign intraepithelial dyskeratosis. *Arch Ophthalmol 1968;79:291–293.*

80. Fraunfelder FT, Wingfield D: Management of intraepithelial conjunctival tumors and squamous cell carcinomas. *Am J Ophthalmol 1983;95:359–363.*

81. Spencer WH: *Ophthalmic Pathology: An Atlas and Textbook,* Vol 1, ed 3. Philadelphia: WB Saunders, 1985, 187–190.

82. Awdry P: Lymphangiectasia haemorrhagica conjunctivae. *Br J Ophthalmol 1969;53:274–278.*

83. Nik NA, Glew WB, Zimmerman LE: Malignant melanoma of the choroid in the nevus of Ota of a black patient. *Arch Ophthalmol 1982;100:1641–1643.*

84. Yanoff M, Fine BS: *Ocular Pathology: A Text and Atlas.* Hagerstown, MD: Harper & Row, 1975, 632.

85. Spencer WH: *Ophthalmic Pathology: An Atlas and Textbook,* Vol 1, ed 3. Philadelphia: WB Saunders, 1985, 199–201.

86. Spencer WH: *Ophthalmic Pathology: An Atlas and Textbook,* Vol 1, ed 3. Philadelphia: WB Saunders, 1985, 201–206.

87. Griffith WR, Green WR, Weinstein GW: Conjunctival malignant melanoma originating in acquired melanosis sine pigmento. *Am J Ophthalmol 1971;72:595–599.*

88. Spencer WH: *Ophthalmic Pathology: An Atlas and Textbook,* Vol 1, ed 3. Philadelphia: WB Saunders, 1985, 217–218.

## CHAPTER 3
## LIMBAL TUMORS

1. Elsas FJ, Green WR: Epibulbar tumors in childhood. *Am J Ophthalmol 1975;79:1001–1007.*

2. Mansour AM, Barber JC, Reinecke RD, et al: Ocular choristomas. *Surv Ophthalmol 1989;33:339–358.*

3. Dailey EG, Lubowitz RM: Dermoids of the limbus and cornea. *Am J Ophthalmol 1962;53:661–665.*

4. Mattos J, Contreras F, O'Donnell FE Jr: Ring dermoid syndrome: A new syndrome of autosomal dominantly inherited, bilateral, annular limbal dermoids with corneal and conjunctival extension. *Arch Ophthalmol 1980;98:1059–1061.*

5. Henkind P, Marinoff G, Manas A, et al: Bilateral corneal dermoids. *Am J Ophthalmol 1973;76:972–977.*

6. Baum JL, Feingold M: Ocular aspects of Goldenhar's syndrome. *Am J Ophthalmol 1973;75:250–257.*

7. Mansour AM, Wang F, Henkind P, et al: Ocular findings in the facioauriculovertebral sequence (Goldenhar-Gorlin syndrome). *Am J Ophthalmol 1985;100:555–559.*

8. Panton RW, Sugar J: Excision of limbal dermoids. *Ophthalmic Surg 1991;22:85-89.*

9. Pokorny KS, Hyman BM, Jakobiec PA, et al: Epibulbar choristomas containing lacrimal tissue: Clinical distinction from dermoids and histologic evidence of an origin from the palpebral lobe. *Ophthalmology 1987;94:1249–1257.*

10. Spencer WH, Zimmerman LE: Conjunctiva, in Spencer WH (ed): *Ophthalmic Pathology: An Atlas and Textbook,* Vol 1, ed 3. Philadelphia: WB Saunders, 1985, 109–228.

11. Waring GO III, Roth AM, Ekins MB: Clinical and pathologic description of 17 cases of corneal intraepithelial neoplasia. *Am J Ophthalmol 1984;97:547–559.*

12. Campbell RJ, Bourne WM: Unilateral central corneal epithelial dysplasia. *Ophthalmology 1981;88:1231–1238.*

13. Jakobiec FA, Folberg R, Iwamoto T: Clinicopathologic characteristics of premalignant and malignant melanocytic lesions of the conjunctiva. *Ophthalmology 1989;96:147–166.*

14. McDonnell JM, Carpenter JD, Jacobs P, et al: Conjunctival melanocytic lesions in children. *Ophthalmology 1989;96:986–993.*

# CHAPTER 4
## THE CORNEAL EPITHELIUM

1. Tisdale AS, Spurr–Michaud SJ, Rodrigues M, et al: Development of the anchoring sutures of the epithelium in rabbit and human fetal corneas. *Invest Ophthalmol Vis Sci 1988;29:727–736.*

2. Sevel D, Isaacs R: A re-evaluation of corneal development. *Trans Am Ophthalmol Soc 1988;86:178–207.*

3. Alvarado J, Murphy C, Juster R: Age-related changes in the basement membrane of the human corneal epithelium. *Invest Ophthalmol Vis Sci 1983;24:1015–1028.*

4. Kaufman HE, McDonald MB, Barron BA, Waltman SR (eds): *The Cornea.* New York, Edinburgh, London, Melbourne: Churchill Livingstone, 1988, 38.

5. Lohman LE, Rao GN, Aquavella JV: Normal human corneal epithelium: In vivo microscopic observations. *Arch Ophthalmol 1982;100:991–993.*

6. Soong HK, Fairley JA: Actin in human corneal epithelium. *Arch Ophthalmol 1985;103:565–568.*

7. Anhalt GJ, Jampel HD, Patel HP, et al: Bullous pemphigoid autoantibodies are markers of corneal epithelial hemidesmosomes. *Invest Ophthalmol Vis Sci 1987;28:903–907.*

8. Yurchenco PD, Schittny JC: Molecular architecture of basement membranes. *FASEB J 1990;4:1577–1590.*

9. Tervo T, Sulonen J, Valtonen S, et al: Distribution of fibronectin in human and rabbit corneas. *Exp Eye Res 1986;42:399–406.*

10. Gipson IK: The epithelial basement membrane zone of the limbus. *Eye 1989;3:132–140.*

11. Griffiths SN, Drasdo N, Barnes DA, Sabell AG: Effect of epithelial and stromal edema on the light scattering properties of the cornea. *Am J Optom Physiol Opt 1986;63:888–894.*

12. Gipson IK: Corneal epithelial and stromal reactions to excimer laser photorefractive keratectomy. *Arch Ophthalmol 1990;108:1539–1540.*

13. Ebato B, Friend J, Thoft R: Comparison of central and peripheral human corneal epithelium in tissue culture. *Invest Ophthalmol Vis Sci 1987;28:1450–1456.*

14. Ebato B, Friend J, Thoft R: Comparison of limbal and peripheral human corneal epithelium in tissue culture. *Invest Ophthalmol Vis Sci 1988;29:1533–1537.*

15. Thoft RA, Friend J: The X, Y, Z hypothesis of corneal epithelial maintenance. *Invest Ophthalmol Vis Sci 1983;24:1442–1443.*

16. Lemp MA, Mathers WD: Corneal epithelial cell movement in humans. *Eye 1989;3:438–445.*

17. Tseng SCG: Concept and application of limbal stem cells. *Eye 1989;3:141–157.*

18. Thoft RA, Wiley LA, Sundarraj N: The multipotential cells of the limbus. *Eye 1989;3:109–113.*

19. Klyce SD, Neufeld AH, Zadunaisky JA: The activation of chloride transport by epinephrine and Db cyclic-AMP in the cornea of the rabbit. *Invest Ophthalmol Vis Sci 1973;12:127.*

20. Redmond TM, Duke EJ, Coles WH, et al: Localization of corneal superoxide dismutase by biochemical and histocytochemical techniques. *Exp Eye Res 1984;38:369–378.*

21. Crouch R, Ling Z, Hayden BJ: Corneal oxygen scavenging systems: Lysis of corneal epithelial cells by superoxide anions. *Basic Life Sci 1988;49:1043–1046.*

22. Abraham NG, Lin JHC, Dunn MW, Schwartzman ML: Presence of heme oxygenase and NADPH cytochrome P-450 (C) reductase in human corneal epithelium. *Invest Ophthalmol Vis Sci 1987;28:1464–1472.*

23. Sweeney DF, Vannas A, Holden BA, et al: Evidence for sympathetic neural influence on human corneal epithelial function. *Acta Ophthalmol 1985;63:215–220.*

24. Ueda S, del Cerro M, LoCascio JA, Aquavella JV: Peptidergic and catecholaminergic fibers in the human corneal epithelium: An immunohistochemical and electron microscopic study. *Acta Ophthalmol 1989;67(suppl 192):80–90.*

25. Treseler PA, Foulks GN, Sanfilippo F: The expression of HLA antigens by cells in the human cornea. *Am J Ophthalmol 1984;98:763–772.*

26. Dreizen NG, Whitsett CF, Austin GE, Stulting RD: Laser densitometric analysis of class I HLA antigen expression by corneal epithelium. *Invest Ophthalmol Vis Sci 1986;27:883–890.*

27. Gillette TE, Chandler JW, Greiner JV: Langerhans cells of the ocular surface. *Ophthalmology 1982;89:700–711.*

28. de Kruijf EJFM, Boot JP, Laterveer L: A simple method for determination of corneal epithelial permeability in humans. *Eye Res 1987;6:1327–1334.*

29. Wong S, Rodrigues MM, Blackman HJ, et al: Color specular microscopy of disorders involving the corneal epithelium. *Ophthalmology 1984;91:1176–1183.*

30. Gipson IK, Anderson RA: Actin filaments in normal and migrating corneal epithelial cells. *Invest Ophthalmol Vis Sci 1977;16:161–166.*

31. Berman M: The pathogenesis of corneal epithelial defects. *Acta Ophthalmol 1989;67(suppl 192):55–64.*

32. Dua HS, Forrester JV: Clinical patterns of corneal epithelial wound healing. *Am J Ophthalmol 1987;104:481–489.*

33. Azar DT, Spurr–Michaud SJ, Tisdale AS, Gipson IK: Decreased penetration of anchoring fibrils into the diabetic stroma. *Arch Ophthalmol 1989;107:1520–1523.*

34. Kenyon KR, Wafai Z, Michels R, et al: Corneal basement membrane abnormality in diabetes mellitus. *Invest Ophthalmol Vis Sci 1978;17(ARVO suppl):245.*

35. Imperia PS, Lazarus HM, Lass JH: Ocular complications of systemic cancer chemotherapy. *Surv Ophthalmol 1989;34:209–230.*

36. Huer DK, Parrish RK, Gressel MG, et al: 5-fluorouracil and glaucoma filtering surgery. *Ophthalmology 1986;93:1537–1546.*

37. Tripathi BJ, Kwait PS, Tripathi RC: Corneal growth factors: A new generation of ophthalmic pharmaceuticals. *Cornea 1990;9:2–9.*

38. Tripathi RC, Raja SC, Tripathi BJ: Prospects for epidermal growth factor in the management of corneal disorders. *Surv Ophthalmol 1990;34:457–462.*

39. Ramselaar JAM, Boot JP, van Haeringen NJ, et al: Corneal epithelial permeability after instillation of ophthalmic solutions containing local anaesthetics and preservatives. *Curr Eye Res 1988;7:947–950.*

40. Boets EPM, van Best JA, Boot JP, Oosterhuis JA: Corneal epithelial permeability and daily contact lens wear as determined by fluorophotometry. *Curr Eye Res 1988;7:511–514.*

41. Lemp MA, Gold JB: The effects of extended-wear hydrophilic contact lenses on the human corneal epithelium. *Am J Ophthalmol 1986;101:274–277.*

## CHAPTER 5
### THE MOLECULAR STRUCTURE OF THE CORNEAL STROMA IN HEALTH AND DISEASE

1. Stepp MA, Spurr–Michaud S, Tisdale A, et al: $a_6b_4$ intergin heterodimer is a component of hemidesmosomes. *Proc Natl Acad Sci USA* 1990;87:8970–8974.

2. Jones JCR, Kurpakus MA, Cooper HM, Quaranta V: A function for the integrin alpha 6 beta 4 in the hemidesmosome. *Cell Regulation* 1991;2:247–438.

3. Kurpakus MA, Quanrata V, Jones JCR: Surface relocation of alpha 6 beta 4 integrin and assembly of hemidesmosomes and in vitro model of wound healing. *J Cell Biol* 1991;115:1737–1750.

4. Stepp MA, Spurr-Michaud S, Tisdale A, et al: Alpha 6 beta 4 integrin heterodimer is a component of hemidesmosomes. *Proc Natl Acad Sci USA* 1990;87:8970–8974.

5. Carter WG, Rayan MC, Gahr PJ: A new cell adhesion ligand for integrin alpha 3 beta 1 in epithelial basement membranes. *Cell* 1991;65:599–610.

6. Rouselle P, Lunstrom GP, Keene DR, Burgeson RE: An epithelium-specific basement membrane adhesion molecule that is a component of anchoring filaments. *J Cell Biol* 1991;114:567–576.

7. Cintron C, Covington HI: Proteoglycan distribution in developing rabbit cornea. *J Histochem Cytochem* 1990;38:675–784.

8. Heremans A, Schueren VD, Cock BD, et al: Matrix-associated heparan sulfate proteoglycan: Core protein-specific monoclonal antibodies decorate the pericelluar matrix of connective tissue cells and the stromal side of basement membranes. *J Cell Biol* 1989;109:3199–3211.

9. Fitch JM, Birk DE, Linsenmayer C, et al: The spatial organization of Descemet's membrane-associated type IV collagen in the avian cornea. *J Cell Biol [in press].*

10. Cintron C, Hong B-S, Covington HI, et al: Heterogeneity of collagens in rabbit cornea: Type III collagen. *Invest Ophthalmol Vis Sci* 1988;29:767–775.

11. Sawada H, Konomi H, Hirosawa K: Characterization of the collagen in the hexagonal lattice of Descemet's membrane: Its relation to type VIII collagen. *J Cell Biol* 1990;110:219–227.

12. Linsenmayer TF, Fitch JM, Birk DE: Heterotypic collagen fibrils and stabilizing collagens. Controlling elements in corneal morphogenesis. *Ann NY Acad Sci* 1990;580:143–160.

13. Birk DE, Fitch JM, Babiarz JP, et al: Collagen fibrillogenesis in vitro: Interaction of types I and V collagen regulates fibril diameter. *J Cell Sci* 1990;95:649–657.

14. Cintron C, Hong B-S, Kublin CK: Quantitative analysis of collagen from normal developing corneas and corneal scars. *Curr Eye Res* 1981;1:1–8.

15. Keene DR, Sakai LY, Bachinger HP, et al: Type III collagen can be present on banded collagen fibrils regardless of fibril diameter. *J Cell Biol* 1987;105:2393–2402.

16. Svoboda KK, Hay ED: Embryonic corneal epithelium interaction with exogenous laminin and basal lamina is F-actin dependent. *Dev Biol* 1987;123:455–469.

17. Sugrue SP: Isolation of collagen binding proteins from embryonic chicken corneal epithelial cells. *J Biol Chem* 1987;262:3338–3343.

18. Gipson IK, Spurr–Michaud SJ, Tisdale AS: Hemidesmosomes and anchoring fibril collagen appear synchronously during devlopment and wound healing. *Dev Biol* 1988;126:253–262.

19. Gipson IK, Spurr–Michaud S, Tisdale AS, et al: Reassembly of the anchoring structures of the corneal epithelium during wound repair in the rabbit. *Invest Ophthalmol Vis Sci* 1989;30:425–434.

20. Linsenmayer TF, Bruns RR, Mentzer A, et al: Type VI collagen: Immunohistochemical identification of a filamentous component of the extracellular matrix of the developing avian corneal stroma. *Dev Biol* 1986;118:425–431.

21. Cintron C, Hong B-S: Heterogeneity of collagens in rabbit cornea: Type VI collagen. *Invest Ophthalmol Vis Sci* 1988;29:760–766.

22. Cho H, Covington HI, Cintron C: Immunolocalization of type VI collagen in developing and healing rabbit cornea. *Invest Ophthalmol Vis Sci 1990;31:1096–1102.*

23. Yamaguchi N, Benya PD, van der Rest M, et al: The cloning and sequencing of alpha 1 (VIII) collagen cDNAs demonstrate that type VIII collagen is a short chain collagen and contains triple-helical and carboxyl-terminal non-triple-helical domains similar to those of type X collagen. *J Biol Chem 1989;264:16022–16029.*

24. Svoboda KK, Nishimura I, Sugrue SP, et al: Embryonic chicken cornea and cartilage synthesize type IX collagen molecules with different amino-terminal domains. *Proc Natl Acad Sci USA 1988;85:7496–7500.*

25. Linsenmayer TF, Gibney E, Gordon MK, et al: Extracellular matrices of the developing chick retina and cornea. Localization of mRNAs for collagen types II and IX by in situ hybridization. *Invest Ophthalmol Vis Sci 1990;31:1271–1276.*

26. Yamagata M, Yamada KM, Yamada SS, et al: The complete primary structure of type XII collagen shows a chimeric molecule with reiterated fibronectin type III motifs, von Willebrand factor A motifs, a domain homologous to a noncollagenous region of type IX collagen, and short collagenous domains with an Arg-Gly-Asp site. *J Cell Biol 1991;115:209–221.*

27. Gerecke DR, Gordon MK, Olsen BR: The amino-terminal regions of homotrimeric type XII collagen molecules and multidomain structures containing von Willbrand factor A and fibronectin type III repeats (abstr). *J Cell Biol 1991;115:106a.*

28. Cintron C, Kublin CL: Regeneration of corneal tissue. *Dev Biol 1977;61:346–357.*

29. Axelsson I, Heinegård D: Characterization of the keratan sulphate proteoglycans from bovine corneal stroma. *Biochem J 1978;169:517–530.*

30. Axelsson I, Heinegård D: Characterization of chondroitin sulfate-rich proteoglycans from bovine corneal stroma. *Exp Eye Res 1980;31:57–66.*

31. Hassell JR, Newsome DA, Hascall VC: Characterization and biosynthesis of proteoglycans of corneal stroma from rhesus monkey. *J Biol Chem 1979;254:12346–12354.*

32. Gregory JD, Cöster L, Damle SP: Proteoglycans of rabbit corneal stroma. *J Biol Chem 1982;257:6965–6970.*

33. Damle SP, Gregory JD: Proteoglycans of mammalian corneal stroma, in Greiling H, Scott JE (eds): *Keratan Sulphate. Chemistry, Biology, Chemical Pathology.* London: The Biochemical Society, 1989, 148–151.

34. Oldberg Å, Antonsson P, Lindblom K, et al: A collagen-binding 59-kd protein (fibromodulin) is structurally related to the small interstitial proteoglycans PG-S1 and PG-S2 (decorin). *EMBO J 1989;8:2601–2604.*

35. Funderburgh JL, Conrad GW: Isoforms of corneal keratan sulfate proteoglycan. *J Biol Chem 1990;265:8297–8303.*

36. Funderburgh JL, Funderburgh ML, Mann MM, Conrad GW: Unique glycosylation of three keratan sulfate proteoglycan isoforms. *J Biol Chem 1990;266:13336–13341.*

37. Nilsson B, Nakazawa K, Hassell JR, et al: Structure of oligosaccharides and the linkage region between keratan sulfate and the core protein on proteoglycans from monkey cornea. *J Biol Chem 1983;258:60056–60063.*

38. Jost CJ, Funderburgh JL, Mann M, et al: Cell-free translation and characterization of corneal keratan sulfate proteoglycan core proteins. *J Biol Chem 1991;266:13336–13341.*

39. Blochberger TC, Vergnes J-P, Hempel J, Hassell JR: cDNA to chick lumican (corneal keratan sulfate proteoglycan) reveals homology to the small interstitial proteoglycan gene family and expression in muscle and intestine. *J Biol Chem 1992;267:345–352.*

40. Li W, Vergnes J-P, Cornuet PK, Hassell JR: cDNA clone to chick corneal chondroitin/dermatan sulfate proteoglycan reveals identity to decorin. *Arch Biochem Biophys 1992;296:190–197.*

41. Midura RJ, Hascall VC: Analysis of the proteoglycans synthesized by corneal explants from embryonic chicken. *J Biol Chem 1989;264:1423–1430.*

42. Gregory JD, Damle SP, Covington HI, et al: Developmental changes in proteoglycans of rabbit corneal stroma. *Invest Ophthalmol Vis Sci* 1988;29:1413–1417.

43. Hassell JR, Cintron C, Kublin C, et al: Proteoglycan changes during restoration of transparency in corneal scars. *Arch Biochem Biophys* 1983;222:362–369.

44. Cintron C, Gregory JD, Damle SP, et al: Biochemical analyses of proteoglycans in rabbit corneal scars. *Invest Ophthalmol Vis Sci* 1990;31:1975–1981.

45. Zimmermann DR, Ruoslahti E: Multiple domains of the large fibroblast proteoglycan. *EMBO J* 1989;8:2975–2981.

46. Castoro JA, Bettelheim AA, Bettelheim FA: Water gradients across bovine cornea. *Invest Ophthalmol Vis Sci* 1988;29:963.

47. Cintron C, Covington HI: Proteoglycan distribution in developing rabbit cornea. *J Histochem Cytochem* 1990;38:675–684.

48. Sundarraj N, Chao J, Gregory JD, et al: Ocular distribution of keratan sulfates during pre- and postnatal development in rabbits. *J Histochem Cytochem* 1986;34:971–976.

49. Funderburgh JL, Cintron C, Covington HI, et al: Immunoanalysis of keratan sulfate proteoglycan from corneal scars. *Invest Ophthalmol Vis Sci* 1988;29:1116–1123.

50. Cintron C, Covington HI, Kulbin CL: Morphologic analyses of proteoglycans in rabbit corneal scars. *Invest Ophthalmol Vis Sci* 1990;31:1789–1798.

51. Scott JE, Haigh M: Identification of specific binding sites for keratan sulphate proteoglycans and chondroitin-dermatan sulphate proteoglycans on collagen fibrils in cornea by the use of Cupromeronic Blue in "critical-electrolyte-concentration" techniques. *Biochem J* 1988;253:607–610.

52. Connor CG, Zagrod ME: Contact lens-induced corneal endothelial poymegathism: Functional significance and possible mechanisms. *Am J Optom Physiol Opt* 1986;63:539–544.

53. Cejková J, Lojda Z, Brunová B, et al: Disturbances in the rabbit cornea after short-term and long-term wear of hydrogel contact lenses. *Histochemistry* 1988;89:91–97.

54. Anseth A: Studies on corneal polysaccharides. V. Changes in corneal glycosaminoglycans in transient stromal edema. *Exp Eye Res* 1969;8:297–301.

55. Kaye GI, Edelhauser HF, Stern ME, et al: Further studies of the effect of perfusion with a $Ca^{++}$-free medium on the rabbit cornea: Extraction of stromal components, in: Hollyfield JG (ed): *The Structure of the Eye.* New York: Elsevier North Holland, 1982, 271–278.

56. Kangas TA, Edelhauser HF, Twining SS, et al: Loss of stromal glycosaminoglycans during corneal edema. *Invest Ophthalmol Vis Sci* 1990;31:1994–2002.

57. Ruoslahti E: Structure and biology of proteoglycans. *Annu Rev Cell Biol* 1988;1:229–255.

58. Hassell JR, Kimura JH, Hascall VC: Proteoglycan core protein families. *Annu Rev Biochem* 1986;55:539–567.

59. Goetinck PL, Stirpe NS, Tsonis PA, et al: The tandemly repeated sequences of cartilage link protein contain the sites for interaction with hyaluronic acid. *J Cell Biol* 1987;105:2403–2408.

60. Pringle G, Dodd C: Immunoelectron microscopic localization of the proteins of decorin near the d and e bands of tendon collagen fibrils by use of monoclonal antibodies. *J Histochem Cytochem* 1990;38:1405–1411.

61. Brown DC, Vogel KG: Characteristics of the in vitro interaction of a small proteoglycan (PG II) of bovine tendon with type I collagen. *Matrix* 1990;9:468–978.

62. Vogel KG, Paulsson M, Heinegard D: Specific inhibition of type I and type II collagen fibrillogenesis by the small proteoglycan of tendon. *Biochem J* 1984;223:587–597.

63. Rada JA, Schrenengost PK, Hassell JR: Regulation of corneal collagen fibrillogenesis by corneal keratan sulfate proteoglycan core protein (abstr). *Invest Ophthalmol Vis Sci* 1991;32:1010.

64. Krusius T, Ruoslahti E: Primary structure of an extracellular matrix proteoglycan core protein deduced from cloned cDNA. *Proc Natl Acad Sci USA 1986;83:7683–7687.*

65. Day AA, Ramis CI, Fisher LW, et al: Characterization of bone PGII cDNA and its relationship to PG II mRNA from other connective tissues. *Nucleic Acids Res 1986;14:9861–9872.*

66. Yamaguchi Y, Mam DM, Ruoslahti E: Negative regulation of transforming growth factor-β by the proteoglycan decorin. *Nature 1990;346:281–284.*

67. Meek KM, Scott JE, Nave C: An X-ray diffraction analysis of rat tail tendons treated with Cupromeronic Blue. *J Microsc 1985;139:205–219.*

68. Young RD: The ultrastructural organization of proteoglycans and collagen in human and rabbit scleral matrix. *J Cell Sci 1985;74:95–104.*

69. Scott JE, Haigh M: "Small"-proteoglycan:collagen interactions: Keratan sulphate proteoglycan associates with rabbit corneal collagen fibrils at the "a" and "c" bands. *Biosci Rep 1985;5:765–774.*

70. Gyi TJ, Meek EM, Elliott GP: Collagen interfibrillar distances in corneal stroma using synchrotron X-ray diffraction: A species study. *Int J Biol Macromol 1988;10:265–274.*

71. Keene DR, Engvall E, Glanville RW: Ultrastructure of type VI collagen in human skin and cartilage suggests and anchoring function for this filamentous network. *J Cell Biol 1988;l07:1995–2006.*

72. Takahashi T, Tohyama K: Electron microscopic study of distribution of proteoglycans in bovine cornea and sclera. *Jpn J Ophthalmol 1991;35:211–225.*

73. Nakamura M, Hirano K, Kobayashi M, et al: Assembly of 100 nm periodic fibrils in the mouse and human infant corneal stroma: Type VI collagen proteoglycan-type I collagen interaction (abstr). *Invest Ophthalmol Vis Sci 1992;33:1192.*

74. Cho H, Kublin CL, Cintron C: Keratan sulfate proteoglycan associates with type VI collagen in fetal rabbit cornea and sclera (abstr). *Invest Ophthalmol Vis Sci 1990;31:101.*

75. Takahashi T, Cintron C: The association of decorin with extracellular matrix of developing rabbit cornea (abstr). *Invest Ophthalmol Vis Sci 1992;33:893.*

76. Bidanset DJ, Guidry C, Rosenberg LC, et al: Binding of the proteoglycan decorin to collagen type VI. *J Biol Chem 1992;267:5250–5256.*

77. Fini ME, Plucinska IM, Mayer AS, et al: A gene for rabbit synovial cell collagenase member of a family of metalloproteinases that degrade the connective tissue matrix. *Biochemistry 1987;26:6156–6165.*

78. Chin JR, Murphy G, Werb Z: Stromelysin, a connective tissue-degrading metalloendopeptidase secreted by stimulated rabbit synovial fibroblasts in parallel with collagenase. Biosynthesis, isolation, characterization, and substrates.*J Biol Chem 1985;260:12367–12376.*

79. Murphy G, Hembry AM, McGarrity AM, et al: Gelatinase (type IV collagenase) immunolocalization in cells and tissues: Use of an antiserum to rabbit bone gelatinase that identifies high and low Mr forms. *J Cell Sci 1989;92:487–495.*

80. Hibbs MS, Hoidal JR, Kang AH: Expression of a metalloproteinase that degrades native type V collagen and denatured collagen by cultured human alveolar macrophages. *J Clin Invest 1987;80:1644–1650.*

81. Collier IE, Wihelm SM, Eisen AZ, et al: H-ras oncogene transformed human bronchial epithelial cells (TBE-1) secrete a single metalloprotease capable of degrading basement membrane collagen. *J Biol Chem 1988;263:6579–6587.*

82. Kenyon KR: Inflammatory mechanisms in corneal ulceration. *Trans Am Ophthalmol Soc 1985;83:610–663.*

83. Yue BYJT, Sugar J, Benveniste K: RNA metabolism in cultures of corneal stromal cells from patients with keratoconus. *Proc Soc Exp Biol Med 1985;178:126–132.*

84. Critchfield JW, Calandra AJ, Nesburn AB, et al: Keratoconus I. Biochemical studies of normal and keratoconus corneas. *Exp Eye Res 1988;46:953–963.*

85. Bron AJ: Keratoconus. *Cornea 1988;7:163–169.*

86. Ihalainen A, Salo T, Forsius H, et al: Increase in type I and type IV collagenolytic activity in primary cultures of keratoconus cornea. *Eur J Clin Invest 1986;16:78–84.*

87. Kenney MC, Chwa M, Escobar M, et al: Altered gelatinolytic activity by keratoconus corneal cells. *Biochem Biophys Res Commun 1989;161:353–357.*

88. Funderburgh JL, Funderburgh ML, Rodriques MM, et al: Altered antigencity of keratan sulfate proteoglycan in selected corneal diseases. *Invest Ophthalmol Vis Sci 1990;31: 419–428.*

89. Sawaguchi S, Yue BYJT, Sugar J, et al: Lysosomal enzyme abnormalities in keratoconus. *Arch Ophthalmol 1989;107:1507–1510.*

90. Sawaguchi S, Twining SS, Yue BYJT, et al: Alpha-1 proteinase inhibitor levels in keratoconus. *Exp Eye Res 1990;50:549–554.*

91. Yang CJ, SundarRaj N, Thonar EJ-MA, et al: Immunohistochemical evidence of heterogeneity in macular corneal dystrophy. *Am J Ophthalmol 1988;106:65–71.*

92. Meek KM, Quantock AJ, Elliott GF, et al: Macular corneal dystrophy: The macromolecular structure of the stroma observed using electron microscopy and synchrotron X-ray diffraction. *Exp Eye Res 1989;49:941–958.*

93. Quantock AJ, Meek KM, Ridgway EA, et al: Macular corneal dystrophy: Reduction in both corneal thickness and collagen interfibrillar spacing. *Curr Eye Res 1990;9:393–398.*

94. Dunn S, Jester JV, Arthur J, et al: Endothelial cell loss following radial keratotomy in a primate model. *Arch Ophthalmol 1984;102:1666–1670.*

95. Marshall J, Trokel S, Rothery S, et al: An ultrastructural study of corneal incisions induced by an excimer laser at 193 nm. *Ophthalmology 1982;92:749–758.*

96. Marshall J, Trokel S, Rothery S, et al: A comparative study of corneal incisions induced by diamond and steel knives and two ultraviolet radiations from an excimer laser. *Br J Ophthalmol 1986;70:482–501.*

97. Berns MW, Liaw L-H, Allison O, et al: An acute light and electron microscopic study of ultraviolet 193-nm excimer laser corneal incisions. *Ophthalmology 1988;95:1422–1433.*

98. Gaster RN, Binder PS, Coalwell K, et al: Corneal surface ablation by 193 nm excimer laser and wound healing in rabbits. *Invest Ophthalmol Vis Sci 1989;30:90–98.*

99. Hanna KD, Pouliquen Y, Waring GO, et al: Corneal stromal wound healing in rabbits after 193-nm excimer laser surface ablation. *Arch Ophthalmol 1989;107:895–901.*

100. Tuft SJ, Zabel RW, Marshall J: Corneal repair following keratectomy. A comparison between conventional surgery and laser photoablation. *Invest Ophthalmol Vis Sci 1989;30:1769–1777.*

101. Malley, DS, Steinert RF, Puliafito CA, et al: Immunofluorescence study of corneal wound healing after excimer laser anterior keratectomy in mokey eye. *Arch Ophthalmol [in press].*

102. Marshall J, Trokel SL, Rothery S, et al: Long-term healing of the central cornea after photorefractive keratectomy using an excimer laser. *Ophthalmology 1988;95:1411–1421.*

103. McDonald MG, Frantz JM, Klyce SD, et al: One-year refractive results of central photorefractive keratectomy for myopia in the nonhuman primate cornea. *Arch Ophthalmol 1990;108:40–47.*

104. Cintron C, Hassinger LC, Kublin CL, et al: Biochemical and ultrastructural changes in collagen during corneal wound healing. *J Ultrstruct Res 1978;65:13–22.*

105. Grierson I, Miller JM, Day JE: Wound repair: The fibroblast and the inhibition of scar formation. *Eye 1988;2:135–148.*

## CHAPTER 6
### THE CORNEAL ENDOTHELIUM

1. Yee RW, Matsuda M, Schultz RO, Edelhauser HF: Changes in the normal corneal endothelial cellular pattern as a function of age. *Curr Eye Res 1985;4:671–678.*

2. Schultz RO, Matsuda M, Yee RW, et al: Corneal endothelial changes in Type I and Type II diabetes mellitus. *Am J Ophthalmol 1984;98:401–410.*

3. Stiemke MM, McCartney M, Cantu–Crouch D, Edelhauser HF: Maturation of the corneal endothelial tight junction. *Invest Ophthalmol Vis Sci 1991;32:2757–2765.*

4. Kim KE, Urken SI, Holley GP, et al: Corneal endothelial cytoskeleton changes in F-actin with age, diabetes and following cytochalasin. *Am J Ophthalmol [in press].*

5. Watsky MA, McCartney MD, McLaughlin BJ, Edelhauser HF: Corneal endothelial functions and the effects of ouabain. *Invest Ophthalmol Vis Sci 1990;31:933–941.*

6. Kaye GI, Tice LW: Studies on the cornea. V. Electron microscopic localization of adenosine triphosphatase activity in the rabbit cornea in relation to transport. *Invest Ophthalmol 1966;5:22–32.*

7. Geroski DH, Edelhauser HF: Quantitation of Na/K ATPase pump sites in the rabbit corneal endothelium. *Invest Ophthalmol Vis Sci 1984;25:1056–1060.*

8. Hull DS, Green K, Boyd M, Wynn HR: Corneal endothelium bicarbonate transport and the effect of carbonic anhydrase inhibitors on endothelial permeability fluxes and corneal thickness. *Invest Ophthalmol Vis Sci 1977;16:883–892.*

9. Watsky MA, McDermott ML, Edelhauser HF: In vitro corneal endothelial permeability in rabbit and human: The effect of age, intraocular surgery and diabetes. *Exp Eye Res 1989;49:751–767.*

10. Stiemke MM, Edelhauser HF, Geroski DH: The developing corneal endothelium: Correlation of morphology, hydration and Na/K ATPase pump site density. *Curr Eye Res 1991;10:145–156.*

11. Burns RR, Bourne WM, Burbaker RF: Endothelial function in patients with corneal guttata. *Invest Ophthalmol Vis Sci 1981;20:77–85.*


1. Mishima S: Clinical investigations on the corneal endothelium. *Ophthalmology 1982;89:525–530.*

2. Waring III GO, Bourne WM, Edelhauser HF, Kenyon KR: The corneal endothelium—normal and pathologic structure and function. *Ophthalmology 1982;89:531–590.*

3. Vogt A: Die Sichtbarkeit des lebenden Hornhautendothels. Ein Beitrog zur Methodik der Spaltlampenmikroskopie. *Graefes Arch Ophthalmol 1920;101:123–144.*

4. Dickstein S, Maurice DM: The metabolic basis to the fluid pump in the cornea. *J Physiol 1972;221:29–41.*

5. Laing RA, Sandstrom MM, Leibowitz HM, et al: In vivo photomicrography of the corneal endothelium. *Arch Ophthalmol 1975;93:143–145.*

6. Bourne WM, Kaufman HE: Specular microscopy of human corneal endothelium. *Am J Ophthalmol 1976;81:319–323.*

7. Laing RA, Sandstrom MM, Leibowitz HM: Clinical specular microscopy. *Arch Ophthalmol 1979;97:1714–1719.*

8. Maurice DM: A scanning slit optical microscope. *Invest Ophthalmol 1974;13:1033–1037.*

9. Lohman LE, Rao GN, Aquavella JA: Optics and clinical applications of wide-field specular microscopy. *Am J Ophthalmol 1981;92:43–48.*

10. Sherrard ES, Buckley RJ: Visualization of the corneal endothelium in the clinic. *Ophthalmologica 1983;187:118–128.*

11. Roberts CW, Koester CJ: Video with wide-field specular microscopy. *Ophthalmology 1981;88:146–149.*

12. Koester CJ, Roberts CW, Donn A, Hoefle FB: Wide field specular microscopy. *Ophthalmology 1980;87:849–860.*

13. Sherrard ES, Buckley RJ: Contact clinical specular microscopy of the corneal endothelium: Optical modifications to the applanating objective cone. *Invest Ophthalmol Vis Sci 1981;20:816–820.*

14. Sherrard ES, Buckley RJ: Relocation of specific endothelial features with the clinical specular microscope. *Br J Ophthalmol 1981;65:820–827.*

15. Laing RA: Specular microscopy of the cornea. *Curr Top Eye Res 1980;3:157–219.*

## CHAPTER 7
WIDEFIELD CLINICAL SPECULAR MICROSCOPY AND COMPUTERIZED MORPHOMETRIC ANALYSIS

16. Langston RHS, Roisman TS: Comparison of endothelial evaluation techniques. *J Am Intraocul Implant Soc 1981;7:239–241.*

17. Holladay JT, Bishop JE, Prager TC: Quantitative endothelial biomicroscopy. *Ophthal Surg 1983;14:33–40.*

18. Yee RW, Matsuda M, Edelhauser HF: Wide-field endothelial counting panels. *Am J Ophthalmol 1985;99:596–597.*

19. Waring III GO, Krohn MA, Ford GE, et al: Four methods of measuring human corneal endothelial cells from specular photomicrographs. *Arch Ophthalmol 1980;98:848–855.*

20. Olsen T: Sampling problems associated with quantitative morphometry of endothelial cells. *Acta Ophthalmol (Copenh) 1981;59:854–862.*

21. Hirst LW, Yamauchi K, Enger C, et al: Quantitative analysis of widefield specular microscopy. *Invest Ophthalmol Vis Sci 1989;30:1972–1979.*

22. Shaw EL, Rao GN, Arthur EJ, Aquavella JV: The functional reserve of corneal endothelium. *Trans Am Acad Ophthalmol Otolaryngol 1978;85:640–649.*

23. Rao GN, Shaw EL, Arthur EJ, Aquavella JV: Endothelial cell morphology and corneal deturgescence. *Ann Ophthalmol 1979;11:885–899.*

24. Schultz RO, Matsuda M, Yee RW, et al: Corneal endothelial changes in type I and type II diabetes mellitus. *Am J Ophthalmol 1984;98:401–410.*

25. Suda T: Mosaic pattern changes in human corneal endothelium with age. *Jpn J Ophthalmol 1984;28:331–338.*

26. Yee RW, Matsuda M, Schultz RO, Edelhauser HF: Changes in the normal corneal endothelial cellular pattern as a function of age. *Curr Eye Res 1985;4:671–678.*

27. Rao GN, Lohman LE, Aquavella JV: Cell size–shape relationships in corneal endothelium. *Invest Ophthalmol Vis Sci 1982;22:271–274.*

28. Laing RA, Sandstrom MM, Berrospi AR, Leibowitz HM: Changes in the corneal endothelium as a function of age. *Exp Eye Res 1976;22:587–594.*

29. Laule A, Cable MK, Hoffman CE, Hanna C: Endothelial cell population changes of human cornea during life. *Arch Ophthalmol 1978;96:2031–2035.*

30. Matsuda M, Suda T, Manabe R: Quantitative analysis of endothelial mosaic pattern changes in anterior keratoconus. *Am J Ophthalmol 1984;98:43–49.*

31. Matsuda M, Yee RW, Glasser DB, et al: Specular microscopic evaluation of donor corneal endothelium. *Arch Ophthalmol 1986;104:259–262.*

32. MacRae SM, Matsuda M, Yee R: The effect of long-term hard contact lens wear on the corneal endothelium. *CLAO J 1985;11:322–326.*

33. Holden BA, Sweeney DF, Vannas A, et al: Effects of long-term extended contact lens wear on the human cornea. *Invest Ophthalmol Vis Sci 1985;26:1489–1501.*

34. MacRae SM, Matsuda M, Shellans S, Rich LF: The effects of hard and soft contact lenses on the corneal endothelium. *Am J Ophthalmol 1986;102:50–57.*

35. Carlson KH, Bourne WM, Brubaker RF: Effect of long-term contact lens wear on corneal endothelial cell morphology and function. *Invest Ophthalmol Vis Sci 1988;29:185–193.*

36. Schoessler JP, Orsborn GN: A theory of corneal endothelial polymegathism and aging. *Curr Eye Res 1987;6:301–305.*

37. Matsuda M, Bourne WM: Long-term morphologic changes in the endothelium of transplanted corneas. *Arch Ophthalmol 1985;103:1343–1346.*

38. Matsuda M, Suda T, Manabe R: Serial alterations in endothelial cell shape and pattern after intraocular surgery. *Am J Ophthalmol 1984;98:313–319.*

39. Schultz RO, Glasser DB, Matsuda M, et al: Response of the corneal endothelium to cataract surgery. *Arch Ophthalmol 1986;104:1164–1169.*

40. Glaser DB, Matsuda M, Gager WE, Edelhauser HF: Corneal endothelial morphology after anterior chamber lens implantation. *Arch Ophthalmol 1985;103:1347–1349.*

41. Glaser DB, Matsuda M, Ellis JG, Edelhauser HF: Effects of intraocular irrigating solutions on the corneal endothelium after in vivo anterior chamber irrigation. *Am J Ophthalmol 1985;99:321–328.*

42. Yee RW, Matsuda M, Kern TS, et al: Corneal endothelial changes in diabetic dogs. *Curr Eye Res 1985;4:759–766.*

43. Meyer LA, Ubels JL, Edelhauser HF: Corneal endothelial morphology in the rat. Effects of aging, diabetes and topical aldose reductase inhibitor treatment. *Invest Ophthalmol Vis Sci 1988;29:940–948.*

44. Matsuda M, Sawa M, Edelhauser HF, et al: Cellular migration and morphology in corneal endothelial wound repair. *Invest Ophthalmol Vis Sci 1985;26:443–449.*

45. Yee RW, Geroski DH, Matsuda M, et al: Correlation of corneal endothelial pump site density, barrier function and morphology in wound repair. *Invest Ophthalmol Vis Sci 1985;26:1191–1201.*

46. Macdonald JM, Geroski DH, Edelhauser HF: Effect of inflammation on the corneal endothelium pump and barrier. *Curr Eye Res 1987;6:1125–1132.*

47. Inaba M, Matsuda M, Shiozaki Y, Kosaki H: Morphologic analysis of human corneal endothelium. *Invest Ophthalmol Vis Sci 1984;25(suppl 1):240.*

48. Rao G, Waldron W, Aquavella J: Morphology of graft endothelium and donor age. *Br J Ophthalmol 1980;64:523–527.*

49. Rao GN, Aquavella JV, Goldberg SH, Berk SL: Pseudophakic bullous keratopathy. Relationship to preoperative corneal endothelial status. *Ophthalmology 1984;91:1135–1140.*

50. Doughty MJ: Toward a quantitative analysis of corneal endothelial cell morphology: A review of techniques and their application. *Optom Vis Sci 1989;66:626–642.*

51. Sperling S: Early morphological changes in organ cultured human corneal endothelium. *Acta Ophthalmol (Copenh) 1978;56:785–792.*

52. Sherrard ES: The corneal endothelium *in vivo:* Its response to mild trauma. *Exp Eye Res 1976;22:347–357.*

53. Olsen T: Variations in endothelial morphology of normal corneas and after cataract extraction. A specular microscopic study. *Acta Ophthalmol 1979;57:1014–1019.*

54. Honda H, Ogita Y, Higuchi S, Kani K: Cell movements in a living mammalian tissue: Long-term observations of individual cells in wounded endothelia of cats. *J Morphol 1982;174:25–39.*

55. Thompson DW: *On Growth and Form.* Vol II, ed 2. Cambridge: Cambridge University Press, 1969, 465–644.

56. Rao GN: Morphometry of corneal endothelium. *Cornea 1984/1985;3:153–154.*

57. Carlson KH, Bourne WM, McLaren JW, Brubaker RF: Variations in human corneal endothelial cell morphology and permeability to fluorescein with age. *Exp Eye Res 1988;47:27–41.*

58. Hoffer KJ: Preoperative cataract evaluation: endothelial cell evaluation. *Int Ophthalmol Clin 1982;22:15–35.*

59. Bigar F: Specular microscopy of the corneal endothelium. *Dev Ophthalmol 1982;6:1–94.*

60. Mayer DJ: *Clinical Wide-field Specular Microscopy.* London: Baillière Tindall, 1984, 1–113.

61. Bigar F: Cornea guttata in donor material. *Arch Ophthalmol 1978;96:653–655.*

62. Roberson MC, Wicheta WE: Endothelial loss in corneal concussion injury. *Ann Ophthalmol 1985;17:457–458.*

63. Markowitz SN, Morin JD: The endothelium in primary angle-closure glaucoma. *Am J Ophthalmol 1984;98:103–104.*

64. Setälä K: Corneal endothelial cell density after an attack of acute glaucoma. *Acta Ophthalmol (Copenh) 1979;57:1004–1013.*

65. Olsen T: The endothelial cell damage in acute glaucoma on the corneal thickness response to intraocular pressure. *Acta Ophthalmol (Copenh) 1980;58:257–266.*

66. Bigar F, Witmer R: Corneal endothelial changes in primary acute angle-closure glaucoma. *Ophthalmology 1982;89:596–599.*

67. Setälä K: Corneal endothelial cell density in iridocyclitis. *Acta Ophthalmol (Copenh) 1979;57:277–286.*

68. Olsen T: Changes in the corneal endothelium after acute anterior uveitis as seen with the specular microscope. *Acta Ophthalmol (Copenh) 1980;58:250–256.*

69. Brooks AMV, Gillies WE: Fluorescein angiography of the iris and specular microscopy of the corneal endothelium in some cases of glaucoma secondary to chronic cyclitis. *Ophthalmology 1988;95:1624–1630.*

70. Brooks AMV, Grant G, Gillies WE: Comparison of specular microscopy and examination of aspirate in phacolytic glaucoma. *Ophthalmology 1990;97:85–89.*

71. Olsen T: The specular microscopic appearance of corneal graft endothelium during an acute rejection episode. A case report. *Acta Ophthalmol (Copenh) 1979;57:882–890.*

72. Olsen T: Variations in endothelial morphology of normal corneas and after cataract extraction. A specular microscopic study. *Acta Ophthalmol (Copenh) 1979;57:1014–1019.*

73. Abbott RL, Forster RK: Clinical specular microscopy and intraocular surgery. *Arch Ophthalmol 1979;97:1476–1479.*

74. Culbertson WW, Abbott RL, Forster RK: Endothelial cell loss in penetrating keratoplasty. *Ophthalmology 1982;89:600–604.*

75. Bigar F, Schimmelpfennig B, Gieseler R: *Graefes Arch Klin Exp Ophthalmol 1976;200:195–200.*

76. Bourne WM: Examination and photography of donor corneal endothelium. *Arch Ophthalmol 1976;94:1799–1800.*

77. Roberts CW, Rosskothen HD, Koester CJ: Wide field specular microscopy of excised donor corneas. *Arch Ophthalmol 1981;99:881–883.*

78. Nesburn AB, Mandelbaum S, Willey DE, et al: A specular microscopic viewing system for donor corneas. *Ophthalmology 1983;90:686–691.*

79. Abbott RL, Fine BS, Webster RG, et al: Specular microscopic and histologic observations in nonguttate corneal endothelial degeneration. *Ophthalmology 1981;88:788–800.*

80. Abbott RL, Fine M, Guillet E: Long-term changes in corneal endothelium following penetrating keratoplasty. *Ophthalmology 1983;90:676–685.*

81. Laing RA, Leibowitz HM, Oak SS, et al: Endothelial mosaic in Fuchs' dystrophy. A qualitative evaluation with the specular microscope. *Arch Ophthalmol 1981;99:80–83.*

82. Brooks AMV, Grant GB, Gillies WE: The identification of corneal guttae. *Cornea 1991;10:249–260.*

83. Brooks AMV, Grant G, Gillies WE: Differentiation of posterior polymorphous dystrophy from other posterior corneal opacities by specular microscopy. *Ophthalmology 1989;96:1639–1645.*

84. Waring GO III: Clinical specular microscopy of posterior polymorphous endothelial dystrophy. *Am J Ophthalmol 1983;95:143–155.*

85. Laganowski HC, Sherrard ES, Kerr Muir MG: The posterior corneal surface in posterior polymorphous dystrophy: A specular microscopical study. *Cornea 1991;10:224–232.*

86. Hirst LW, Quigley HA, Stark WJ, Shields MB: Specular microscopy of iridocorneal endothelial syndrome. *Am J Ophthalmol 1980;89:11–21.*

87. Sherrard ES, Frangoulis MA, Kerr Muir MG: On the morphology of cells of posterior cornea in the iridocorneal endothelial syndrome. *Cornea 1991;10:233–243.*

88. Kupfer C, Kaiser-Kupfer MI, Datiles M, McCain L: The contralateral eye in the iridocorneal endothelial (ICE) syndrome. *Ophthalmology 1983;90:1343–1350.*

## CHAPTER 8
PATHOPHYSIOLOGY OF CORNEAL ENDOTHELIAL DYSFUNCTION

1. Beesly RD, Olson RJ, Brady SE: The effects of prolonged phacoemulsification time on the corneal endothelium. *Ann Ophthalmol 1986;18:216–222.*

2. Craig MT, Olson RJ, Mamalis N, Olson RJ: Air bubble endothelial damage during phacoemulsification in human eye bank eyes: The protective effects of Healon and Viscoat. *J Cataract Refract Surg 1990;16:597–602.*

3. Yee RW, Geroski DH, Matsuda M, et al: Correlation of corneal endothelial pump site density, barrier function, and morphology in wound repair. *Invest Ophthalmol Vis Sci 1985;26:1191–1201.*

4. Matsuda M, Sawa M, Edelhauser HF, et al: Cellular migration and morphology in corneal endothelial wound repair. *Invest Ophthalmol Vis Sci 1985;26:443–449.*

5. Schultz RO, Glasser DB, Matsuda M, et al: Response of the corneal endothelium to cataract surgery. *Arch Ophthalmol 1986; 104:1164–1169.*

6. Mishima S: Clinical investigations on the corneal endothelium. XXXVIII Edward Jackson Memorial Lecture. *Am J Ophthalmol 1982;93:1–29.*

7. Rao GN, Shaw EL, Arthur EJ, Aquavella JV: Endothelial cell morphology and corneal deturgescence. *Ann Ophthalmol 1979;11:885–899.*

8. Rao GN, Aquavella JV, Goldberg SH, Berk SL: Pseudophakic bullous keratopathy. Relationship to preoperative corneal endothelial status. *Ophthalmology 1984;91:1135–1140.*

9. Foulks GN, Thoft RA, Perry HD, Tolentino FI: Factors related to corneal epithelial complications after closed vitrectomy in diabetics. *Arch Ophthalmol 1979;97:1076–1078.*

10. Schultz RO, Matsuda M, Yee RW, et al: Corneal endothelial changes in type I and type II diabetes mellitus. *Am J Ophthalmol 1984;98:401–410.*

11. Nirankari VS, Baer JC: Persistent corneal edema in aphakic eyes from daily-wear and extended-wear contact lenses. *Am J Ophthalmol 1984;98:329–335.*

12. Edelhauser HF, Hanneken AM, Pederson HJ, Van Horn DL: Osmotic tolerance of rabbit and human corneal endothelium. *Arch Ophthalmol 1981;99:1281–1287.*

13. Gonnering R, Edelhauser HF, Van Horn DL, Durant W: The pH tolerance of rabbit and human corneal endothelium. *Invest Ophthalmol Vis Sci 1979;18:373–390.*

14. Stern ME, Edelhauser HF, Pederson HJ, Staatz WD: Effects of ionophores X537A and A23187 and calcium-free medium on corneal endothelial morphology. *Invest Ophthalmol Vis Sci 1981;20:497–507.*

15. Kaye GI, Mishima S, Cole JD, Kaye NW: Studies on the cornea. VII. Effects of perfusion with a $Ca^{++}$-free medium on the corneal endothelium. *Invest Ophthalmol Vis Sci 1968;7:53–66.*

16. Whikehart DR, Edelhauser HF: Glutathione in rabbit corneal endothelia: The effects of selected perfusion fluids. *Invest Ophthalmol Vis Sci 1978;17:455–464.*

17. Ng MC, Riley MV: Relation of intracellular levels and redox state of glutathione to endothelial function in the rabbit cornea. *Exp Eye Res 1980;30:511–517.*

18. Mishima S, Kudo T: In vitro incubation of rabbit cornea. *Invest Ophthalmol 1967;6:329–339.*

19. McDermott ML, Edelhauser HF, Hack HM, Langston RHS: Ophthalmic irrigants: A current review and update. *Ophthalmic Surg 1988;19:724–733.*

20. Glasser DB, Matsuda M, Ellis JG, Edelhauser HF: Effects of intraocular irrigating solutions on the corneal endothelium after in vivo anterior chamber irrigation. *Am J Ophthalmol 1985;99:321–328.*

21. Merrill DL, Fleming TC, Girard LJ: The effects of physiologic balanced salt solutions and normal saline on intraocular and extraocular tissues. *Am J Ophthalmol 1960;49:895–898.*

22. Glasser DB, Matsuda M, Edelhauser HF: Comparison of corneal endothelial structural and functional integrity after irrigation with bicarbonate-buffered andacetate-citrate-buffered solutions, in Cavanagh HD (ed): *The Cornea: Transactions of the World Congress on the Cornea III.* New York: Raven Press, 1988;101–106.

23. Dikstein S, Maurice DM: The metabolic basis to the fluid pump in the cornea. *J Physiol 1972;221:29–41.*

24. Edelhauser HF, Van Horn DL, Hyndiuk RA, Schultz RO: Intraocular irrigating solutions: Their effect on the corneal endothelium. *Arch Ophthalmol 1975;93:648–657.*

25. Edelhauser HF, Van Horn DL, Schultz RO, Hyndiuk RA: Comparative toxicity of intraocular irrigating solutions on the corneal endothelium. *Am J Ophthalmol 1976;81:473–481.*

26. Edelhauser HF: Intraocular irrigating solutions, in: Lamberts DW, Potter DE (eds): *Clinical Ophthalmic Pharmacology. Boston: Little, Brown, 1987, 431–444.*

27. Edelhauser HF, Gonnering R, Van Horn DL: Intraocular irrigating solutions: A comparative study of BSS Plus and lactated Ringer's solution. *Arch Ophthalmol 1978;96:516–520.*

28. Araie M: Barrier function of corneal endothelium and the intraocular irrigating solutions. *Arch Ophthalmol 1986;104:435–438.*

29. Kline OR, Symes DJ, Lorenzetti OJ, deFaller JM: Effect of BSS Plus on the corneal endothelium with intraocular lens implantation. *J Toxicol Cutan Ocular Toxicol 1983;2:243–247.*

30. Bourne WM, Liesegang TJ, Waller RR, Ilstrup DM: The effect of sodium hyaluronate on endothelial cell damage during extracapsular cataract extraction and posterior chamber lens implantation. *Am J Ophthalmol, 1984;98:759–762.*

31. Rosenfeld SI, Waltman SR, Olk RJ, Gordon M: Comparison of intraocular irrigating solutions in pars plana vitrectomy. *Ophthalmology 1986;93:109–114.*

32. Bourne WM: Morphologic and functional evaluation of the endothelium of transplanted human corneas. *Trans Am Ophthalmol Soc 1983;81:403–450.*

33. Hirst LW, Auer C, Abbey H, et al: Quantitative analysis of wide-field endothelial specular photomicrographs. *Am J Ophthalmol 1984;97:488–495.*

34. Isenberg RA, Weiss RL, Apple DJ, Lowry DB: Fungal contamination of balanced salt solution. *J Am Intraocul Implant Soc 1985;11:485–486.*

35. Samples JR, Binder PS: Contamination of irrigating solution used for cataract surgery. *Ophthal Surg 1984;15:66.*

36. O'Day DM: Special note. *Am J Ophthalmol 1984;97:128.*

37. Stern WH, Tamura E, Jacobs RA, et al: Epidemic postsurgical Candida parapsilosis endophthalmitis. Clinical findings and management of 15 consecutive cases. *Ophthalmology 1985;92:1701–1709.*

38. Googe JM, Mamalis N, Apple DJ, Olson RJ: BSS Warning. *J Am Intraocul Implant Soc 1984;10:202.*

39. Briggs RB, McCartney DL: Balanced salt solution infusion alert. *Arch Ophthalmol 1988;106:718.*

40. Glasser DB, Matsuda M, Edelhauser HF: A comparison of the efficacy and toxicity of and intraocular pressure response to viscous solutions in the anterior chamber. *Arch Ophthalmol 1986;104:1819–1824.*

41. McDermott ML, Edelhauser HF: Drug binding of ophthalmic viscoelastic agents. *Arch Ophthalmol 1989;107:261–263.*

42. Binkhorst CD: Inflammation and intraocular pressure after the use of Healon in intraocular lens surgery. *J Am Intraocul Implant Soc 1980;6:340–341.*

43. Pape LG: Intracapsular and extracapsular technique of lens implantation with Healon. *J Am Intraocul Implant Soc 1980;6:342–343.*

44. Percival P: Protective role of Healon during lens implantation. *Trans Ophthalmol Soc UK 1981;101:77–78.*

45. Lazenby GW, Broocker G: The use of sodium hyaluronate (Healon) in intracapsular cataract extraction with insertion of anterior chamber intraocular lenses. *Ophthalmic Surg 1981;12:646–649.*

46. Cherfan GM, Rich WJ, Wright G: Raised intraocular pressure and other problems with sodium hyaluronate and cataract surgery. *Trans Ophthalmol Soc UK 1983;103:227–232.*

47. Barron BA, Busin M, Page C, et al: Comparison of the effects of Viscoat and Healon on postoperative intraocular pressure. *Am J Ophthalmol 1985;100:377–384.*

48. MacRae SM, Edelhauser HF, Hyndiuk RA, et al: The effects of sodium hyaluronate, chondroitin sulfate, and methylcellulose on the corneal endothelium and intraocular pressure. *Am J Ophthalmol 1983;95:332–341.*

49. Rich WJ, Radtke ND, Cohan BE: Early ocular hypertension after cataract extraction. *Br J Ophthalmol 1974;58:725–731.*

50. Berson FG, Patterson MM, Epstein DL: Obstruction of aqueous outflow by sodium hyaluronate in enucleated human eyes. *Am J Ophthalmol 1983;95:668–672.*

51. Iwata S, Miyauchi S: Biochemical studies on the use of sodium hyaluronate in the anterior eye segment: III. Histological studies on distribution and efflux process of 5-amino fluorescein-labeled hyaluronate. *Jpn J Ophthalmol 1985;29:187–197.*

52. West DR, Lischwe TD, Thompson VM, Ide CH: Comparative efficacy of the β-blockers for the prevention of increased intraocular pressure after cataract extraction. *Am J Ophthalmol 1988;106:168–173.*

53. McCulley JP, Stern ME, Meyer DR: In vitro assessment of the comparative toxicity of viscoelastic substances. *Invest Ophthalmol Vis Sci 1985;(suppl 26):239.*

54. Nevyas AS, Raber IM, Eagle RC, et al: Acute band keratopathy following intracameral Viscoat. *Arch Ophthalmol 1987;105:958–964.*

55. Binder PS, Deg JK, Kohl FS: Calcific band keratopathy after intraocular chondroitin sulfate. *Arch Ophthalmol 1987;105:1243–1247.*

56. Slack JW, Hyndiuk RA: Toxicology of surgical solutions and drugs, in Albert D, Jakobiec F (eds): *Textbook of Ophthalmology: The Harvard System.* New York: WB Saunders, in press.

57. Richter W: Non-immunogenicity of purified hyaluronic acid preparations tested by passive cutaneous anaphylaxis. *Int Arch Allerg Appl Immunol 1974;47:211–217.*

58. Richter W, Ryde M, Zetterstrom O: Non-immunogenicity of purified sodium hyaluronate preparation in man. *Int Arch Allerg Appl Immunol 1979;59:45–48.*

59. Hoover DL, Giangiacomo J, Benson RL: Descemet's membrane detachment by sodium hyaluronate. *Arch Ophthalmol 1985;103:805–808.*

60. McKnight SJ, Giangiacomo J, Adelstein E: Inflammatory response to viscoelastic materials. *Ophthalmic Surg 1987;18:804–806.*

61. Hultsch E: The scope of hyaluronic acid as an experimental intraocular implant. *Ophthalmology 1980;87:706–712.*

62. Fleming TC, Merrill DL, Girard LJ: Studies of the irritating action of methylcellulose. *Arch Ophthalmol 1959;61:565–567.*

63. American Academy of Ophthalmology: Recall of CooperVision Viscoat. *Clin Alert Nov 25, 1967, 6/1.*

64. Machemer R: Vitrectomy—A Pars Plana Approach. New York: Grune & Stratton, *1975, 51.*

65. Edelhauser HF, Hine JE, Pederson H, et al: The effect of phenylephrine on the cornea. *Arch Ophthalmol 1979;97:937–947.*

66. Cohen KL, Van Horn DL, Edelhauser HF, Schultz RO: Effect of phenylephrine on normal and regenerated endothelial cells in cat cornea. *Invest Ophthalmol Vis Sci 1979;18:242–249.*

67. Hull DS, Chemotti MT, Edelhauser HF, et al: Effect of epinephrine on the corneal endothelium. *Am J Ophthalmol 1975;79:245–250.*

68. Edelhauser HF, Hyndiuk RA, Zeeb A, Schultz RO: Corneal edema and the intraocular use of epinephrine. *Am J Ophthalmol 1982;93:327–333.*

69. Slack JW, Edelhauser HF, Helenek MJ: A bisulfite-free intraocular epinephrine solution. *Am J Ophthalmol 1990;110:77–82.*

70. Coles WH: Pilocarpine toxicity. *Arch Ophthalmol 1975;93:36–41.*

71. Grehn F: Intraocular thymoxamine for miosis during surgery. *Am J Ophthalmol 1987;103:709–711.*

72. Prosdocimo G, De Marco D: Intraocular dapiprazole to reverse mydriasis during extracapsular cataract extraction. *Am J Ophthalmol 1988;105:321–322.*

73. Hollands RH, Drance SM, Schulzer M: The effect of acetylcholine on early postoperative intraocular pressure. *Am J Ophthalmol 1987;103:749–753.*

74. Hollands RH, Drance SM, Schulzer M: The effect of intracameral carbachol on intraocular pressure after cataract extraction. *Am J Ophthalmol 1987;104:225–228.*

75. Ruiz RS, Rhem MN, Prager TC: Effects of carbachol and acetylcholine on intraocular pressure after cataract extraction. *Am J Ophthalmol 1989;107:7–10.*

76. Yee RW, Edelhauser HF: Comparison of intraocular acetylcholine and carbachol. *J Cataract Refract Surg 1986;12:18–22.*

77. Birnbaum DR, Hull DS, Green K, Frey NP: Effect of carbachol on rabbit corneal endothelium. *Arch Ophthalmol 1987;105:253–255.*

78. Green K, Livingston V, Bowman K, Hull DS: Chlorhexidine effects on corneal epithelium and endothelium. *Arch Ophthalmol 1980;98:1273–1281.*

79. Gasset AR, Ishii Y, Kaufman HE, Miller T: Cytotoxicity of ophthalmic preservatives. *Am J Ophthalmol 1974;78:98–105.*

80. Coles WH: Effects of antibiotics on the in vitro rabbit corneal endothelium. *Invest Ophthalmol 1975;14:246–250.*

81. Van Horn DL, Edelhauser HF, Prodanovich G, et al: Effect of the ophthalmic preservative thimerosal on the rabbit and human corneal endothelium. *Invest Ophthalmol Vis Sci 1977;16:273–280.*

82. Green K, Hull DS, Vaughn ED, et al: Rabbit endothelial response to ophthalmic preservatives. *Arch Ophthalmol 1977;95:2218–2221.*

83. Weinreb RN, Wood I, Tomazzoli L, Alvarado J: Subconjunctival injections. Preservative-related changes in the corneal endothelium. *Invest Ophthalmol Vis Sci 1986;27:525–531.*

84. Lemp MA, Zimmerman LE: Toxic endothelial degeneration in ocular surface disease treated with topical medications containing benzalkonium chloride. *Am J Ophthalmol 1988;105:670–673.*

85. American Academy of Ophthalmology: Corneal toxicity with antibiotic steroid-soaked collagen shields. *Clin Alert Nov 9, 1990, 11/1.*

86. Nuyts RMMA, Edelhauser HF, Pels E, Breebaart AC: Toxic effects of detergents on the corneal endothelium. *Arch Ophthalmol 1990;108:1158–1162.*

87. Edelhauser HF, Antoine ME, Pederson HJ, et al: Intraocular safety evaluation of ethylene oxide and sterilant residues. *J Toxicol (Cutan Ocular Toxicol) 1983;2:7–39.*

88. Stark WJ, Rosenblum P, Maumenee AE, Cowan CL: Postoperative inflammatory reactions to intraocular lenses sterilized with ethylene oxide. *Ophthalmology 1980;87:385–389.*

89. Kim JH: Intraocular inflammation of denatured viscoelastic substance in cases of cataract extraction and lens implantation. *J Cataract Refract Surg 1987;13:537–542.*

90. Breebaart AC, Nuyts RMMA, Pels E, et al: Toxic endothelial cell destruction of the cornea after routine extracapsular cataract surgery. *Arch Ophthalmol 1990;108:1121–1125.*

91. Hamed LM, Ellis FD, Boudreault G, et al: Hibiclens keratitis. *Am J Ophthalmol 1987;104:50–56.*

92. Phinney RB, Mondino BJ, Hofbauer JD, et al: Corneal edema related to accidental Hibiclens exposure. *Am J Ophthalmol 1988;106:210–215.*

93. Apt L, Isenberg SJ: Hibiclens keratitis (correspondence). *Am J Ophthalmol 1987;104:670.*

94. Shore JW: Hibiclens keratitis (correspondence). *Am J Ophthalmol 1987;104:670–671.*

95. Apt L, Isenberg SJ: Chemical preparation of skin and eye in ophthalmic surgery: An international survey. *Ophthalmic Surg 1982;13:1026–1029.*

96. MacRae SM, Brown B, Edelhauser HF: The corneal toxicity of presurgical skin antiseptics. *Am J Ophthalmol 1984;97:221–232.*

97. Apt L, Isenberg S, Yoshimori R, Paez JH: Chemical preparation of the eye in ophthalmic surgery. III. Effect of povidone-iodine on the conjunctiva. *Arch Ophthalmol 1984;102:728–729.*

98. Haimann MH, Abrams GW, Edelhauser HF, Hatchell DL: The effect of intraocular irrigating solutions on lens clarity in normal and diabetic rabbits. *Am J Ophthalmol 1982;94:594–605.*

99. Haimann MH, Abrams GW: Prevention of lens opacification during diabetic vitrectomy. *Ophthalmology 1984;91:116–121.*

100. Lambrou FH, Snyder RW, Williams GA: Use of tissue plasminogen activator in experimental hyphema. *Arch Ophthalmol 1987;105:995–997.*

101. Snyder RW, Lambrou FH, Williams GA: Intraocular fibrinolysis with recombinant human tissue plasminogen activator. *Arch Ophthalmol 1987;105:1277–1280.*

102. Lambrou FH, Snyder RW, Williams GA, Lewandowski M: Treatment of experimental intravitreal fibrin with tissue plasminogen activator. *Am J Ophthalmol 1987;104:619–623.*

103. Johnson RN, Olsen K, Hernandez E: Tissue plasminogen activator treatment of postoperative intraocular fibrin. *Ophthalmology 1988;95:592–596.*

104. Williams GW, Lambrou FH, Jaffe GA, et al: Treatment of postvitrectomy fibrin formation with intraocular tissue plasminogen activator. *Arch Ophthalmol 1988;106:1055–1058.*

105. Ortiz JR, Walker SD, McManus PE, et al: Filtering bleb thrombolysis with tissue plasminogen activator. *Am J Ophthalmol 1988;106:624–625.*

106. Rowland FN, Donovan MJ, Gillies C, et al: Fibrin: Mediator of in vivo and in vitro injury and inflammation. *Curr Eye Res 1985;4:537–553.*

107. Dabbs CK, Aaberg TA, Aquilar HE, et al: Complications of tissue plasminogen activator therapy after vitrectomy for diabetes. *Am J Ophthalmol 1990;110:354–360.*

108. Thompson JT, Glaser BM, Michels RG, de Bustros S: The use of intravitreal thrombin to control hemorrhage during vitrectomy. *Ophthalmology 1986;93:279–282.*

109. Blacharski PA, Charles ST: Thrombin infusion to control bleeding during vitrectomy for stage V retinopathy of prematurity. *Arch Ophthalmol 1987;105:203–205.*

110. Mannis MJ, Sweet E, Landers MB, Lewis RA: Uses of thrombin in ocular surgery. Effect on the corneal endothelium. *Arch Ophthalmol 1988;106:251–253.*

111. McDermott ML, Edelhauser HF, Mannis MJ: Intracameral thrombin and the corneal endothelium. *Am J Ophthalmol 1988;106:414–422.*

112. Creel DJ, Wang JM, Wong KC: Transient blindness associated with transurethral resection of the prostate. *Arch Ophthalmol 1987;105:1537–1539.*

113. de Bustros S, Glaser BM, Johnson MA: Thrombin infusion for the control of intraocular bleeding during vitreous surgery. *Arch Ophthalmol 1985;103:837–839.*

114. Verdoorn C, Hendrikse F: Intraocular human thrombin infusion in diabetic vitrectomies. *Ophthalmic Surg 1989;20:278–279.*

115. Aaberg TA: Balancing the benefits and risks of intracameral thrombin. *Am J Ophthalmol 1988;106:485–486.*

116. Refojo MF, Dohlman CH, Koliopoulos J: Adhesives in ophthalmology. A review. *Surv Ophthalmol 1971;15:217–236.*

117. Leonard F, Kulkarni RK, Brandes G: Synthesis and degradation of poly (alkyl alpha-cyanoacrylates). *J Appl Polymer Sci 1966;10:259–266.*

118. Nesburn AB, Ziniti P: Cell culture toxicity of two cyanoacrylate adhesives. *Invest Ophthalmol 1969;(suppl 8):648.*

119. Aaronson SB, McMaster PRB, Moore TE Jr, Coon MA: Toxicity of the cyanoacrylates. *Arch Ophthalmol 1970;84:342–349.*

120. Ferry AP, Barnert AH: Granulomatous keratitis resulting from use of cyanoacrylate adhesive for closure of perforated corneal ulcer. *Am J Ophthalmol 1971;72:538–541.*

121. Sani BP, Refojo MF: 14C-isobutyl 2-cyanoacrylate adhesive. Determination of absorption in the cornea. *Arch Ophthalmol 1972;87:216–221.*

122. Hanna C, Shibley S: Tissue reaction to intracorneal silicone rubber (Silastic RTV 382) and methyl-2-cyanoacrylate (Eastman 910 adhesive). *Am J Ophthalmol 1965;60:323–327.*

123. Bloomfield S, Barnert AH, Kanter PD: The use of Eastman 910 monomer as an adhesive in ocular surgery. I. Biologic effects on ocular tissue. *Am J Ophthalmol 1963;55:742–748.*

124. Gasset AR, Hood CI, Ellison ED, Kaufman HE: Ocular tolerance to cyanoacrylate monomer tissue adhesive analogues. *Invest Ophthalmol 1970;9:3–11.*

125. Girard LJ, Cobb S, Reed T: Surgical adhesives and bonded contact lenses: An experimental study. *Ann Ophthalmol 1969;1:65–73.*

126. Siegal JE, Zaidman GW: Surgical removal of cyanoacrylate adhesive after accidental instillation in the anterior chamber. *Ophthalmic Surg 1989;20:179–181.*

127. Hyndiuk RA, Hull DS, Kinyoun JL: Free tissue patch and cyanoacrylate in corneal perforations. *Ophthalmic Surg 1974;5:50–55.*

128. Sternberg P, Hatchell DL, Foulks GN, Landers MB: The effect of silicone oil on the cornea. *Arch Ophthalmol 1985;103:90–94.*

129. Leaver PK, Grey RHB, Garner A: Silicone oil injection in the treatment of massive preretinal retraction. II. Late complications in 93 eyes. *Br J Ophthalmol 1979;63:361–367.*

130. Haut J, Ullern M, Chermet M, Van Effenterre: Complications of intraocular injections of silicone combined with vitrectomy. *Ophthalmologica 1980;180:29–35.*

131. Federman JL, Schubert HD: Complications associated with the use of silicone oil in 150 eyes after retina–vitreous surgery. *Ophthalmology 1988;95:870–876.*

132. Beekhuis WH, van Rij G, Zivojnovic R: Silicone oil keratopathy: indications for keratoplasty. *Br J Ophthalmol 1985;69:247–253.*

133. Bennett SR, Abrams GW: Band keratopathy from emulsified silicone oil. *Arch Ophthalmol 1990;108:1387.*

134. Van Horn DL, Edelhauser HF, Aaberg TM, Pederson HJ: In vivo effects of air and sulfur hexafluoride gas on rabbit corneal endothelium. *Invest Ophthalmol 1972;11:1028–1036.*

135. Olson RJ: Air and the corneal endothelium. An in vivo specular microscopic study in cats. *Arch Ophthalmol 1980;98:1283–1284.*

136. Leibowitz HM, Laing RA, Sandstrom M: Corneal endothelium. The effect of air in the anterior chamber. *Arch Ophthalmol 1974;92:227–230.*

137. Brubaker S, Peyman GA, Vygantas C: Toxicity of octofluorocyclobutane after intracameral injection. *Arch Ophthalmol 1974;92:324–328.*

138. Nabih M, Peyman GA, Clark LC, et al: Experimental evaluation of perfluorophenanthrene as a high specific gravity vitreous substitute: A preliminary report. *Ophthalmic Surg 1989;20:286–293.*

139. Foulks GN, de Juan E, Hatchell DL, et al: The effect of perfluoropropane on the cornea in rabbits and cats. *Arch Ophthalmol 1987;105:256–259.*

140. Olsen T: Changes in the corneal endothelium after acute anterior uveitis as seen with the specular microscope. *Acta Ophthalmol 1980;58:250–256.*

141. Macdonald JM, Geroski DH, Edelhauser HF: Effect of inflammation on the corneal endothelial pump and barrier. *Curr Eye Res 1987;6:1125–1132.*

142. Davis KL, Conners M, Dunn MW, Schwartzmann ML: Contact lens mediated hypoxia stimulates novel cytochrome P450 arachidonate metabolites. *Invest Ophthalmol Vis Sci 1990;(suppl 31):406.*

143. Maurice D: The cornea and sclera, in Davson H (ed): The Eye. New York: Academic Press, 1984, 1–158.

144. Klyce SD: Stromal lactate accumulation can account for corneal oedema osmotically following epithelial hypoxia in the rabbit. *J Physiol (Lond) 1981;321:49–64.*

145. Bonnano JA, Polse KA: Corneal acidosis during contact lens wear: Effects of hypoxia and $CO_2$. *Invest Ophthalmol Vis Sci 1987;28:1514–1520.*

146. Holden BA, Williams L, Zantos SG: The etiology of transient endothelial changes in the human cornea. *Invest Ophthalmol Vis Sci 1985;26:1354–1359.*

147. Schoessler JP, Woloschak MJ: Corneal endothelium in veteran PMMA contact lens wearers. *Int Contact Lens Clinics 1981;8:19–25.*

148. Schoessler JP: Corneal endothelial polymegethism associated with extended wear. *Int Contact Lens Clinics 1982;10:148–155.*

149. Hirst LW, Auer C, Cohn J, et al: Specular microscopy of hard contact lens wearers. *Ophthalmology 1984;91:1147–1153.*

150. Stocker EG, Schoessler JP: Corneal endothelial polymegathism induced by PMMA contact lens wear. *Invest Ophthalmol Vis Sci 1985;26:857–863.*

151. MacRae SM, Matsuda M, Yee RW: The effect of long-term hard contact lens wear on the corneal endothelium. *CLAO J 1985;11:322–326.*

152. MacRae SM, Matsuda M, Shellans S, Rich LF: The effects of hard and soft contact lenses on the corneal endothelium. *Am J Ophthalmol* 1986;102:50–57.

153. MacRae SM, Matsuda M, Shellans S: Corneal endothelial changes associated with contact lens wear. *CLAO J* 1989;15:82–87.

154. Holden BA, Sweeney DF, Vannas A, et al: Effects of long-term extended contact lens wear on the human cornea. *Invest Ophthalmol Vis Sci* 1985;26:1489–1501.

155. Polse KA, Brand RJ, Cohen SR, Guillon M: Hypoxic effects on corneal morphology and function. *Invest Ophthalmol Vis Sci* 1990;31:1542–1554.

156. Matsuda M, Inaba M, Suda T, MacRae SM: Corneal endothelial changes associated with aphakic extended contact lens wear. *Arch Ophthalmol* 1988;106:70–72.

157. Lass JH, Dutt RM, Spurney RV, et al: Morphologic and fluorophotometric analysis of the corneal endothelium in long-term hard and soft contact lens wearers. *CLAO J* 1988;14:105–109.

158. Carlson KH, Bourne WM, Brubaker RF: Effect of long-term contact lens wear on corneal endothelial cell morphology and function. *Invest Ophthalmol Vis Sci* 1988;29:185–193.

159. MacDonald JM, McCarey BE: Hypoxic stress of contact lens wear on the pump site density of the corneal endothelium. *Invest Ophthalmol Vis Sci,* 1988;(suppl 29):419.

160. Dutt RM, Stocker EG, Wolff CH, et al: A morphologic and fluorophotometric analysis of the corneal endothelium in long-term extended wear soft contact lens wearers. *CLAO J* 1989;15:121–123.

161. Yee RW, Matsuda M, Kern TS, et al: Corneal endothelial changes in diabetic dogs. *Curr Eye Res* 1985;4:759–766.

162. Matsuda M, Awata T, Ohashi Y, et al: The effects of aldose reductase inhibitor on the corneal endothelial morphology in diabetic rats. *Curr Eye Res* 1987;6:391–397.

163. Meyer LA, Ubels JL, Edelhauser HF: Corneal endothelial morphology in the rat. Effects of aging, diabetes, and topical aldose reductase inhibitor treatment. *Invest Ophthalmol Vis Sci* 1988;29:940–948.

1. Barchiesi BJ, Eckel RH, Ellis PP: The cornea and disorders of lipid metabolism. *Surv Ophthalmol* 1991;36:1–22.

2. Gass JDM: The iron lines of the superficial cornea: Hudson-Stähli line, Stocker's line, and Fleischer's ring. *Arch Ophthalmol* 1964;71:348–358.

3. Barraquer-Somers E, Chan CC, Green WR: Corneal epithelial iron deposition. *Ophthalmology* 1983;90:729–734.

4. Norn MS: Hudson-Stähli's line of cornea. I. Incidence and morphology. *Acta Ophthalmol (Copenh)* 1968;46:106–118.

5. Norn MS: Hudson-Stähli's line of cornea. II. Aetiological studies. *Acta Ophthalmol (Copenh)* 1968;46:119–128.

6. Ferry AP: A "new" iron line of the superficial cornea: Occurrence in patients with filtering blebs. *Arch Ophthalmol* 1968;79:142–145.

7. Vogt A: Corneal degenerations of various etiology, in *Textbook and Atlas of Slit Lamp Microscopy of the Living Eye.* Vol 1. Bonn: Wayenborgh, c 1930, reprint 1981, 92–121.

8. Sugar HS, Kobernick S: The white limbus girdle of Vogt. *Am J Ophthalmol* 1960;50:101–107.

9. Cogan DG, Kuwabara T: Arcus senilis, its pathology and histochemistry. *Arch Ophthalmol* 1959;61:553–560.

10. Walton KW: Studies on the pathogenesis of corneal arcus formation. The human corneal arcus and its relation to atherosclerosis as studied by immunofluorescence. *J Pathol* 1973;111:263–274.

11. Walton KW, Dunkerley DJ: Studies on the pathogenesis of corneal arcus formation. II. Immunofluorescent studies on lipid deposition in the eye of the lipid-fed rabbit. *J Pathol* 1974;114:217–229.

12. Andrews JS: The lipids of arcus senilis. *Arch Ophthalmol* 1962;68:264–266.

13. Rifkind BM: Corneal arcus and hyperlipoproteinaemia. *Surv Ophthalmol* 1972;16:295–304.

# CHAPTER 9
## DEGENERATIVE CHANGES OF THE CORNEA

14. Vinger PF, Sachs BA: Ocular manifestations of hyperlipoproteinaemia. *Am J Ophthalmol 1970;70:563–573.*

15. Winder AF: Factors influencing the variable expression of xanthelasmata and corneal arcus in familial hypercholesterolemia. *Birth Defects 1982;18:449–462.*

16. Pe'er J, Vidaurri J, Halfon S-T, et al: Association between corneal arcus and some of the risk factors for coronary artery disease. *Br J Ophthalmol 1984;67:795–798.*

17. Smith JL, Susac JO: Unilateral arcus senilis: Sign of occlusive disease of the carotid artery. *JAMA 1973;226:676.*

18. Rosenman RH, Brand RJ, Sholtz BJ, Jenkins CD: Relation of corneal arcus to cardiovascular risk factors and incidence of coronary disease. *N Engl J Med 1979;29:1322–1324.*

19. Horven I, Egge K, Gjone E: Corneal and fundus changes in familial LCAT deficiency. *Acta Ophthalmol (Copenh) 1974;52:201–210.*

20. Fredrickson DS, Gotto AM, Levy RI: Familial lipoprotein deficiency, in Stanbury JB, Wyngaarden JB, Fredrickson DS (eds): *The Metabolic Basis of Inherited Disease,* ed 6. New York: McGraw-Hill, 1989, 493–530.

21. Paufique L, Etienne R: La cornea farinata. *Bull Soc Ophtalmol Fr 1950;50:522–526.*

22. Curran RE, Kenyon KR, Green WR: Pre-Descemet's membrane corneal dystrophy. *Am J Ophthalmol 1974;77:711–716.*

23. Bron AJ, Tripathi RC: Anterior corneal mosaic: Further observations. *Br J Ophthalmol 1969;53:760–764.*

24. Tripathi RC, Bron AJ: Secondary anterior crocodile shagreen of Vogt. *Br J Ophthalmol 1975;59:59–63.*

25. Krachmer JH, Dubord PJ, Rodrigues MM, et al: Corneal posterior crocodile shagreen and polymorphic amyloid degeneration: A histopathologic study. *Arch Ophthalmol 1983;101:54–59.*

26. Sturrock G: Glassy corneal striae. *Albrecht Graefes Arch Clin Ophthalmol 1973;188:245–252.*

27. Feeney ML, Garron LK: Descemet's membrane in the human peripheral cornea: A study by light and electron microscopy, in Smelser GK (ed): *Structure of the Eye. Proceedings of the Seventh International Congress of Anatomists, New York, 1960.* New York: Academic Press, 1961, 367–380.

28. Klintworth GK: Chronic actinic keratopathy: A condition associated with conjunctival elastosis (pingueculae) and typified by characteristic extracellular concretions. *Am J Pathol 1972;67:327–348.*

29. Moran DJ, Hollows FC: Pterygium and ultraviolet radiation: A positive correlation. *Br J Ophthalmol 1984;68:343–346.*

30. Taylor HR, West SK, Rosenthal FS, et al: Corneal changes associated with chronic UV irradiation. *Arch Ophthalmol 1989;107:1481–1484.*

31. Cameron ME: *Pterygium Throughout the World.* Springfield, Ill: Charles C Thomas, 1965.

32. Mackenzie FD, Hirst LW, Battistutta D, Green A: Risk analysis in the development of pterygia. *Ophthalmoloy 1992;99:1056–1061.*

33. Austin P, Jakobiec HA, Iwamoto T: Elastodysplasia and elastodystrophy as pathologic bases of ocular pterygia and pinguecula. *Ophthalmology 1983;90:96–109.*

34. Zauberman H: Pterygium and its recurrence. *Am J Ophthalmol 1967;63:1780–1786.*

35. Youngson RM: Recurrence of pterygium after excision. *Br J Ophthalmol 1972;56:120–125.*

36. Alaniz-Camino F: The use of postoperative beta radiation in the treatment of pterygia. *Ophthalmic Surg 1982;13:1022–1025.*

37. Cooper JS, Lerch IA: Postoperative irradiation of pterygia. *Radiology 1980;135:743–745.*

38. Harrison M, Kelly A, Ohlrich J: Pterygium: Thiotepa versus beta radiation, a double-blind trial. *Trans Aust Coll Ophthalmol 1969;1:64–66.*

39. Asregadoo ER: Surgery, thio-tepa, and corticosteroid in the treatment of pterygium. *Am J Ophthalmol 1972;74:960–963.*

40. Singh G, Wilson MR, Foster CS: Mitomycin eye drops as treatment for pterygium. *Ophthalmology 1988;95:813–821.*

41. Hayasaka S, Noda S, Yamamoto Y, et al: Postoperative instillation of low-dose mitomycin C in the treatment of primary pterygium. *Am J Ophthalmol 1988;106:715–718.*

42. Kenyon KR, Wagoner MD, Hettinger ME: Conjunctival autograft transplantation for advanced and recurrent pterygium. *Ophthalmology 1985;92:1461–1470.*

43. Pearlman G, Susal AL, Hushaw J, et al: Recurrent pterygium and treatment with lamellar keratoplasty with presentation of a technique to limit recurrences. *Ann Ophthalmol 1970;2:763–771.*

44. Poirier RH, Fish JR: Lamellar keratoplasty for recurrent pterygium. *Ophthalmic Surg 1976;7:38–41.*

45. Laughrea PA, Arentsen JJ: Lamellar keratoplasty in the management of recurrent pterygium. *Ophthalmic Surg 1986;17:106–108.*

46. Busin M, Halliday BL, Arffa RC, et al: Precarved lyophilized tissue for lamellar keratoplasty in recurrent pterygium. *Am J Ophthalmol 1986;102:222–227.*

47. Bietti GB, Guerra P, Ferraris de Gaspare PF: La dystrophie corneene nodulaire en ceinture des pays tropicaux à sol aride. *Bull Soc Fr Ophtalmol 1955;68:101-129.*

48. Freedman A: Labrador keratopathy. *Arch Ophthalmol 1965;74:198-202.*

49. Gray RH, Johnson GJ, Freedman A: Climatic droplet keratopathy. *Surv Ophthalmol 1992;36:241-253.*

50. Klintworth GK: Lattice corneal dystrophy. An inherited variety of amyloidosis restricted to the cornea. *Am J Pathol 1967;50:371–399.*

51. Meretoja J: Familial systemic paramyloidosis with lattice dystrophy of the cornea, progressive cranial neuropathy, skin changes and various internal symptoms: A previously unrecognized heritable syndrome. *Ann Clin Res 1969;1:314–324.*

52. Mannis MJ, Krachmer JH, Rodrigues MM, Pardos GJ: Polymorphic amyloid degeneration of the cornea. A clinical and histopathologic study. *Arch Ophthalmol 1981;99:1217–1223.*

53. Vannas A, Hogan MJ, Wood I: Salzmann's nodular degeneration of the cornea. *Am J Ophthalmol 1975;79:211–219.*

54. O'Connor GR: Calcific band keratopathy. *Trans Am Ophthalmol Soc 1972;70:58–81.*

55. Coats G: Two cases showing a small superficial opaque white rings in the cornea. *Trans Ophthalmol Soc UK 1912;32:53–56.*

56. Krachmer JH: Pellucid marginal corneal degeneration. *Arch Ophthalmol 1978;96:1217–1221.*

57. Rodrigues MM, Newsome DA, Krachmer JH, et al: Pellucid marginal corneal degeneration: A clinicopathologic study of two cases. *Exp Eye Res 1981;33:277–288.*

58. Barraquer F: Results of the crescent resection in keratotorus. *Dev Ophthalmol 1981;5:49–51.*

59. Schanzlin DJ, Sarno EM, Robin JB: Crescentic lamellar keratoplasty for pellucid marginal degeneration. *Am J Ophthalmol 1983;96:253–254.*

60. Terrien F: Dystrophie marginale symétrique des cornées avec astigmatisme. *Arch Ophtalmol 1900;20:12–21.*

61. Austin P, Brown SI: Inflammatory Terrien's marginal corneal disease. *Am J Ophthalmol 1981;92:189–202.*

62. Süveges I, Levai G, Alberth B: Pathology of Terrien's disease. *Am J Ophthalmol 1972;74:1191–1200.*

63. Iwamoto T, DeVoe AG, Farris RL: Electron microscopy in cases of marginal degeneration of the cornea. *Invest Ophthalmol 1972;11:241–257.*

64. Brown AC, Rao GN, Aquavella JV: Peripheral corneal grafts in Terrien's marginal degeneration. *Ophthalmic Surg 1983;14:931–934.*

65. Caldwell DR, Insler MS, Boutros G, et al: Primary surgical repair of severe peripheral marginal ectasia in Terrien's marginal degeneration. *Am J Ophthalmol 1984;97:332–336.*

66. Bierly JR, Dunn JP, Dawson CR, et al: Fuchs' superficial marginal keratitis. *Am J Ophthalmol 1992;113:541–545.*

67. Fine BS, Townsend WM, Zimmerman LE: Primary lipoidal degeneration of the cornea. *Am J Ophthalmol 1974;78:12–23.*

68. Jack RL, Luse SA: Lipid keratopathy, an electron microscopic study. *Arch Ophthalmol 1970;83:678–691.*

69. Baum JL: Cholesterol keratopathy. *Am J Ophthalmol 1969;67:372–375.*

70. Sturrock GD: Nocturnal lagophthalmos and recurrent erosion. *Br J Ophthalmol 1976;60:97–103.*

71. Cavanagh DW, Pihlaja D, Thoft RA, et al: Pathogenesis and treatment of persistent epithelial defects. *Trans Am Acad Ophthalmol Otolaryngol 1976;81:754–769.*

72. Chandler PA: Recurrent erosion of the cornea. *Am J Ophthalmol 1945;28:355–363.*

73. Mcllean EN, MacRae SM, Rich LF: Recurrent erosion: Treament by anterior stromal puncture. *Ophthalmology 1986;93:784–788.*

74. Alper MG: The anesthetic eye: An investigation of changes in the anterior ocular segment of the monkey caused by interrupting the trigeminal nerve at various levels along its course. *Trans Am Ophthalmol Soc 1975;73:323–365.*

75. Sigelman S, Friedenwald JS: Mitotic and wound healing activities of the corneal epithelium: Effect of sensory denervation. *Arch Ophthalmol 1954;52:46–57.*

76. Mishima S: The effects of the denervation and the stimulation of the sympathetic and the trigeminal nerve on the mitotic rate of the corneal epithelium in the rabbit. *Jpn J Ophthalmol 1957;1:56–73.*

77. Mittag TW, Mindel JS, Green JP: Choline acetyltransferase in familial dysautonomia. *Ann NY Acad Sci 1974;228:301–306.*

## CHAPTER 10
### CONGENITAL ANOMALIES AND INHERITED DYSTROPHIES OF THE CORNEA

1. Waring GO III, Rodrigues MM, Laibson PR: Corneal dystrophies I. Dystrophies of the epithelium, Bowman's layer and stroma. *Surv Ophthalmol 1978;23:71–122.*

2. Cook CS: Experimental models of anterior segment dysgenesis. *Ophthalmic Paediatr Genet 1989;10:33–46.*

3. Salmon JF, Wallis CE, Murray ADN: Variable expressivity of autosomal dominant microcornea with cataract. *Arch Ophthalmol 1988;106:505–510.*

4. Skuta GL, Sugar J, Ericson ES: Corneal endothelial cell measurements in megalocornea. *Arch Ophthalmol 1983;101:51–53.*

5. Biglan AW, Brown SI, Johnson BL: Keratoglobus and blue sclera. *Am J Ophthalmol 1977;83:225–233.*

6. Shields MB, Buckley E, Klintworth GK, Thresher R: Axenfeld-Rieger syndrome: A spectrum of developmental disorders. *Surv Ophthalmol 1985;29:387–409.*

7. Townsend WM, Font RL, Zimmerman LE: Congenital corneal leukomas II. Histopathologic findings in 19 eyes with central defect in Descemet's membrane. *Am J Ophthalmol 1974;77:192–206.*

8. Miller MT, Epstein RJ, Sugar J, et al: Anterior segment anomalies associated with the fetal alcohol syndrome. *J Pediatr Ophthalmol Strabismus 1984;21:8–18.*

9. Laibson PR: Microcystic corneal dystrophy. *Trans Am Ophthalmol Soc 1976;74:488–531.*

10. Cogan DG, Donaldson DD, Kuwabara T, Marshall D: Microcystic dystrophy of the corneal epithelium. *Trans Am Ophthalmol Soc 1964;62:213–225.*

11. Laibson PR, Krachmer JH: Familial occurrence of dot (microcystic), map, fingerprint dystrophy of the cornea. *Invest Ophthalmol 1975;14:397–399.*

12. Werblin TP, Hirst LW, Stark WJ, Maumenee IH: Prevalence of map-dot-fingerprint changes in the cornea. *Br J Ophthalmol 1981;65:401–409.*

13. Buxton JN, Fox ML: Superficial epithelial keratectomy in the treatment of epithelial basement membrane dystrophy. *Arch Ophthalmol 1983;101:392–395.*

14. Wood TO, Griffith ME: Surgery for corneal epithelial basement membrane dystrophy. *Ophthalmic Surg 1988;19:20–24.*

15. Fine BS, Yanoff M, Pitts E, Slaughter FD: Meesmann's epithelial dystrophy of the cornea. *Am J Ophthalmol 1977;83:633–642.*

16. Bourne WM: Soft contact lens wear decreases epithelial microcysts in Meesmann's corneal dystrophy. *Trans Am Ophthalmol Soc 1986;84:170–182.*

17. Lisch W, Steuhl K-P, Lisch C, et al: A new, band-shaped and whorled microcystic dystrophy of the corneal epithelium. *Am J Ophthalmol 1992;114:35–44.*

18. Reis W: Familiäre fleckige Hornhautentartung. *Dtsch Med Wochenschr 1917;43:575.*

19. Bücklers M: Uber eine weitere familiäre Hornhautdystrophie (Reis). *Klin Monatsbl Augenheilkd 1949;114:386–397.*

20. Wittebol-Post D, Pels E: The dystrophy described by Reis and Bücklers: Separate entity or variant of the granular dystrophy? *Ophthalmologica 1989;199:1–9.*

21. Moller HU: Granular corneal dystrophy Groenouw type I (GrI) and Reis-Bücklers' corneal dystrophy (R-B): One entity? *Acta Ophthalmol 1989;67:678–684.*

22. Sajjadi SH, Javadi MA: Superficial juvenile granular dystrophy. *Ophthalmology 1992;99:95–102.*

23. Grayson M, Wilbrandt H: Dystrophy of the anterior limiting membrane of the cornea (Reis-Bückler type). *Am J Ophthalmol 1966;61:345–349.*

24. Wittebol-Post D, van Schooneveld MJ, Pels E: The corneal dystrophy of Waardenburg and Jonkers. *Ophthalmic Paediatr Genetics 1989;10:249–255.*

25. Weidle EG: Differentialdiagnose der Hornhautdystrophien vom Typ Groenouw I, Reis-Bücklers und Thiel-Behnke. *Fortschr Ophthalmol 1989;86:265–271.*

26. Duke-Elder S, Leigh AG: *System of Ophthalmology.* Vol VIII, Part 2. *Diseases of the outer eye.* St. Louis: CV Mosby, 1965, 898–900.

27. Meier S: The distribution of cranial neural crest cells during ocular morphogenesis. *Prog Clin Biol Res 1982;82:1–15.*

28. Hay ED: Development of the vertebrate cornea. *Int Rev Cytol 1980;63:263–322.*

29. Freiberger M: Corneal dystrophy in three generations with a genealogical chart. *Arch Ophthalmol 1936;16:257–270.*

30. Jones ST, Zimmerman LE: Histopathologic differentiation of granular, macular and lattice dystrophies of the cornea. *Am J Ophthalmol 1961;51:394–410.*

31. Teng CC: Granular dystrophy of the cornea: A histochemical and electron microscopic study. *Am J Ophthalmol 1967;63:772–791.*

32. Garner A: Histochemistry of corneal granular dystrophy. *Br J Ophthalmol 1969;53:799–807.*

33. Kanai A, Yamaguchi T, Nakajima A: The histochemical and analytical electron microscopic studies of the corneal granular dystrophy. *Acta Soc Ophthalmol Jpn 1977;81:145–154.*

34. Rodrigues MM, Streeten BW, Krachmer JH, et al: Microfibrillar protein and phospholipid in granular corneal dystrophy. *Arch Ophthalmol 1983;101:802–810.*

35. Folberg R, Alfonso E, Croxatto JO, et al: Clinically atypical granular corneal dystrophy with pathologic features of lattice-like amyloid deposits. *Ophthalmology 1988;95:46–51.*

36. Ramsay RM: Familial corneal dystrophy lattice type. *Trans Am Ophthalmol Soc 1957;60:701–739.*

37. Klintworth GK: Lattice corneal dystrophy: An inherited variety of amyloidosis restricted to the cornea. *Am J Pathol 1967;50:371–399.*

38. Rabb MF, Blodi F, Boniuk M: Unilateral lattice dystrophy of the cornea. *Trans Am Acad Ophthalmol Otolaryngol 1974;78:440–444.*

39. Kanai A, Tanaka M, Kaneko H, et al: Clinical and histopathological studies of the lattice dystrophy of the cornea. *Acta Soc Ophthalmol Jpn 1973;77:357–367.*

40. Francois J, Feher J: Light microscopical and polarisation optical study of the lattice dystrophy of the cornea. *Ophthalmologica 1972;164:1–18.*

41. Francois J, Hanssens M, Teuchy H, et al: Ultrastructural changes in lattice dystrophy of the cornea. *Ophthalmic Res 1975;7:321–344.*

42. McTigue JW, Fine BS: The stromal lesion in lattice dystrophy of the cornea. A light and electron microscopic study. *Invest Ophthalmol 1964;3:355–365.*

43. Meretoja J: Familial systemic paramyloidosis with lattice dystrophy of the cornea, progressive cranial neuropathy, skin changes and various internal symptoms. A previously unrecognized heritable syndrome. *Ann Clin Res 1969;1:314–324.*

44. Gorevic PD, Munoz PC, Gorgone G, et al: Amyloidosis due to a mutation of the gelsolin gene in an American family with lattice corneal dystrophy Type II. *N Engl J Med 1991;325:1780–1785.*

45. Loeffler KU, Edward DP, Tso MOM: An immunohistochemical study of gelsolin immunoreactivity in corneal amyloidosis. *Am J Ophthalmol 1992;113:546–554.*

46. Hida T, Tsubota K, Kigasawa K, et al: Clinical features of a newly recognized type of lattice corneal dystrophy. *Am J Ophthalmol 1987;104:241–248.*

47. Hida T, Proia AD, Kigasawa K, et al: Histopathologic and immunochemical features of lattice corneal dystrophy type III. *Am J Ophthalmol 1987;104:249–254.*

48. Stock EL, Feder RS, O'Grady RB, et al: Lattice corneal dystrophy Type IIIA: Clinical and histopathologic correlations. *Arch Ophthalmol 1991;109:354–358.*

49. Herman SJ, Hughes WF: Recurrence of hereditary corneal dystrophy following keratoplasty. *Am J Ophthalmol 1973;75:689–694.*

50. Lorenzetti DWC, Kaufman HE: Macular and lattice dystrophies and their recurrences after keratoplasty. *Trans Am Acad Ophthalmol Otolaryngol 1967;71:112–118.*

51. Klintworth GK, Vogel FS: Macular corneal dystrophy: An inherited acid mucopolysaccharide storage disease of the corneal fibroblast. *Am J Pathol 1964;45:565–586.*

52. Nakazawa K, Hassell JR, Hascall VC, et al: Defective processing of keratan sulfate in macular corneal dystrophy. *J Biol Chem 1984;259:13751–13757.*

53. Thonar EJ-MA, Meyer RF, Dennis RF, et al: Absence of normal keratan sulfate in the blood of patients with macular corneal dystrophy. *Am J Ophthalmol 1986;102:561–569.*

54. Edward DP, Yue BYJT, Sugar J, et al: Heterogeneity in macular corneal dystrophy. *Arch Ophthalmol 1988;106:1579–1583.*

55. Edward DP, Thonar EJ-MA, Srinivasan M, et al: Macular dystrophy of the cornea: A systemic disorder of keratan sulfate metabolism. *Ophthalmology 1990;97:1194–1200.*

56. Yang CJ, SunderRaj N, Thonar EJ-MA, Klintworth GK: Immunohistochemical evidence of heterogeneity in macular corneal dystrophy. *Am J Ophthalmol 1988;106:65–71.*

57. Jones ST, Zimmerman LE: Histopathologic differentiation of granular, macular and lattice dystrophies of the cornea. *Am J Ophthalmol 1961;51:394–410.*

58. Garner A: Histochemistry of corneal macular dystrophy. *Invest Ophthalmol 1969;8:475–483.*

59. Hassell JR, Newsome DA, Krachmer J, et al: Macular corneal dystrophy: Failure to synthesize a mature keratan sulfate proteoglycan. *Proc Natl Acad Sci USA 1980;77:3705–3709.*

60. Teng CC: Macular dystrophy of the cornea: A histochemical and electron microscopic study. *Am J Ophthalmol 1966;62:436–454.*

61. Snip R, Kenyon K, Green W: Macular corneal dystrophy. Ultrastructural pathology of corneal endothelium and Descemet's membrane. *Invest Ophthalmol 1973;12:88–97.*

62. Klintworth GK, Reed J, Stainer GA, Binder PS: Recurrence of macular corneal dystrophy with grafts. *Am J Ophthalmol 1983;95:60–72.*

63. Luxenberg M: Hereditary crystalline dystrophy of the cornea. *Am J Ophthalmol 1967;63:507–511.*

64. Grop K: Clinical and histologic findings in crystalline corneal dystrophy. *Acta Ophthalmol Suppl (Copenh) 1973;120:52–57.*

65. Bron AJ, Williams HP, Carruthers ME: Hereditary crystalline stromal dystrophy of Schnyder. I. Clinical features of a family with hyperlipoproteinaemia. *Br J Ophthalmol 1972;56:383–399.*

66. Weller RO, Rodger FC: Crystalline stromal dystrophy: Histochemistry and ultrastructure of the cornea. *Br J Ophthalmol 1980;64:46–52.*

67. Rodrigues MM, Kruth HS, Krachmer JH, Willis R: Unesterified cholesterol in Schnyder's corneal crystalline dystrophy. *Am J Ophthalmol 1987;104:157–163.*

68. Ghosh M, McCulloch C: Crystalline dystrophy of the cornea: A light and electron microscopic study. *Can J Ophthalmol 1977;12:321–329.*

69. Karseras AG, Price DC: Central crystalline corneal dystrophy. *Br J Ophthalmol 1970;54:659–662.*

70. Weiss JS: Schnyder's dystrophy of the cornea: A Swede-Finn connection. *Cornea 1992;11:93–101.*

71. Streeten BW, Falls HF: Hereditary fleck dystrophy of the cornea. *Am J Ophthalmol 1961;51:275–278.*

72. Nicholson DH, Green WR, Cross HE, et al: A clinical and histopathological study of Francois-Neetens speckled corneal dystrophy. *Am J Ophthalmol 1977;83:554–560.*

73. Byers PH, Holbrook KA, Hall JG, et al: A new variety of spondyloepiphyseal dysplasia characterized by punctate corneal dystrophy and abnormal dermal collagen fibrils. *Hum Genet 1978;40:157–169.*

74. Carpel EF, Sigelman RJ, Doughman DJ: Posterior amorphous corneal dystrophy. *Am J Ophthalmol 1977;83:629–632.*

75. Johnson AT, Folberg R, Vrabec MP, et al: The pathology of posterior amorphous dystrophy. *Ophthalmology 1990;97:104–109.*

76. Roth SI, Mittelman D, Stock EL: Posterior amorphous corneal dystrophy: An ultrastructural study of a variant with histological features of an endothelial dystrophy. *Cornea 1992;11:165–172.*

77. Strachan IM: Pre-Descemetic corneal dystrophy. *Br J Ophthalmol 1968;52:716–717.*

78. Bramsen T, Ehlers N, Baggesen LH: Central cloudy corneal dystrophy of Francois. *Acta Ophthalmol 1976;54:221–226.*

79. Witschel H, Fine BS, Grützner P, McTigue JW: Congenital hereditary stromal dystrophy of the cornea. *Arch Ophthalmol 1978;96:1043–1051.*

80. Grayson M, Wilbrandt H: Pre-Descemet dystrophy. *Am J Ophthalmol 1967;64:276–282.*

81. Johnston MC, Noden DM, Hazelton RD, et al: Origins of avian ocular and periocular tissues. *Exp Eye Res 1979;29:27–43.*

82. Hay ED: Development of the vertebrate cornea. *Int Rev Cytol 1980;63:263–322.*

83. Meier S: The distribution of cranial neural crest cells during ocular morphogenesis. *Prog Clin Biol Res 1982;82:1–15.*

84. Bahn CF, Falls HF, Varley GA, et al: Classification of corneal endothelial disorders based on neural crest origin. *Ophthalmology 1984;91:558–563.*

85. Kupfer C, Kaiser-Kupfer MI, Datiles M, McCain L: The contralateral eye in the iridocorneal endothelial (ICE) syndrome. *Ophthalmology 1983;90:1343–1350.*

86. Goar EL: Dystrophy of the corneal endothelium (cornea guttata): With report of a histological examination. *Am J Ophthalmol 1934;17:215–221.*

87. Dohlman C-H: Familial congenital cornea guttata in association with anterior polar cataract. *Acta Ophthalmol (Kbh) 1951;29:445–473.*

88. Lorenzetti DWC, Uotila MH, Parikh N, Kaufman HE: Central cornea guttata. Incidence in the general population. *Am J Ophthalmol 1967;1155–1158.*

89. Krachmer JH, Purcell JJ Jr, Young CW, Bucher KD: Corneal endothelial dystrophy: A study of 64 families. *Arch Ophthalmol 1976;96:2036–2039.*

90. Fuchs E: Dystrophia epithelialis corneae. *Graefes Arch Clin Exp Ophthalmol 1910;76:478–508.*

91. Cross HE, Maumenee AE, Cantolino SJ: Inheritance of Fuchs' endothelial dystrophy. *Arch Ophthalmol 1971;85:268–272.*
92. Waring GO, Laibson PR, Rodrigues M: Clinical and pathologic alterations of Descemet's membrane with emphasis on endothelial metaplasia. *Surv Ophthalmol 1974;18:325–368.*
93. Iwamoto T, DeVoe AG: Electron microscopic studies on Fuchs' combined dystrophy: II. Anterior portion of the cornea. *Invest Ophthalmol 1971;10:29–40.*
94. Hamada R, Giraud JP, Pouliquen Y: Electron microscopic study on the Fuchs' dystrophy. *Acta Soc Ophthalmol Jpn 1973;77:531–545.*
95. Arentsen JJ, Laibson PR: Penetrating keratoplasty and cataract extraction. Combined vs. nonsimultaneous surgery. *Arch Ophthalmol 1978;96:75–76.*
96. Koeppe L: Klinische Beobachtungen mit der Nernstspaltlampe und dem Hornhautmikroskop. *Graefes Arch Clin Exp Ophthalmol 1916;91:363–379.*
97. Theodore FH: Congenital type of endothelial dystrophy. *Arch Ophthalmol 1939;21:626–638.*
98. Kanai A, Waltman S, Polack FM, Kaufman HE: Electron microscopic study of hereditary corneal edema. *Invest Ophthalmol 1971;10:89–99.*
99. Kanai A, Kaufman HE: Further electron microscopic study of hereditary corneal edema. *Invest Ophthalmol 1971;10:545–554.*
100. Levenson JE, Chandler JW, Kaufman HE: Affected asymptomatic relatives in congenital hereditary endothelial dystrophy. *Am J Ophthalmol 1973;76:967–971.*
101. Grayson M: The nature of hereditary deep polymorphous dystrophy of the cornea: Its association with iris and anterior chamber dysgenesis. *Trans Am Ophthalmol Soc 1974;72:516–559.*
102. Richardson WP, Hettinger ME: Endothelial and epithelial-like cell formations in a case of posterior polymorphous dystrophy. *Arch Ophthalmol 1985;103:1520–1524.*
103. Krachmer JH: Posterior polymorphous corneal dystrophy: A disease characterized by epithelial-like endothelial cells which influence management and prognosis. *Trans Am Ophthalmol Soc 1985;83:413–475.*
104. Harboyan G, Mamo J, Dei KV, Koram F: Congenital corneal dystrophy: Progressive sensorineural deafness in a family. *Arch Ophthalmol 1971;85:27–32.*
105. Judisch GF, Maumenee IH: Clinical differentiation of recessive congenital hereditary endothelial dystrophy and dominant hereditary endothelial dystrophy. *Am J Ophthalmol 1978;85:606–612.*
106. Kenyon KR, Maumenee AE: The histological and ultrastructural pathology of congenital hereditary corneal dystrophy: A case report. *Invest Ophthalmol 1968;7:475–500.*
107. Kenyon KR, Maumenee AE: Further studies of congenital endothelial dystrophy of the cornea. *Am J Ophthalmol 1973;76:419–439.*

## CHAPTER 11
### KERATITIS AND ENDOPHTHALMITIS

1. Waring GO III, Laibson PR: A systematic method of drawing corneal pathologic conditions. *Arch Ophthalmol 1977;95:1540–1542.*
2. Asbell P, Stenson S: Ulcerative keratitis: Survey of 30 years' laboratory experience. *Arch Ophthalmol 1982;100:77–80.*
3. Liesegang TJ, Forster RK: Spectrum of microbial keratitis in South Florida. *Am J Ophthalmol 1980;90:38–47.*
4. Musch DC, Sugar A, Meyer RF: Demographic and predisposing factors in corneal ulceration. *Arch Ophthalmol 1983;101:1545–1548.*
5. Chandler JW, Milam DF: Diphtheria corneal ulcers. *Arch Ophthalmol 1978;96:53–56.*
6. Plaut AG: Microbial IgA proteases. *N Engl J Med 1978;298:1459–1463.*
7. Schein OD, Glynn RJ, Poggio EC, et al: The relative risk of ulcerative keratitis among users of daily-wear and extended-wear soft contact lenses. *N Engl J Med 1989;321:773–778.*
8. Poggio EC, Glynn RJ, Schein OD, et al: The incidence of ulcerative keratitis among users of daily-wear and extended-wear soft contact lenses. *N Engl J Med 1989;321:779–783.*

9. Benson WH, Lanier JD: Comparison of techniques for culturing corneal ulcers. *Ophthalmology 1992;99:800–804.*

10. Glasser DB, Gardner S, Ellis JG, et al: Loading doses and extended dosing intervals in topical gentamicin therapy. *Am J Ophthalmol 1985;99:329–332.*

11. Davis SD, Sarff LD, Hyndiuk RA: Corticosteroid in experimentally induced *Pseudomonas* keratitis: Failure of prednisolone to impair the efficacy of tobramycin and carbenicillin therapy. *Arch Ophthalmol 1978;96:126–128.*

12. Leibowitz HM, Kupferman A: Topically administered corticosteroids: Effect on antibiotic-treated bacterial keratitis. *Arch Ophthalmol 1980;98:1287–1290.*

13. Bohigian GM, Foster CS: Treatment of *Pseudomonas* keratitis in the rabbit with antibiotic-steroid combinations. *Invest Ophthalmol Vis Sci 1977;16:553–556.*

14. Smolin G, Okumoto M, Leong-Sit L: Combined gentamicin-tobramycin-corticosteroid treatment. II. Effect on gentamicin-resistant *Pseudomonas* keratitis. *Arch Ophthalmol 1980;98:473–474.*

15. Okumoto M, Smolin G: Pneumococcal infections of the eye. *Am J Ophthalmol 1974;77:346–352.*

16. O'Day DM, Smith RS, Gregg CR, et al: The problem of Bacillus species infection with special emphasis on the virulence of *Bacillus cereus. Ophthalmology 1981;88:833–838.*

17. Stern GA, Lubniewski A, Allen C: The interaction between *P. aeruginosa* and the corneal epithelium. *Arch Ophthalmol 1985;103:1221–1225.*

18. Watt PJ: Pathogenic mechanisms of organisms virulent to the eye. *Trans Ophthalmol Soc UK 1986;195:26–31.*

19. Kessler E, Mondino BJ, Brown SI: The corneal response to *Pseudomonas aeruginosa:* Histopathological and enzymatic characterization. *Invest Ophthalmol Vis Sci 1977;16:116–125.*

20. Reiss GR, Campbell RJ, Bourne WM: Infectious crystalline keratopathy. *Surv Ophthalmol 1986;31:69–72.*

21. Liesegang TJ, Forster RK: Spectrum of microbial keratitis in South Florida. *Am J Ophthalmol 1980;90:38–47.*

22. Kaufman HE, Wood RM: Mycotic keratitis. *Am J Ophthalmol 1965;59:993–1000.*

23. Forster RK, Wirta MG, Solis M, Rebell G: Methenamine-silver-stained corneal scrapings in keratomycosis. *Am J Ophthalmol 1976;82:261–265.*

24. Arffa RC, Avni I, Ishibashi Y, et al: Calcofluor and ink-potassium hydroxide preparations for identifying fungi. *Am J Ophthalmol 1985;100:719–723.*

25. Liesegang TJ: Biology and molecular aspects of herpes simplex and varicella-zoster virus infections. *Ophthalmology 1992;99:781–799.*

26. Pepose JS: External ocular infections in immunodeficiency. *Curr Eye Res 1991;10 (suppl):87–95.*

27. Pepose JS: Herpes simplex keratitis: Role of viral infection versus immune response. *Surv Ophthalmol 1991;35:345–352.*

28. Liesegang TJ: Epidemiology of ocular herpes simplex: Natural history in Rochester, Minn, 1950 through 1982. *Arch Ophthalmol 1989;107:1160–1165.*

29. Cloque CMP, Menage MJ, Easty DL: Severe herpetic keratitis. I. Prevalence of visual impairment in a clinic population. *Br J Ophthalmol 1988;72:530–533.*

30. Schwab IR: Oral acyclovir in the management of herpes simplex ocular infections. *Ophthalmology 1988;95:423–430.*

31. Foster CS, Duncan J: Penetrating keratoplasty for herpes simplex keratitis. *Am J Ophthalmol 1981;92:336–343.*

32. Pfister RR, Richards JS, Dohlman CH: Recurrence of herpetic keratitis in corneal grafts. *Am J Ophthalmol 1972;73:192–196.*

33. Liesegang TJ: The varicella-zoster virus: Systemic and ocular features. *J Am Acad Dermatol 1984;11:165–191.*

34. Ragozzino MW, Melton LJ III, Kurland LT, et al: Population-based study of herpes zoster and its sequelae. *Medicine (Baltimore) 1982;61:310–316.*

35. Cobo M, Foulks GN, Liesegang T, et al: Observations on the natural history of herpes zoster ophthalmicus. *Curr Eye Res 1987;6:195–199.*

36. Liesegang TJ: Corneal complications from herpes zoster ophthalmicus. *Ophthalmology 1985;92:316–324.*

37. Cobo LM, Foulks GN, Liesegang TJ, et al: Oral acyclovir in the therapy of acute herpes zoster ophthalmicus. *Ophthalmology 1985; 92:1574–1583.*

38. Van Der Spuy S, Levy DW, Levin W: Cimetidine in the treatment of herpes virus infections. *S Afr Med J 1980;58:112–116.*

39. Levy DW, Banerjee AK, Glenny HP: Cimetidine in the treatment of herpes zoster. *J R Coll Physicians Lond 1985;19:96–98.*

40. Matoba AY: Ocular disease associated with Epstein-Barr virus infection. *Surv Ophthalmol 1990;35:145–150.*

41. Pflugfelder SC, Tseng SCG, Pepose JS, et al: Epstein-Barr virus infection and immunologic dysfunction in patients with aqueous tear deficiency. *Ophthalmology 1990;97:313–323.*

42. Meisler DM, Bosworth DE, Krachmer JH: Ocular infectious mononucleosis manifested as Parinaud's oculoglandular syndrome. *Am J Ophthalmol 1981;92:722–726.*

43. Wilhelmus KR: Ocular involvement in infectious mononucleosis. *Am J Ophthalmol 1981;91:117–118.*

44. Matoba AY, Wilhelmus KR, Jones DB: Epstein-Barr viral stromal keratitis. *Ophthalmology 1986;93:746–751.*

45. Matoba AY, Jones DB: Corneal subepithelial infiltrates associated with systemic Epstein-Barr viral infection. *Ophthalmology 1987; 94:1669–1671.*

46. Jawetz E: Adenovirus type 8 and the story of epidemic keratoconjunctivitis. *Trans Ophthalmol Soc UK 1962;82:613–619.*

47. O'Day DM, Guyer B, Hierholzer JC, et al: Clinical and laboratory evaluation of epidemic keratoconjunctivitis due to adenovirus types 8 and 19. *Am J Ophthalmol 1976;81:207–215.*

48. Thygeson P: Office and dispensary transmission of epidemic keratoconjunctivitis. *Am J Ophthalmol 1957;43:98–101.*

49. D'Angelo LJ, Hierholzer JC, Holman RC, Smith JD: Epidemic keratoconjunctivitis caused by adenovirus type 8: Epidemiologic and laboratory aspects of a large outbreak. *Am J Epidemiol 1981;113:44–49.*

50. Dawson CR, Hanna L, Wood TR, Despain R: Adenovirus type 8 keratoconjunctivitis in the United States. *Am J Ophthalmol 1970;69:473–480.*

51. Nesburn AB, Lowe GH III, Lepoff NJ, Maguen E: Effect of topical trifluridine on Thygeson's superficial punctate keratitis. *Ophthalmology 1984;91:1188–1192.*

52. Naginton J, Watson PG, Playfair TJ, et al: Amoebic infection of the eye. *Lancet 1974;2:1537–1540.*

53. Moore MB: Management of *Acanthamoeba* keratitis, in: Cavanagh HD (ed): *The Cornea: Transactions of the World Congress on the Cornea III.* New York: Raven Press, 1988, 517–521.

54. Gillette TE, Chandler JW, Greiner JV: Langerhans cells of the ocular surface. *Ophthalmology 1982;89:700–711.*

55. Epstein RJ, Hendricks RL, Stulting RD: Interleukin-2 induces corneal neovascularization in A/J mice. *Cornea 1990;9:318–323.*

56. Cogan DG, Dickersin GR: Nonsyphilitic interstitial keratitis with vestibuloauditory symptoms: A case with fatal aortitis. *Arch Ophthalmol 1964;71:172–175.*

57. Ridley DS, Jopling WH: Classification of leprosy according to immunity. A five group system. *Int J Lepr 1966;34:255–273.*

58. Ridley DS: Histological classification and the immunological spectrum of leprosy. *Bull WHO 1974;51:451–465.*

59. Winterkorn JMS: Lyme disease: Neurologic and ophthalmic manifestations. *Surv Ophthalmol 1990;35:191–204.*

60. Tabbara KF, Butrus SI: Vernal keratoconjunctivitis and keratoconus. *Am J Ophthalmol 1983;95:704–705.*

61. Mondino BJ, Laheji AK, Adamu SA: Ocular immunity to *Staphylococcus aureus*. *Invest Ophthalmol Vis Sci 1987;28:560–564.*

62. Bierly JR, Dunn JP, Dawson CR, et al: Fuchs' superficial marginal keratitis. *Am J Ophthalmol 1992;113:541–545.*

63. Speaker MG, Milch FA, Shah MK, et al: Role of external bacterial flora in the pathogenesis of acute postoperative endophthalmitis. *Ophthalmology 1991;98:639–650.*

64. Joondeph BC, Flynn HW Jr, Miller D, Joondeph HC: A new culture method for infectious endophthalmitis. *Arch Ophthalmol 1989;107:1334–1337.*

65. Kattan HM, Flynn HW Jr, Pflugfelder SC, et al: Nosocomial endophthalmitis survey: Current incidence of infection after intraocular surgery. *Ophthalmology 1991;98:227–238.*

66. Javitt JC, Vitale S, Canner JK, et al: National outcomes of cataract extraction. Endophthalmitis following in-patient surgery. *Arch Ophthalmol 1991;109:1085–1089.*

67. Menikoff JA, Speaker MG, Marmor M, Raskin EM: A case-control study of risk factors for postoperative endophthalmitis. *Ophthalmology 1991;98:1761–1768.*

68. Meisler DM, Mandelbaum S: Propionibacterium-associated endophthalmitis after extracapsular cataract extraction. Review of reported cases. *Ophthalmology 1989;96:54–61.*

69. Moffett DG Jr, Edward DP: Anterior segment necrosis associated with endogenous endophthalmitis secondary to group C streptococcal septicemia. *Can J Ophthalmol 1991;26:283–287.*

70. Algan M, Jonon B, George JL, et al: *Listeria monocytogenes* endophthalmitis in a renal-transplant patient receiving cyclosporin. *Ophthalmologica 1990;201:23–27.*

71. Schmid S, Martenet AC, Oelz O: Candida endophthalmitis: Clinical presentation, treatment and outcome in 23 patients. *Infection 1991;19:21–24.*

72. Venditti M, De Bernardis F, Micozzi A, et al: Fluconazole treatment of catheter-related right-sided endocarditis caused by *Candida albicans* and associated with endophthalmitis and folliculitis. *Clin Infect Dis 1992;14:422–426.*

73. Denning DW, Armstrong RW, Fishman M, Stevens DA: Endophthalmitis in a patient with disseminated cryptococcosis and AIDS who was treated with itraconazole. *Rev Infect Dis 1991;13:1126–1130.*

# CHAPTER 12
## CORNEAL SURGERY

1. Van Rij G, Waring GO III: Configuration of corneal trephine opening using five different trephines in human donor eyes. *Arch Ophthalmol 1988;106:1228–1233.*

2. Olson RJ: Variation in corneal graft size related to trephine technique. *Arch Ophthalmol 1979;97:1323–1325.*

3. Girard LJ, Eguez I, Esnaola N, et al: Effect of penetrating keratoplasty using grafts of various sizes on keratoconic myopia. *J Cataract Refract Surg 1988;14:541–547.*

4. Bertram BA, Drews C, Gemmill M, et al: Inadequacy of a polyester (Mersilene) suture for the reduction of astigmatism after penetrating keratoplasty. *Trans Am Ophthalmol Soc 1990;88:237–249.*

5. Cravy TV: Long-term corneal astigmatism related to selected elastic, monofilament nonabsorbable sutures. *J Cataract Refract Surg 1989;15:61–69.*

6. McNeil JI, Wessels IF: Adjustment of single continuous suture to control astigmatism after penetrating keratoplasty. *Refract Corneal Surg 1989;5:216–223.*

7. Musch DC, Meyer RF: Prospective evaluation of a regression-determined formula for use in triple procedure surgery. *Ophthalmology 1998;95:79–85.*

8. Lass JH, DeSantis DM, Reinhart WJ, et al: Clinical and morphometric results of penetrating keratoplasty with one-piece anterior-chamber or suture-fixed posterior-chamber lenses in the absence of lens capsule. *Arch Ophthalmol 1990;108:1427–1431.*

9. Gunderson T: Conjunctival flaps in the treatment of corneal disease with reference to a new technique of application. *Arch Ophthalmol 1958;60:880–888.*

10. Paton D, Milauskas AT: Indications, surgical techniques, and results of thin conjunctival flaps on the cornea. *Int Ophthalmol Clin 1970;10:329–345.*

11. Maguire LJ, Shearer DR: A simple method of conjunctival dissection for Gunderson flaps. *Arch Ophthalmol 1991;109:1168–1169.*

12. McDonald MB, Kaufman HE, Aquavella JV, et al: The nationwide study of epikeratophakia in adults. *Am J Ophthalmol 1987;103:358–365.*

13. Kaufman HE, Werblin TP: Epikeratophakia for the treatment of keratoconus. *Am J Ophthalmol 1982;93:342–347.*

14. Arffa RC, Marvelli TL, Morgan KS, et al: Keratometric and refractive results of pediatric epikeratophakia. *Arch Ophthalmol 1985;103:1656–1659.*

15. Morgan KS, McDonald MB, Hiles DA, et al: The nationwide study of epikeratophakia for aphakia in children. *Am J Ophthalmol 1987;102:366–374.*

16. Uozato H, Guyton DL: Centering corneal procedures. *Am J Ophthalmol 1987;103:264–275.*

17. Mandel MR, Shapiro MB, Krachmer JH: Relaxing incisions with augmentation sutures for the correction of postkeratoplasty astigmatism. *Am J Ophthalmol 1987;103:441–447.*

18. Krachmer JH, Fenzl RE: Surgical correction of high postkeratoplasty astigmatism. *Arch Ophthalmol 1980;98:1400–1402.*

19. Casebeer JC: *A System of Precise, Predictable Keratorefractive Surgery. A System for Success.* (Chiron Ophthalmic Educational Series.) Irvine, CA: Chiron Corporation, 1992.

20. Waring GO III: *Refractive Keratotomy for Myopia and Astigmatism.* St. Louis: Mosby Year Book, 1992.

21. Berkeley RG, Sanders DR, Picolo MG: Effect of incision direction on radial keratotomy outcome. *J Cataract Refract Surg 1991;17:819–823.*

22. Waring GO III, Lynn MJ, Fielding B, et al: Results of the Prospective Evaluation of Radial Keratotmy (PERK) Study 4 years after surgery for myopia. PERK Study Group. *JAMA 1990;263:1083–1091.*

23. Waring GO: Preliminary phase IIb results of PRK using Summit laser. *Argus 1992;15:12.*

24. Thoft RA: Keratoepithelioplasty. *Am J Ophthalmol 1984;97:1–6.*

25. Speaker MG, Guerriero PN, Met JA, et al: A case-control study of risk factors for intraoperative suprachoroidal expulsive hemorrhage. *Ophthalmology 1991;98:202–210.*

26. Wilson SE, Kaufman HE. Graft failure after penetrating keratoplasty. *Surv Ophthalmol 1990;34:325–356.*

## CHAPTER 13
### THE SCLERA

1. Sainz de la Maza M, Dutt JE, Foster CS: Distribution of collagens and fibronectin in human adult and fetal sclera (abstr). *Invest Ophthalmol Vis Sci 1992;33(suppl):711.*

2. Snell RS, Lemp MA: *Clinical Anatomy of the Eye.* Boston: Blackwell Scientific Publications, 1989, 125–127.

3. Johnston MC, Noden DM, Hazelton RD, et al: Origins of avian ocular and periocular tissues. *Exp Eye Res 1979;29:27–43.*

4. Ozanics V, Rayborn M, Sagun D: Some aspects of corneal and scleral differentiation in the primate. *Exp Eye Res 1976;22:305–327.*

5. Harrison SA, Mondino BJ, Mayer FJ: Scleral fibroblasts: Human leukocyte antigen expression and complement production. *Invest Ophthalmol Vis Sci 1991;31:2412–2419.*

6. Torcyznski E, Jakobiec FA, Madewell J, et al: Synophthalmia: An histopathological organogenetic and radiographic analysis. *Doc Ophthalmol 1977;44:311–378.*

7. Brockhurst RJ: Nanophthalmos with uveal effusion: A new clinical entity. *Trans Am Ophthalmol Soc 1974;72:371–403.*

8. Mietz H, Kasner L, Green WR: The ultrastructure of the cornea and sclera in osteogenesis imperfecta type III (abstr). *Invest Ophthalmol Vis Sci 1992;33(suppl):772.*

9. Watson PG, Hayreh SS: Scleritis and episcleritis. *Br J Ophthalmol 1976;60:163–191.*

10. Watson PG: The diagnosis and management of scleritis. *Ophthalmology 1980;87:716–720.*

11. Benson WE: Posterior scleritis. *Surv Ophthalmol 1988;32:297–316.*

12. Pulido JS, Goeken JA, Nerad JA, et al: Ocular manifestations of patients with circulating antineutrophil cytoplasmic antibodies. *Arch Ophthalmol 1990;108:845–850.*

13. Nussenblatt RB, Palestine AG: Cyclosporine: Immunology, pharmacology and therapeutic uses. *Surv Ophthalmol 1986;31:159–169.*

## CHAPTER 14
## LACRIMAL SYSTEM: DRY-EYE STATES AND OTHER CONDITIONS

1. Duke–Elder S, Cook C: Embryology, in Duke–Elder S (ed): *System of Ophthalmology,* Vol III, Part 1. St. Louis: CV Mosby, 1963, 239–246.

2. Busse H, Muller KM, Kroll P: Radiological and histological findings of the lacrimal passage of the newborn. *Arch Ophthalmol 1980;98:528.*

3. Murube-del-Castillo J: Development of the lacrimal apparatus, in Milder B, Weil BA (eds): *The Lacrimal System.* Norwalk, CT: Appleton-Century-Crofts, 1983.

4. Wolff E: *The Anatomy of the Eye and Orbit,* ed 4. New York, Toronto: Blakiston, 1954, 194–196.

5. Sjögren H, Kroning E: Keratoconjunctivitis sicca after partial extirpation of the palpebral lacrimal gland. *Acta Ophthalmol 1951;29:355–360.*

6. Duke–Elder S, Wybar KC: The anatomy of the visual system, in Duke–Elder S (ed): *System of Ophthalmology,* Vol III, Part 3. St. Louis: CV Mosby, 1963, 562–576.

7. Jones LT: Anatomy and physiology of the ocular appendages, in Rech MJ (ed): *Treatment of Lid and Epibulbar Tumors.* Springfield, IL: Charles C Thomas, 1963.

8. McEwen WK, Goodner EK: Secretion of tears and blinking, in Dauson H (ed): *The Physiology of the Eye,* Vol E. New York: Academic Press, 1969.

9. Whitwell J: Denervation of the lacrimal gland. *Br J Ophthalmol 1958;42:518–525.*

10. Bothelho SY, Hisada M, Fuenmayor N: Functional innervation of the lacrimal gland in the cat. *Arch Ophthalmol 1966;76:581–588.*

11. Goldstein AM, Palau A, Bothelho SY: Inhibition and facilitation of pilocarpine-induced lacrimal flow by norepinephrine. *Invest Ophthalmol 1967;6:498–511.*

12. Balik J, Pavlova D, Urbanova S: The effect of atropine and pilocarpine on the secretion of sodium into tears. *Cesk Oftal 1966;22:263–267.*

13. Gottesfeld BH, Leavitt FH: "Crocodile tears" treated by injection into the sphenopalatine ganglion. *Arch Neurol 1942;47:314–315.*

14. deHass EBH: Lacrimal gland response to parasympathetic denervation. *Arch Ophthalmol 1960;64:34–43.*

15. Mishima S, Gasset A, Klyce SD, Baum JL: Determination of tear volume and tear flow. *Invest Ophthalmol 1966;5:264–276.*

16. Iwata S, Lemp MA, Holly FJ, Dohlman CH: Evaporation rate of water from precorneal tear film and cornea in rabbit. *Invest Ophthalmol 1969;8:613–619.*

17. Doane MG: Blinking and the mechanics of the lacrimal drainage system. *Ophthalmology 1981;88(8):844–850.*

18. Doane MG: Turnover and drainage of tears. *Am J Opthalmol 1984;16(2):111–114.*

19. Andrews JS: Human tearfilm lipids: I. Composition of the principal non-polar component. *Exp Eye Res 1970;10:223–227.*

20. Holly FJ, Lemp MA: Tear physiology and dry eyes. *Surv Ophthalmol 1977;22:69–87.*

21. Rexed U: The pH of the lacrimal fluid determined by a capillary micro-glass electrode. *Acta Ophthalmol 1958;36:711–718.*

22. Norm MS: Bromothymol blue vital staining of conjunctiva and cornea. *Acta Ophthalmol 1968;46:231–242.*

23. Mastman GL, Blades EJ, Henderson JW: The total osmotic pressure of tears in normal and various pathological conditions. *Arch Ophthalmol 1961;65:509–513.*

24. Reim M, Lax F, Lichte H, Truss R: Steady state levels of glucose in different layers of the cornea, aqueous humor, blood, and tears in vivo. *Ophthalmologica 1967;154:39–50.*

25. Thoft RA, Friend J: Corneal epithelial glucose utilization. *Arch Ophthalmol 1972;88:58–62.*

26. Tapaszto I, Vass Z: The demonstration of protein fractions of human tears by means of micro electrophoresis. *Acta Ophthalmol 1965;43:796–801.*

27. Bonavida B, Sapse AT, Sercarz EE: A unique lacrimal protein absent from serum and other secretions: Specific tear prealbumin. *Nature 1969;221:375.*

28. Allansmith MR: Immunology of the tears. *Int Ophthalmol Clin 1973;13(1):47–72.*

29. Mackie IA, Seal DV: Tear fluid lysozyme concentration: Guide to practolol toxicity. *Br Med J 1975;2:732.*

30. Avisar R, Menache R, Shaked P, et al: Lysozyme content of tears in patients with Sjögren's syndrome and rheumatoid arthritis. *Am J Ophthalmol 1979;87:148–151.*

31. Watson RR, Reyes MA, McMurray DN: Influence of malnutrition on the concentration of IgA, lysozyme, amylase and aminopeptidase in children's tears. *Proc Soc Exp Biol Med 1978;157:215–219.*

32. Sapse AT, Bonavida B, Stone WJ, Sercarz EE: Human tear lysozyme; III. Preliminary studies on lysozyme levels in subjects with smog eye irritation. *Am J Ophthalmol 1968;66:76–80.*

33. McClellan BH, Whitney CR, Newman LP, Allansmith MR: Immunoglobulins in tears. *Am J Ophthalmol 1973;76:89–101.*

34. Franklin RM, Kenyon KR, Tomasi TB: Immunohistologic studies of human lacrimal gland: Localization of immunoglobulins, secretory component and lactoferrin. *J Immunol 1973;110:984–992.*

35. Broekhuyse RM: Tear lactoferrin: A bacteriostatic and complexing protein. *Invest Ophthalmol 1974;13:550–554.*

36. Lemp MA, Holly FJ, Iwata S, Dohlman CH: The precorneal tear film. I. Factors in spreading and maintaining a continuous tear film over the corneal surface. *Arch Ophthalmol 1970;83:89–94.*

37. Duke–Elder S: Normal and abnormal development, in Duke–Elder S (ed): *System of Ophthalmology,* Vol III, Part 2. St. Louis: CV Mosby, 1963, 911–923.

38. Bowen R: Hereditary ectodermal dysplasia of the anhidrotic type. *South Med J 1957;50:1018–1021.*

39. Davidoff E, Friedman AH: Congenital alacrima. *Surv Opthalmol 1977;22:113–119.*

40. Howard R: Familial dysautonomia (Riley–Day syndrome). *Am J Ophthalmol 1967;64:392–398.*

41. Dunnington JH: Congenital alacrima in familial autonomic dysfunction. *Arch Ophthalmol 1954;52:925–931.*

42. Smith AA, Dancis J, Breinin G: Ocular responses to autonomic drugs in familial dysautonomia. *Invest Ophthalmol 1965;4:358–361.*

43. Blanksma LJ, Pol BA: Congenital fistulae of the lacrimal gland. *Br J Ophthalmol 1980;64:515–517.*

44. Green WR, Zimmerman LE: Ectopic lacrimal gland tissue. *Arch Opthalmol 1967;78:318–327.*

45. Hornblass A, Herschorn B: Lacrimal gland duct cysts. *Ophthalmic Surg 1988;16:301–306.*

46. Jones LT: The cure of epiphora due to canalicular disorders, trauma and surgical failures on the lacrimal passages. *Trans Am Acad Ophthalmol Otolaryngol 1962;66:506–524.*

47. Paul TO: Medical management of congenital nasolacrimal duct obstruction. *J Pediatr Ophthalmol Strabismus 1985;22:68–70.*

48. Petersen RA, Robb RM: The natural course of congenital obstruction of the nasolacrimal duct. *J Pediatr Ophthalmol Strabismus 1978;15:246–250.*

49. Katowitz JA, Welsh MG: Timing of initial probing and irrigation in congenital nasolacrimal duct obstruction. *Ophthalmology 1987;94:698–705.*

50. Weinstein GS, Biglin AW, Patterson JH: Congenital lacrimal sac mucoceles. *Am J Ophthalmol 1982;94:106–110.*

51. Duke–Elder S: The ocular adnexa, in Duke–Elder S (ed): *System of Ophthalmology,* Vol XIII, Part 2. St. Louis: CV Mosby, 1974, 601–609.

52. Jakobiec FA, Iwamoto T, Knowles DM: Ocular adnexal lymphoid tumours: Correlative ultrastructural and immunological markers studies. *Arch Ophthalmol 1982;100:84–98.*

53. Obenauf CD, Shaw HE, Sydnor CF, Klintworth GK: Sarcoidosis and its ophthalmic manifestations. *Am J Ophthalmol 1978;86:648–655.*

54. Hurwitz JJ, Rodgers KJA: Management of acquired dacryocystitis. *Can J Ophthalmol 1983;13:213–216.*

55. Sood NN, Ratnaraj A, Balarman G, et al: Chronic dacryocystitis: A clinicobacteriologic study. *J All India Ophthalmol Soc 1967;15:107–110.*

56. Hornblass A: A simple taste test for lacrimal obstruction. *Arch Ophthalmol 1973;90:435–436.*

57. Baum J: Clinical manifestation of dry eye states. *Trans Ophthalmol Soc UK 1985;104:415–423.*

58. Tabbara KF, Ostler MB, Daniel TF, et al: Sjögren's syndrome: A correlation between ocular findings and labial salivary gland histology. *Trans Am Acad Ophthalmol Otol 1974;78:467–478.*

59. Lamberts DW, Foster CS, Perry HD: Schirmer test after topical anesthesia and the tear meniscus height in normal eyes. *Arch Ophthalmol 1979;97:1082–1085.*

60. Lemp MA, Hamill J: Factors affecting tear breakup in normals. *Arch Ophthalmol 1973;89:103–105.*

61. Lemp MA, Dohlman CH, Kuwabara T, et al: Dry eye secondary to mucus deficiency. *Trans Am Acad Ophthalmol Otolaryngol 1971;75:1223–1227.*

62. Norm MS: Rose bengal vital staining—staining of corneas and conjunctivas by 10 per cent rose bengal, compared with 1 per cent. *Acta Ophthalmol 1970;48:546–559.*

63. Feenstra RPG, Tseng SCG: Comparison of fluorescein and rose bengal staining. *Ophthalmology 1992;99:605–617.*

64. Jordan A, Baum J: Basic tear flow. Does it exist? *Ophthalmology 1980;87:920–930.*

65. Gilbard JP, Farris RL: Tear osmolarity and ocular surface disease in keratoconjunctivitis sicca. *Arch Ophthalmol 1979;97:1642–1646.*

66. Gilbard JP, Farris RL, Santamaria J II: Osmolarity of tear microvolumes in keratoconjunctivitis sicca. *Arch Ophthalmol 1978;96:677–681.*

67. McCulley JP, Dougherty JM, Deneau DG: Classification of chronic blepharitis. *Ophthalmology 1982;89:1173–1180.*

68. Sommer A. *Nutritional Blindness: Xerophthalmia and Keratomalacia.* New York: Oxford University Press, 1982.

69. Brooks HL, Driebe WT, Schemmer GG: Xerophthalmia and cystic fibrosis. *Arch Ophthalmol 1990;108:354–357.*

70. Suan EP, Bedrossian EH, Eagle RC, Laibson P: Corneal perforation in patients with vitamin A deficiency in the United States. *Arch Ophthalmol 1990;108:350–353.*

71. Abdel-Khalek LMR, Williamson J, Lee WR: Morphological changes in human conjunctival epithelium: II, in keratoconjunctivitis sicca. *Br J Ophthalmol 1978;62:800–806.*

72. Nelson JD, Havener VR, Cameron JD: Cellulose acetate impressions of the ocular surface. *Arch Ophthalmol 1983;101:1869–1872.*

73. Lemp MA, Gold JB, Wong S, et al: An in vivo study of corneal surface morphologic features in patients with keratoconjunctivitis sicca. *Am J Ophthalmol 1984;98:426–428.*

74. Wright P: Filamentary keratitis. *Trans Ophthalmol Soc UK 1975;95:260–266.*

75. Pfister RR, Murphy GE: Corneal ulceration and perforation associated with Sjogren's syndrome. *Arch Ophthalmol 1980;98:89–94.*

76. Sommer A, Green R, Kenyon KR: Clinicohistopathologic correlations in xerophthalmic ulceration and necrosis. *Arch Ophthalmol 1980;100:953–963.*

77. Wilson WS, Duncan AJ, Jay JL: Effect of benzalkonium chloride on the stability of the precorneal tear film in rabbit and man. *Br J Ophthalmol 1975;59:667–669.*

78. Norm MS, Opauszki A: Effects of ophthalmic vehicles on the stability of the precorneal film. *Acta Ophthalmol 1977;55:23–24.*

79. Lemp MA, Zimmerman LE: Toxic endothelial degeneration in ocular surface disease treated with topical medication containing benzalconium chloride. *Am J Ophthalmol 1988;105:670–673.*

80. Absolon MJ, Brown CA: Acetylcystein in keratoconjunctivitis sicca. *Br J Ophthalmol 1968;52:310–316.*

81. Jones DB: Prospects in the management of tear deficiency states. *Trans Am Acad Ophthalmol Otolaryngol 1977;83:693–700.*

82. Freeman JM: The punctum plug; evaluation of new treatment for dry eye. *Trans Am Acad Ophthalmol Otolaryngol 1975;79:874–879.*

83. Foulds WS: Intra-canalicular gelatin implants in treatment of keratoconjunctivitis sicca. *Br J Ophthalmol 1961;45:625–627.*

84. Tuberville AW, Frederik WR, Wood TO: Punctal oclusion in tear deficiency syndromes. *Ophthalmology 1982;89:1170–1172.*

85. Dohlman CH, Boruchoff A, Mobilia EF: Complication in use of soft contact lenses in corneal disease. *Arch Ophthalmol 1973;90:367–371.*

86. Haeringen NJV: Clinical biochemistry of tears. *Surv Ophthalmol 1981;26:84–96.*

## CHAPTER 15
### CORNEAL AND EXTERNAL EYE MANIFESTATIONS OF SYSTEMIC DISEASE

1. Howard RO: Classification of chromosomal eye syndromes. *Int Ophthalmol 1981;4:77–91.*

2. Chrousos GA, et al: Ocular findings in Turner syndrome. *Ophthalmology 1984;91:926–928.*

3. Mets MB, Maumenee IH: The eye and the chromosome. *Surv Ophthalmol 1983;28:20–32.*

4. Sugar J: Metabolic disorders of the cornea, in Kaufman HE, Barron BA, McDonald MB, Waltman SR (eds): *The Cornea.* New York: Churchill Livingstone, 1988, 361–382.

5. Barchiesi BJ, Eckel RH, Ellis PP: The cornea and disorders of lipid metabolism. *Surv Ophthalmol 1991;36:1–22.*

6. Sabates R, Krachmer JH, Weingeist TA: Ocular findings in Alport's syndrome. *Ophthalmologica 1983;186:204–210.*

7. Nelson LB, Spaeth GL, Nowinski TS, et al: Aniridia. A review. *Surv Ophthalmol 1984;28:621–642.*

8. Cohen SMZ, et al: Ocular histopathologic and biochemical studies of the cerebrohepatorenal syndrome (Zellweger's syndrome) and its relationship to neonatal adrenoleukodystrophy. *Am J Ophthalmol 1983;96:488–501.*

9. Sasaki T, Tsukahara S: New ocular findings in Gaucher's disease: A report of two brothers. *Ophthalmologica 1985;191:206–209.*

10. Williams ML: Ichthyosiform erythroderma, atypical with deafness, in Buyse ML (ed): *Birth Defects Encyclopedia.* Cambridge, MA: Blackwell Scientific Publ, 1990, 935–936.

11. McDonnell PJ, Schofield OMV, Spalton DJ, Eady RAJ: Eye involvement in junctional epidermolysis bullosa. *Arch Ophthalmol 1989;107:1635–1637.*

12. Sierhut M, et al: Ocular involvement in epidermolysis bullosa acquisita. *Arch Ophthalmol 1989;107:398–401.*

13. Proia AD, Anderson KE: The porphyrias, in Gold DH, Weingeist TA (eds): *The Eye in Systemic Disease.* Philadelphia: JB Lippincott, 1990, 398–401.

# INDEX

**NUMBERS IN BOLD REFER TO FIGURES**